Advancing Health Through Education

MAYFIELD PUBLISHING COMPANY
PALO ALTO AND LONDON

Advancing Health Through Education

A Case Study Approach

EDITED BY

Helen P. Cleary, D.Sc.
Department of Family and Community Medicine
University of Massachusetts Medical School

Jeffrey M. Kichen, M.S.
PRE Associates
Natick, Massachusetts

Phyllis G. Ensor, M.S., Ph.D.
Department of Health Education
Towson State University

VAUGHAN
RA440.3
.U5A45
1985

To
BETTY P. MATHEWS,
ELENA SLIEPCEVICH,
AND
MARY E. SPENCER,

WHOSE GENEROSITY IN SHARING THEIR GIFTS
HAS ENRICHED ALL OF US

Copyright © 1985 by Mayfield Publishing Company
First edition

All rights reserved. No portion of this book may be reproduced
in any form or by any means without written permission
of the publisher.

Library of Congress Catalog Card Number: 84-060884
International Standard Book Number: 0-87484-569-6

Manufactured in the United States of America
10 9 8 7 6 5 4 3 2

Mayfield Publishing Company
285 Hamilton Avenue
Palo Alto, California 94301

Sponsoring editor: C. Lansing Hays
Manuscript editor: Lieselotte Hofmann
Managing editor: Pat Herbst
Production editors: Jan deProsse, Deborah Cogan
Art director/designer: Nancy Sears
Cover designer: Deborah Hopping
Production manager: Cathy Willkie
Compositor: Publisher's Typography
Printer and binder: Malloy Lithographing

Contents

Preface	xiii
Introduction	1
Perspectives on Critical Issues in the Practice of Health Education	5

PART ONE
Case Studies in School Settings — 15

Elementary School Health Education — 20
Charlotte Owens
    Analysis 22

Health Counseling: "I Think I'm . . ." — 25
James F. McKenzie and Roberta Ogletree
    Analysis 28

The Development and Implementation of a Women's
Health Course — 32
Denise Hope Amschler
    Analysis 38

Curriculum Development with the Pima Indians of Arizona — 42
*Kerry J. Redican, Larry K. Olsen, Charles R. Baffi,
and Thomas L. Dezelsky*
    Analysis 50

Organizational Dissonance   54
   Valorie E. Nybo
      Analysis   64

Health Education Required for High School Graduation:
From Resolution and Action to Law   68
   Mabel Crenshaw Robinson
      Analysis   74

The Seaside Story   79
   Judy Drolet
      Analysis   83

PART TWO
Case Studies in Medical Care Settings   89

Organizing Patient Education   95
   Kolleen M. Biel
      Analysis   100

Interdisciplinary Team-Building for Hypertension
Patient Education in an HMO   103
   Paul A. Davis
      Analysis   107

Liaisons: Using Health Education Resources Effectively   112
   Judith R. Miller
      Analysis   114

A Self-Care Unit for Management of the Common Cold in a
Prepaid Setting   117
   Barbara B. Estabrook
      Analysis   121

Patient Education in a Rural Ambulatory-Care Setting:
The Patient Education Reimbursement Project   125
   Randy H. Schwartz and Paula Sanofsky Morris
      Analysis   131

Health Hazard Appraisal in a Family Practice Residency   134
   Edward E. Bartlett
      Analysis   140

A Health Education Service in an Acute Care Hospital   143
   Anna W. Skiff
      Analysis   151

Management Functions of the Health Education Director: Examples of Data Management Activities ... 156
   Jane G. Zapka
      Analysis 174

PART THREE
Case Studies in Community Settings ... 177

The Vermont Connection ... 181
   Marjorie Hamrell and Amy Raiser
      Analysis 187

The Practice of Health Education with a Chicano Population ... 191
   Yolanda Santos
      Analysis 196

Telling Stories of Health ... 199
   Jean E. Morehead
      Analysis 204

Arthritis Self-Management; or, The Chocolate-Chip-Cookie Caper ... 208
   Kate R. Lorig and Janette Laurin
      Analysis 213

East Side Health District's Cervical Cytology Demonstration Project ... 216
   Stanley G. Rosenberg
      Analysis 221

Cooperative Problem Solving: The Neighborhood Self-Help Project ... 225
   Rosalind P. Thomas, Barbara A. Israel, and Guy W. Steuart
      Analysis 235

Planning for Effective Health Education ... 240
   Zora Travis Salisbury
      Analysis 246

Consumer-Planned Health Education in Comprehensive Health Planning ... 250
   Marcia Pinkett-Heller and Noreen M. Clark
      Analysis 258

Changing Tuberculosis Treatment from Inpatient to Outpatient Care and from Sanatorium to General Hospital Care ... 262
   Frances R. Ogasawara
      Analysis 269

Planning and Evaluation of Public Health Education Programs in
Rural Settings: Theory into Practice   273
   Richard A. Windsor
      Analysis   285

Prevention Through Consumer Education   288
   Miriam M. Campbell and Phyllis S. Williams
      Analysis   296

Establishing a Primary Care Clinic in a Traditional Public
Health Organization   301
   Jeanne I. Semura
      Analysis   310

PART FOUR
Case Studies in Worksite Settings   313

Occupational Health Education: A Nontraditional Role for a
Health Educator   319
   Beverly G. Ware
      Analysis   324

The Total Life Concept   327
   Molly McCauley
      Analysis   329

Reach Out for Health   332
   Angelica Cantlon
      Analysis   338

Promoting Worksite Wellness: A Community-Based Project   341
   Brenda Lindemann
      Analysis   348

Organizing a Health Promotion Program at a University
Medical Center   352
   Gary J. Donnelly
      Analysis   358

Initiating a Health Promotion Program for Public School Personnel   362
   Vilma T. Falck
      Analysis   368

PART FIVE
Professional Development 373

A Participant-Observer in a Period of Professional Change 374
   Lawrence W. Green
     Analysis 380

Glossary 383
Author Index 387
Subject Index 391

Preface

This book was born as the result of a casual conversation between two of the editors who were concerned about the wide gap between learning about and practicing health education. We spoke to our colleagues and asked them to write about their experiences. Through articles in professional publications, we invited others who wished to submit a case study to do so.

The response was overwhelming. We were inundated with case studies, and the process of deciding what to omit was painful. Each study offered a valuable lesson in the practice of health education. Our criterion for selection was to try to maintain an appropriate balance of authors representing both academia and practice.

The selected cases illustrate various types of health education practice in schools, communities, medical care facilities, and worksites. We have not attempted to provide an in-depth view of practice in any one setting, but merely to present a glimpse of cases that represent all types of situations from all sections of the United States and a sample (one case) that represents practice overseas. The backgrounds of the authors range all the way from the novice at a first job to the veteran with many valuable years of experience.

To round out this presentation of case studies in specific settings, we conclude with an experienced health educator's trenchant reflections on his career, a narrative that can serve as a guide for reaching personal and professional goals.

The isolated study of facts and theories does not adequately prepare students to practice health education. The use of case studies in professional preparation offers an opportunity to bridge the gap between theory and its practical application. A field experience or internship also offers this opportunity. We suggest that a combination of these two methods is essential for professional preparation because each provides a different way to learn.

The case study approach to education is used by those who teach medicine, law, and business. In many business and law schools it is the underlying educational approach. Health educators have not used this method as often as these other professions have.

In the case study approach, the student is presented with a record of steps taken to achieve a given goal. The goal may or may not be clear; the steps taken may or may not be appropriate. Case studies don't always present the best alternatives for achieving a goal. They do present what happens. Case studies provide a thought-provoking preview of practice experience, which will help the health educator be more knowledgeable and better prepared to face job realities.

Instructors using case studies often question the students in the Socratic method. This method requires a structured discussion with definite purposes to facilitate learning. Instructors will develop their own style and appropriate levels in presenting individual case studies. Students may need to be taught the basic rules of analyzing cases. In the more complicated case studies, it may be essential to provide background information to aid case analysis.

Effective use of the case method will help students develop the ability to apply previously learned concepts and facts. Each case should be examined for the role of the health educator, for the knowledge and skills required, and for theories and strategies. The student should evaluate the case and suggest alternative solutions.

Students must understand that there are not always "right answers." Given human nature and the fact that all organizations are made up of people, there is not always a tidy, orderly solution. In the analyses of case studies, several theories and strategies may work equally well for the same problem, whereas at other times there will be one theory and strategy that clearly will be the best fit. Students who can make the transition from looking for the right answers to looking for the *best feasible alternatives* are making professional progress.

The case studies in this textbook reflect the imperfect state of the health education environment. There is seldom an orderly progression of events, and often professionals are faced with inadequate data and resources to handle their responsibilities. Health educators must develop the ability to foresee problems and to create the best *possible* solutions. The case method, because it reflects reality, will contribute to developing this ability and thereby promote professional competency.

Each case study can be most effectively examined by using the health education framework, illustrated in the Introduction, as a guide. The editors' analysis (including annotated references/selected resources and discussion questions following each case) has been formulated to generate an initial discussion. The purpose here is not to be all-inclusive, but rather to trigger additional discussion, exploration, and learning—in sum, to stimulate an active involvement with the problem.

This book could not have been published without the many dedicated persons who were willing to write the case studies that they hoped would provide beneficial information to the student and the practitioner. Our most profound thanks to every one of them. Our regrets and sincere apologies to those whose cases we could not publish.

The editors are indebted to a number of others who have assisted in the preparation of this book: Chester Kennedy, who worked out the design for the frame of reference; Cindy Simpson and Carol Bikofsky, who assisted with editing the early copy; Barry Portnoy, Ph.D., and Susan Radius, Ph.D., from Towson State University, who reviewed and commented on cases; and Terry Perry and Janice Sohigian, who typed much of the manuscript.

Our thanks are extended also to the health educators who reviewed the manuscript and offered valuable advice: Edward E. Bartlett of the University of Alabama in Birmingham; Moon S. Chen of Ohio State University; Peter A. Cortese of California State University at Long Beach; Larry K. Olsen of Arizona State University; and James H. Price of the University of Toledo.

Finally, there would not have been a book had it not been for the encouragement of C. Lansing Hays, who has become the Maxwell Perkins of health education, the skilled editing of Lieselotte Hofmann, and the ability of Pat Herbst, Jan de Prosse, and Deborah Cogan to shepherd the book through the production process.

Although we thought we understood the entire field of health education before editing this book, this venture has been a humbling experience. We have had to face our own areas of ignorance. We have been impressed with the knowledge and skills required of the practitioner. We realize that future development of the field calls for an increase in professionalization so that we can meet the demands of, and compete successfully in, a market filled with specialized areas that often neglect comprehensive educational needs.

We must admit it has been surprisingly rewarding to work on this book. Reading the cases, discussing them with the authors, and writing the analyses have been exercises in learning. We hope you will find this book of genuine help in grasping some of the realities in the practice of health education.

Helen P. Cleary
Jeffrey M. Kichen
Phyllis G. Ensor

Advancing Health Through Education

Introduction

This textbook of case studies is written for students interested in pursuing a career in health education, for teachers and practitioners faced with the daily responsibility for health education programming, and for administrators whose job responsibilities intersect health education. Our purpose is to facilitate an understanding of how theories and principles learned in the classroom can be transferred to the real world of practice.

In the past, each body of health education literature was aimed at one particular setting. From 1947 to 1972 the Health Education Department of the University of North Carolina's School of Public Health published health educators' reports on their work in the community. A series of case studies dealing with health education issues in the schools was assembled by Hamburg and Hamburg (1968). Simmons (1975) and Carlaw (1982) have approached the considerations involved in the success of health education by focusing on issues within the context of the community. Our approach differs from all the previous literature because it does not limit its scope to one particular setting; it is our view that the knowledge, skills, and issues involved in health education are generic and applicable to any context.

The central issues in the practice of health education have been discussed by Ross and Mico (1980) and by Green and his co-workers (1980). This textbook goes one step further by illustrating the interrelatedness of health education theories and strategies and the potential benefits to be gained by skillfully combining and utilizing them in daily practice.

The cases selected portray a variety of professional health educators who function in diverse settings. Not all the studies represent optimum practice, nor do they all claim great success. They do, however, reflect the current state of the art and raise issues that are fundamental to the training of the health educator. A broader understanding of these critical issues should contribute to the general well-being of the entire population, for it is our belief that the health of people can be immeasurably improved through education.

HOW TO USE THIS BOOK

The case studies are grouped into four parts, each dealing with the practice of health education in a different context: schools, medical care facilities, community agencies, and worksites. This arbitrary division is used only for convenience, and it is essential to remember that the knowledge, skills, and issues are generic and applicable to all settings.

To assist you to better understand each case as well as the comprehensive practice of health education, you should examine the case studies within the HE (health education) framework shown in the accompanying figure. This framework encompasses the role of the health educator, the knowledge and skills needed for successful practice, the theories and strategies that underlie practice, the health/disease concept that requires education services, and the professional operating procedures and practice management techniques that facilitate practice.

ROLE

Seven major responsibilities for entry-level health education personnel have been described and verified by the Health Education Role Delineation Project (U.S. Department of Commerce 1982):

1. Assessing the need for health education
2. Planning health education programs
3. Coordinating planned education programs
4. Providing direct health education services
5. Evaluating health education programs
6. Promoting organizational and social development
7. Continuing personal professional development

The following additional responsibilities are most often assumed by senior-level practitioners:

1. Training
2. Basic research and theory development
3. Staff supervision and management
4. Grant writing and fund development
5. Policy making

Each case study will present the health educators's involvement in at least one or more of these roles.

KNOWLEDGE AND SKILLS

Essential knowledge and skills are drawn from a variety of disciplines that provide diverse capabilities. You are urged to examine each case to determine the base of knowledge and skills that underlies the health educator's activities. This base is not always explicitly stated in each case, so it is useful to review some of the bases here.

The knowledge and skills required by all health educators at any level of practice or in any setting fall into several broad categories, which include those pertaining to educational methods, health behavior determinants, health topics, program administration, structure of organizations, theories of learning, social and behavior change, professionalism, and systems analysis. A tentative list of the bases of knowledge and skills needed by entry-level health educators is provided in the role verified section of the Role Delineation Project (U.S. Department of Commerce 1982). Of course, the senior-level practitioner must have additional knowledge and skills.

THEORIES AND STRATEGIES

Behavioral science and learning theories provide the assumptions and accepted principles that establish the explanations and predictions of human behavior. Theories commonly used by health education professionals include field theories and theories of individual behavior, communications, social learning, and organizational behavior. Ross and Mico (1980) provide a concise introduction to many of these theories.

Strategies supply the methods of intervention used to establish the desired human behavior. Community organization may be one strategy for effecting change in a community's use of pesticides; group discussion may be a strategy for assisting hypertension patients to cope better with their illness. The strategy of a fifth-grade teacher may be to use a game to teach his or her class the effects of drugs on the human system; the strategy of an industry may be to run a media campaign to raise awareness of the need for preventive practices. Detailed discussions of strategies are given by Green and his colleagues (1980).

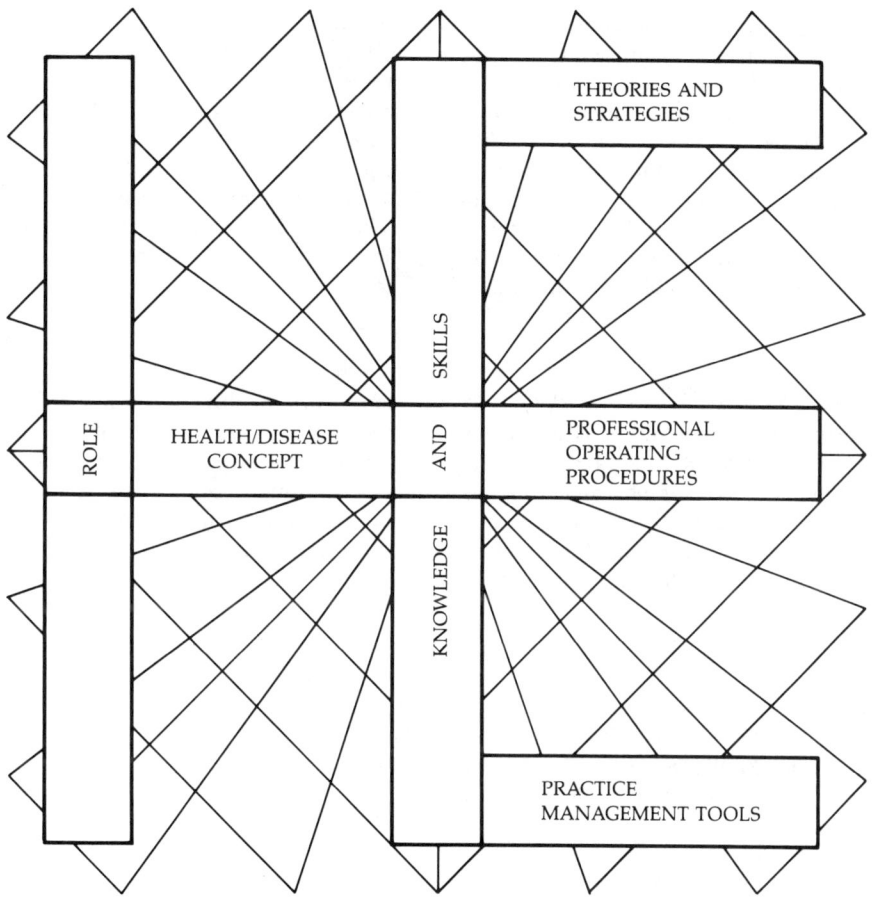

Practice of Health Education

HEALTH/DISEASE CONCEPT

Each case study should be read with a view toward determining if a health/disease concept is involved. Not every case focuses on a specific disease such as cervical cancer or diabetes, but instead may be concerned with broad concepts such as general nutrition or child health. If a health/disease concept does exist, it is important to consider the health educator's role concerning it. Is the health educator viewed as the expert or does he or she work as a coordinator or trainer or evaluator? Depending on the answer to this question, the activities involved will vary considerably.

PROFESSIONAL OPERATING PROCEDURES

Establishing professional conduct in carrying out one's daily activities is essential to good practice. Such conduct allows successful interaction with staff for increased credibility and also encourages increased support for health education within the organization.

Reading the case studies should result in a greater awareness of professional operating methods. What procedures does the health educator use in developing a working group? For example, has the agenda been carefully prepared prior to the meeting with the committee chairperson? Does the health educator interact with other personnel on the medical staff? Does the health educator function as a peer advocating her or his area of expertise? What has the health educator done, or perhaps should she or he have done, to build credibility? For example, did the health educator offer assistance with an agency program, even though unasked, if it seemed that she or he could make a contribution? Obviously, the examples are too numerous to mention, but establishing an aura of professionalism is of prime importance.

PRACTICE MANAGEMENT TECHNIQUES

Systematic procedures for obtaining and dispensing information and data are integral to achieving optimum results. What type of record-keeping system does the health educator use, and how does that aid in the completion of tasks? What channels of communication are established with administration, other staff, and consumers? Management techniques may not be explicitly stated in each case study; some ferreting may have to be done. It is important for the new health education practitioner to be aware of practice management techniques and to understand how they can facilitate the accomplishment of tasks. Certainly, it is better to become aware of them while a student than to face them unprepared while learning on the job.

ADDITIONAL FACTORS

In addition to the six components listed in the HE framework, health educators will find a number of miscellaneous issues that often occur outside of their control but that may be crucial to effective programming. Issues such as funding and staff continuity, for example, may directly or indirectly determine whether the programs succeed or fail.

REFERENCES

Carlaw, R. W., ed. 1982. *Perspectives on Community Health Education: A Series of Case Studies.* Vol. 1, *United States.* Oakland, Calif.: Third Party Publishing.

Green, L. W.; Kreuter, M. W.; Deeds, S. G.; and Partridge, K. B. 1980. *Health Education Planning: A Diagnostic Approach.* Palo Alto, Calif.: Mayfield.

Hamburg, M., and Hamburg, M. W. 1968. *Health and Social Problems in the Schools: Case Studies for School Personnel.* Philadelphia: Lea & Feiger.

Ross, H. S., and Mico, P. R. 1980. *Theory and Practice in Health Education.* Palo Alto, Calif.: Mayfield.

Simmons, J., ed. 1975. "Making Health Education Work." *American Journal of Public Health* 65 (October, suppl.):1–49.

University of North Carolina. Department of Health Education. 1947–1972. *Health Educators at Work.* Chapel Hill.

U.S. Department of Commerce. National Technical Information Service. 1982. *Role Refinement and Verification for Health Educators; Final Report.* Access no. (HRP) 09–04273. Springfield, Va.

Perspectives on Critical Issues in the Practice of Health Education

Both the budding and the seasoned health educator should be aware of and informed about current issues in the practice of health education. As this book is about the practice of health education in all settings, we will identify and discuss here some current outstanding issues.

THEORY

Health education does not have a theoretical base separate and distinct from other professions that deal with human services. It is drawn from education and the social and behavioral sciences. All human service professions operate on a similar theoretical base because they all deal with human behavior. Many of their social, behavioral, and educational theories have been derived from observations and maxims of human behavior that were described by ancient masters, that is, the biblical writers and the Greek and Roman philosophers (Ulich 1971). Each of the professions has adapted, refined, and expanded these descriptions and formulated principles based on the language of its own specialty.

Kurt Lewin is reported to have said there is nothing as practical as a good theory, yet few health education practitioners use theory as a guide to establish explanations and predictions of human behavior. Possibly this invaluable aid is ignored because many practitioners neither understand theory nor know how to apply it. This neglect also may be due to the confusion created by the multitude of theories that could be applied to the practice of health education. Establishing the use of theory in health education could further our understanding and be invaluable in teaching us why suggested strategies do or do not work.

Health educators work in a variety of settings with people at all levels and on all types of issues. Therefore it is appropriate for the health educator to select an available theory that is most applicable to the given population and setting. In addition, the health educator can develop a more specific theory for a particular situation, which Mullen (1978) calls a "middle range theory" in her study of post–myocardial infarction patients. This type of literature provides the practitioner with precise guides for individual, group, and community responses to issues related directly to personal or community health. It is imperative that the profession continue to develop these theories specific to the practice of health education.

Theories can be utilized in many different ways. An examinination of the assumptions and accepted principles of human behavior may help us better understand a population's response to a particular program. Although one theory may determine why a specific population responded in a certain way, that theory may not tell us how to deal with that particular response. It may be necessary to explore other theories before finding one that is appropriate to guide us in taking action. The cognitive dissonance theory, for example, explains why some members of a population may flatly reject ideas or programs that, from an objective viewpoint, should be of interest to them (Festinger 1957). Maslow's (1968) hierarchy of needs is a theory that helps us understand why a population's response to a program may not be as enthusiastic as the professionals expected. Assumptions derived from adoption-diffusion theory will help explain individual and community responses to a new practice and provide a valuable guide for program planning and implementation (Rogers 1983).

Because health education draws its theoretical base from education and the social and behavioral sciences, a large resource of developed theory is already available to the health educator. To eliminate potential confusion, it is important to remember three facts about theory development:

1. Theories relevant to the practice of health education deal with human behavior (individual, group, and organizational) and with ways that people learn/change.
2. Theories are formulated from different perspectives; for example, psychologists look at individuals, sociologists look at communities, and anthropologists look at cultures.
3. Theories formulated by the various branches of education and the behavioral and social sciences often deal with identical or similar concepts at different levels of abstraction.

Theories can be applied to either a specific or a broad-based area. Mullen's (1978) work, which explains the specific responses of post–myocardial infarction patients to their disease, is an example of a specific application, and Rogers's explanation of the phenomenon of adoption-diffusion concepts covers a wide spectrum.

Ross and Mico (1980) describe diffusion-adoption from the perspective of a communication theory previously developed by Katz and Lazarsfeld (1955). They suggest that ideas are adopted by a community's opinion leaders, or "gatekeepers," who then pass them on to others: "Opinion leaders, then, constitute the first step in the communication process, and those influenced by them constitute the second step" (Ross and Mico 1980:164). This concept reinforces Rogers's (1983) theory that innovators and early adopters are the first two groups to assume a new practice in a community. It is interesting to note other similarities between the findings established by Rogers, a sociologist who focused on diffusion of a practice through communities, and Katz and Lazarsfeld, psychologists who focused on diffusion of a practice from individual to individual.

Students must learn to recognize similarities among theories and to select those most applicable for a given situation. It is vital for the entry-level practitioner to have a fundamental grasp of the theories that can best facilitate the planning and implementation of programs.

LEARNING/SOCIAL CHANGE (PLANNED)

It is important for the health educator to understand that there are certain similarities between the learning process and the social change process. Lack of this understanding undermines the goals of health education, for it may result in destructive divisiveness and lessen the opportunity for the sharing and mutual support needed by health education professionals.

A brief review of definitions and characteristics

concerning learning and social change will support our thesis that there are definite similarities between the two processes.

In discussing a definition of learning, Kidd (1977:24, 15, 16) suggests that although

> we cannot pin down anything as dynamic as learning . . . we can observe it, note its course and its character. . . .
> Learning . . . is not simply a matter of accretion—of adding something. . . .
> . . . Learning involves a change in behavior: [it] may make us respond differently. . . .
> . . . These [responses] may be primarily "intellectual" changes—the acquiring of new ideas or some reorganization of presently held ideas. . . . The changes may be in attitude where we hope that people will come to a different appreciation and more positive feelings about a subject. Or they may be changes in skill where we expect the learner to become more efficient in performing certain acts. . . .
> Much of learning is related to shifts in the tasks or roles that a person performs.

Other educators agree with Kidd's position (Darkenwald and Merriam 1982:8; Knowles 1970: 50–52).

Zaltman and Duncan (1977:6,9) state that "perhaps the most difficult conceptual issue in studying social change is to adequately define social change. There is a wide array of theories focusing on the process of social change, leaving the definition implicit in the theory." Further, persons or groups change their behavior "when they define the situation as being different and now requiring different behavior." Rogers (1971:7) defines social change as "the process by which alterations occur in the structure and function of a social system. . . . The structure of a social system is provided by the various individual and group statuses which compose it. The functioning element within this structure of status is a role, or the actual behavior of the individual in a given status."

Although both processes, learning and social change, require individual change, they differ significantly in their central focus: learning tends to focus on change as it relates to the individual; social change tends to focus on change as it occurs in groups or social systems or society. There are, however, social change theories about individual change (Weber 1958). Both perspectives recognize that individual learning can result in societal change, and that societal change does require that a certain number of individuals have learned. The similarity between these two concepts is clear. It is also obvious that, in regard to health education activities, in the community setting it is usually more appropriate to adopt social change principles rather than learning principles, whereas in a school setting, learning principles are apt to be more useful than social change principles.

Learning theories are usually espoused by educational psychologists, and social change theories by sociologists. Kidd (1977) has identified theories of learning stated by psychologists. The three classes of theories we believe are most useful in the practice of health education are cognitive theories, field theories, and social learning theories. Bruner's (1966) theory of instruction, his concepts of the process of education, his views on curriculum development, and his ideas about readiness to learn offer guides and explanations for practitioners. Lewin's (1951) field theory of learning, including the concepts of life space and "learned" learning versus "imposed" learning (discussed in the next section), offers explanations and guides for the health educator. Bandura's (1977) social learning theory formalizes the concept of modeling, long recognized as a way by which people learn.

The sociological theory of social change most useful in the practice of health education is that of adoption-diffusion (Rogers 1983). We reviewed the literature on social change theory and agree with Martindale (1972:18) that social action theorists have not generated a well-formulated theory of social change but have "produced a large number of generalizations usually employed by sociology at present to account for various special changes without anchoring these ideas in a single identifiable theory of social change."

In addition to these theories that have been drawn from the behavioral and social sciences and have proven useful in the practice of health education, there are several principles of learning and social change that can be applied in the case studies of this textbook. Taba (1962) and others identified principles of learning derived from well-developed learning theory. Pine and Horne (1969) identified a similar set of principles through their experience in working with antipoverty aids. Zaltman and

Table 1
Principles of Learning and Social Change and Their Application in Health Education

Principles of Learning	Principles of Social Change	Synthesis of Principles Applicable to the Practice of Health Education
1. "An individual learns by imitation and identification" (Taba 1962:132).	". . . in addition to planned change . . . , unplanned change occurs as the result of interaction among forces . . . brought about with no apparent deliberateness" (Zaltman and Duncan 1977:379).	People learn and people change as a result of informal as well as formal processes.
2. "Transfer to new tasks will be better if . . . he (the learner) has experience during learning of applying principles within a variety of tasks" (Taba 1962:87).	". . . stimulate word-of-mouth communication to augment other channels" (Zaltman and Duncan, 1977:381).	People learn and people change as the result of a number of different experiences.
3. What they want to learn, what they are ready to learn, what they are curious about, meaningful material (Pine and Horne 1969; Bruner 1966).	What meets their needs better than their current practices; or those practices which they feel they can do better (Zaltman and Duncan: 380–381).	People will learn about or will change those things they perceive to be meaningful and useful to them.
4. "The personal history of the individual may hamper or enhance his ability to learn" (Taba 1962:87).	What is compatible with their "existing values, beliefs, capabilities"; what is acceptable to their social relationships (Zaltman and Duncan 1977:381)	People will learn or change those things acceptable to their social group.
5. "Learning is a consequence of experience" (Pine and Horne 1969:109).	People will change those things they can try out to see if they work for them (Zaltman and Duncan 1977:381).	People will learn or change those things they have an opportunity to explore.

Duncan (1977) developed a set of principles of social change derived from the experiences of many people.

By combining the principles found in the literature with our own experiences, we have synthesized in Table 1 the learning and social change concepts directly related to the practice of health education.

LEARNING VERSUS COMPLIANCE

The issue of compliance is directly related to our discussion of learning/social change. The practicing health educator must understand the similarity and difference between the learning/social change and compliance processes. Health educators working in medical care settings are familiar with the

Table 1 *continued*

Principles of Learning	Principles of Social Change	Synthesis of Principles Applicable to the Practice of Health Education
6. "The process of learning [is] as important as what is transmitted directly or the content of learning. In this process feelings in turn direct action and conduct" (Taba 1962:132).	"Change agents should avoid the rationalistic bias in designing change programs. . . . [W]hat the change target considers rational may not be the same as what the change agent considers rational" (Zaltman and Duncan 1977:380).	Learning and change have an affective as well as a cognitive component.
7. "Students should be in on where they are trying to go, what they are trying to get hold of and how much pertinent progress they are making" (Bigge 1982:241).	"In planning for change, innovation, the change agent and the client system should try to be clear about the change objectives . . . otherwise ambiguity and uncertainty can occur and can cause resistance" (Zaltman and Duncan 1977:380).	Involve the learners or those who are to change in the process of learning or changing.
8. "Any idea or problem or body of knowledge can be presented in a form simple enough so that any particular learner can understand it in recognizable form" (Bruner 1966:44).	"Every effort should be made to simplify the change to make it less complex or difficult to understand" (Zaltman and Duncan 1977:381).	Begin where the learner or the target population is.
9. The fact that learning takes time is a basic assumption of all literature of learning (Editors).	"The change agent should think in terms of optimum rather than minimum time for introducing change" (Zaltman and Duncan 1977:381).	People learn and people change over time; learning and change take time.

difference. Although Haynes and colleagues (1979) have written a valuable literature review on compliance, nothing in the literature links the compliance process with the learning/change process. Lewin (1951:77–81) provides us with an explanation of this relationship. He speaks of "imposed" learning and "learned" learning. Imposed learning is applied to those individuals who either are not interested in change or are learning against their will. Kelman (1958) calls this process "forced compliance." People can be forced to comply if they feel that the reward or punishment is great enough, that the proposed action is the lesser of two evils, that they face legal constraints, or that they are not totally aware of the end result of the involvement.

Compliance is sometimes the only course by

which people can be helped to alter their behavior in order to protect the public health or welfare or to defend human dignity. If the time bought by compliance helps people learn the relevance of a new behavior to their goals, it may lead to the acceptance of the new behavior. Adoption of a practice, therefore, does not necessarily mean that individuals have learned. It may mean they are complying merely because they have no other choice.

Lewin's "learned" learning refers to the process that occurs when someone decides he or whe *wants* to learn/change. An individual changes because the new behavior is seen as consonant with personal goals, it is identified with a person or thing that he or she admires and wishes to imitate, or the locus of the behavior changes so that the meaning of the behavior takes on a new significance.

THE DISCIPLINE OF HEALTH EDUCATION

The basic discipline of the health educator is education, helping others to learn through planned learning experiences. Some health educators call themselves change agents as opposed to educators. You can pick your title because education results in change, and change results from education.

Some health educators consider their expertise to be in health rather than in education or social change. All health educators are knowledgeable about general health/disease processes, specific health/disease topics, and generic process skills. Some choose to work in specialized areas, such as nutrition, human sexuality, family planning, or cardiovascular disease. Others prefer to concentrate on process skills, such as community organization or group process.

All health educators, however, apply learning/social change theories and principles to health/disease issues or topics in an effort to help people learn positive health practices. All health educators should be able to use process skills and be knowledgeable about the health/disease content in the area in which they are working. If a health educator wishes to emphasize knowledge of content over process skills or process skills over knowledge or content, that is her or his choice. Health educators of both types can be identified in the case studies.

Some health educators resist associating themselves with the field of education; others resist association with social change. Some of this resistance may be due to the traditional training that separates programs for school health educators from those for community health educators or from health educators who do not work in schools. This system has resulted in a dichotomy between these two branches.

HISTORICAL SUMMARY

School health education in the United States extends as far back as the early national period. By the 1840s Horace Mann, the leading figure in the public education movement, was calling for instruction in physiology and hygiene. In addition, the normal schools began requiring future teachers to complete courses in physiology and hygiene. By the 1850s many private higher education institutions were adopting such courses.

As Means (1962) states, during the period 1850–1900 many developments at the national, state, and local levels stimulated school health education. As public health began to organize, particularly in the states, it had a significant influence, along with other forces such as the child study movement.

This impetus set the stage for the fairly rapid growth of school health education during the first quarter of the twentieth century. Many of the voluntary health organizations that sprang up directed their attention to the schools. Groups such as the Joint Committee on Health Problems in Education were formed to study and make recommendations on all aspects of teaching health in schools. There was now more emphasis on individual habits in health instruction, and the use of supplementary materials in the schools greatly expanded. Research and demonstration projects to influence health habits were conducted around the country.

Professionally trained school health educators also came on the scene during this time. The early professional preparation programs were the province of the normal schools. Gradually universities offered bachelor's and master's degree programs. The first doctoral degree in school health education was awarded by Columbia University in 1921 to Mary E. Spencer.

The next 35 years (1926–1969) saw the consolidation and expansion of the activities that occurred during the previous period. Spencer (1933) produced a comprehensive review of the state of the art of teacher preparation during the early part of this period. She also developed a set of standards for teacher preparation that are as applicable today as they were in the early 1930s. Many new training programs began at the college level after World War II. Research continued and a number of organizations that adopted school health as an active interest were formed.

In the sixties, concern over illicit drug use among the young triggered a rapid expansion of school health education efforts. Many school health education programs were separated from physical education, and the issue of how best to teach health resurfaced. Should it be integrated with academic courses or be a separate course?

The late 1960s and 1970s saw enormous activity by the federal government in training school health educators, in sponsoring the development of materials and curricula, and in supporting research (Means 1975).

The 1980s appear to be another period of consolidation, but one in which school health education has to compete more intensely for its share of the education dollar. Concerns over what to teach and how to teach it remain and will probably exist as long as health education is taught in the schools.

Courses in Health Education The first course in health education in a school of public health was given in 1921–1922 at the combined Harvard–MIT School of Public Health. It was not, however, a course in community health education as we know it today but rather a course in school health education. The course grew out of the interest of a physician, Dr. W. T. Sedgwick, and a biologist, Dr. Claire Turner. It included both didactic and practicum components. The practicum was carried out for the most part in the Malden School System in Massachusetts. In later years, Dr. Mary Spencer, the 1921 doctoral candidate at Columbia, played a major role in developing the school health program in Malden.

In 1923 the Harvard School of Public Health was organized. The MIT program continued until 1945. In the late 1930s and early 1940s this program began to train community health educators but still emphasized school health education in its courses. At about the time the MIT program closed, the Harvard School of Public Health instituted a course in health education. This course retained the school health component, although over time this component received less emphasis and gradually disappeared from the curriculum (Turner 1974).

Other schools of public health (e.g., those at Yale and the University of North Carolina) introduced a course or even a major in health education during this same period. By the 1950s most such courses were process-oriented and became rooted largely in the social sciences, often limiting the emphasis on health/disease content. One reason for this may be that many of the students came from the health field and already had a background in health/disease issues.

The two branches of the field, school health education and public (or community) health education, continued to grow independently of each other. Until very recently, there was very little dialogue between them, but, fortunately, this situation is beginning to change. University programs preparing health educators now offer courses in school health even though the emphasis of the programs is community health; and the reverse is also true. Those who had spurned education because it did not enjoy a good reputation as a scientific discipline are beginning to realize that the practicing health educator needs to know the theories and principles of education. Those who had dissociated themselves from the notion of social change, because they related that to social activism, are now learning how valuable the social change literature can be to the health educator.

The gap between the two is closing now; nevertheless, the divisiveness that has existed over the years has taken its toll. The contributions that health educators have made to the health of consumers, to health policy, and to legislation are far less than they might have been. Too much energy has been wasted defending the turf and maintaining the status quo.

CONCLUSION

All the substantive issues of health education relating to theory, learning/social change, compliance, and the discipline must be discussed and carefully considered by health educators. Examination of these issues will assist us in developing a positive professional identity. It will also help us understand the differences and similarities between our profession and the professions of psychology, sociology, social work, and physical education.

Finally, we are proud of the contribution our profession has already made, and can continue to make, to improve the health of all people. We must, however, continually assess and improve our practice.

REFERENCES

Bandura, A. 1977. *Social Learning Theory.* Englewood Cliffs, N.J.: Prentice-Hall.

Bigge, M. L. 1982. *Learning Theories for Teachers.* New York: Harper & Row.

Bruner, J. S. 1966. *Towards a Theory of Instruction.* Cambridge: Harvard University Press.

Darkenwald, G. G., and Merriam, S. B. 1982. *Adult Education: Foundations of Practice.* New York: Harper & Row.

Festinger, L. 1957. *A Theory of Cognitive Dissonance.* Stanford: Stanford University Press.

Haynes, R. B.; Taylor, D. W.; and Sackett, D. L. 1979. *Compliance in Health Care.* Baltimore: Johns Hopkins University Press.

Katz, E., and Lazarsfeld, P. F. 1955. *Personal Influence: The Part Played by People in the Flow of Mass Communication.* Glencoe, Ill.: Free Press.

Kelman, H. C. 1958. "Compliance, Identification and Internalization: Three Processes of Attitude Change." *Journal of Conflict Resolution* 2 (1):51–60.

Kidd, J. R. 1977. *How Adults Learn.* New York: Association Press.

Knowles, M. 1970. *The Modern Practice of Adult Education.* New York: Association Press.

Lewin, K. 1951. *Field Theory in Social Science.* New York: Harper.

Martindale, D. 1972. "Perspectives on the Process of Social Change." In *Creating Social Change,* edited by G. Zaltman, P. Kotler, and I. Kaufman. New York: Holt, Rinehart & Winston.

Maslow, A. H. 1968. *Toward a Psychology of Being.* 2d ed. New York: Van Nostrand Reinhold.

Means, R. K. 1962. *A History of Health Education in the United States.* Philadelphia: Lea & Febiger.

Means, R. K. 1975. *Historical Perspectives on School Health.* Thorofare, N.J.: Charles B. Slack.

Mullen, P. D. 1978. "Cutting Back after a Heart Attack." *Health Education Monographs* 6:295–311.

Pine, G. J., and Horne, P. J. 1969. "Principles and Conditions for Learning in Adult Education." *Adult Leadership* 18(4):108–134.

Rogers, E. M. 1983. *Diffusion of Innovations.* 3d ed. New York: Free Press.

Rogers, E., and Shoemaker, F. 1971. *Communication of Innovations: A Cross-Cultural Approach.* 2d ed. New York: Free Press.

Ross, H. S., and Mico, P. R. 1980. *Theory and Practice in Health Education.* Palo Alto, Calif.: Mayfield.

Spencer, M. E. 1933. *Health Educators for Teachers: A Critical Study of the Pre-service Preparation of Classroom Teachers for the School Health Program.* New York: Columbia University, Teachers College, Bureau of Publications.

Taba, H. 1962. *Curriculum Development: Theory and Practice.* New York: Harcourt Brace Jovanovich.

Turner, C. E. 1974. *I Remember.* New York: Vantage Press.

Ulich, R., ed. 1971. *Three Thousand Years of Educational Wisdom.* Cambridge: Harvard University Press.

Weber, M. 1958. *The Protestant Effort and the Spirit of Capitalism.* New York: Scribner.

Zaltman, G., and Duncan, R. 1977. *Strategies for Planned Change.* New York: Wiley.

PART ONE

Case Studies in School Settings

Schools were the first setting in which health was taught in an organized way. The history of school health education goes back to 1850 (see p. 8 for a historical summary).

THE STATE OF THE ART

At times it may seem that there are as many underlying philosophies and ways to organize health education in the schools as there are school systems. To a great extent this is the result of (1) the decentralized nature of school systems in the United States and (2) the ongoing development of health education as a discipline.

Local school systems have traditionally developed the underlying philosophy and organized curricula for specific disciplines. Usually state education authorities, through legislation and regulations, prescribe what should be taught at what grade level and for how long. This situation generally applies to the basic disciplines (English, mathematics, social studies, and science). In contrast, state education authorities are less prescriptive about subject areas that are not termed "basics."

Health education in many states is either now making or has only recently made the transition from a nonbasic to a basic discipline. This transition is largely the result of top-down efforts by policymakers from both the public sector (state and federal agencies) and the private sector (American School Health Association, American Medical Association, and the National Education Association); but at the local level, grass-roots efforts by interested parents, teachers, and students have also played a part.

Currently, all the states mandate instruction in certain health topics, most often alcohol, tobacco, and drugs. Twenty states require students to pass a health class for graduation. In 37 states, there is a health certification or endorsement for teachers at the elementary and/or secondary level. The Education Commission of the States (1982:27) comments that usually "states recommend or suggest topics to be included in the health education curriculum, but local districts make the final determination regarding the scope of the program. Thus it is not uncommon to find greater or lesser interest and commitment at the local level than exists at the state level."

Some local school systems have instituted what has been termed comprehensive school health education. Although the content areas may vary from system to system, the Education Commission of the States generally considers the minimum elements for a comprehensive program to be as follows:

Personal health
Mental and emotional health
Prevention and control of disease
Nutrition
Substance use and abuse
Accident prevention and safety
Community health
Environmental health
Family life education

Some systems offer significant administrative support by providing a systemwide health education coordinator, whose functions and resources are similar to those granted to the coordinators of other basic disciplines.

ROLE OF THE SCHOOL HEALTH EDUCATOR

The health educator in a school system can be a classroom teacher or a coordinator, and in either capacity he or she may also function as a counselor (McKenzie/Ogletree case). If health education is not considered a basic in a school system, both the coordinator and the teacher may have to advocate for health education, which may require working within and outside the school system. Both must also develop relationships with health resources in the community and work with the community in curriculum development.

Because of sensitive health issues and multi-ethnic communities, it is particularly critical for the school health educator to know the community. Cooperative efforts are possible only if he or she understands and respects the local culture. This is obvious in the case study of the Pima Indian Reservation by Redican, Olsen, Baffi, and Dezelsky. Although less obvious, it was equally important in the Robinson case. The counseling case by McKenzie and Ogletree shows how essential the knowledge of community values is for the classroom teacher who counsels students.

The need for the school health educator, especially at the secondary level, to have elementary counseling skills is also illustrated by the McKenzie/Ogletree case. Counseling is an educational method that should be part of the skill package of every health educator.

Very often the community will demand that the curriculum reflect its own values and culture. In the case by Redican and his colleagues we see this as a prime concern of the planners. However, although the curriculum required many elements specific to the culture, the curriculum planners utilized a number of well-accepted approaches, such as the traditional unit approach and the School Health Curriculum Project (U.S. DHEW 1978). It is clear, then, that a curriculum can respond to local needs without having a totally new conceptual framework.

In some ways the teaching of health can be more demanding than the teaching of other disciplines. The health teacher finds early on that he or she must be a role model for health. Young people's health practices are to a great extent a result of role modeling or social learning. In contrast, the teacher of mathematics or social studies is certainly less likely to have to be a role model for his or her subject. The Seaside program, documented in the Drolet case, is a good example of how a continuing education program can be sensitive to the role modeling issue by helping the participants make changes in their own health behavior.

In addition to the role of the health educator, a number of other issues should be considered: How should health be taught? Who should teach it? What should be taught? Why should health be taught in the schools?

HOW SHOULD HEALTH BE TAUGHT?

According to Kime, Schlaadt, and Tritsch (1977), health instruction at the classroom level can be implemented through three different plans:

1. *Integration*—health is taught as part of the core curriculum, usually within a thematic context.
2. *Correlation*—health is taught with another subject, such as science, physical education, or social studies.
3. *Separate course*—health is taught at regular designated times just as other separate subjects are.

Integration is most commonly used at the elementary level. At the secondary level—middle school, junior high, and high school—either correlation or a separate course is employed; rarely are both used in the same system.

What are the best methods of teaching health? The "how" of teaching can be a volatile issue. Some communities opt for health topics; others find a values and decision-making approach acceptable. Communities that have rejected the latter have felt that it imposed values contrary to those of the community, as the Nybo case illustrates. The preferred curriculum should include both health topics, that is, information, and the skill to make decisions on how to use this information (Kime, Schlaadt, and Tritsch 1977).

WHO SHOULD TEACH HEALTH?

The commitment of the school system to teaching health determines whether health is taught by a teacher who is certified to do so or by one who is certified to teach some other subject but has in-service education in health. As noted earlier, this is a local decision. Whether a school system chooses to hire a teacher certified in health has little to do with budget or time; it is a matter of commitment. Usually, systems that elect to have certified health education teachers teach health as a separate course commit more of their available resources to health education than do systems that choose not to do so.

Requirements for certification of health teachers vary among the states. Rash and Pigg (1979:12) suggest that health should be taught by a "special person, with specialized background of education uniquely equipping him or her for the task of providing health instruction and of fostering the process of health education in the several aspects of the school health program." They suggest minimum preparation should be 24 semester hours in health and safety education, along with preparation in the behavioral sciences. The issue here is not whether health is a separate course or a part of the science or social studies curriculum. The issue is whether the teacher *is prepared to teach health*. To be a convincing teacher, she or he must be committed to the subject.

Teachers can be committed to health issues even though they are not prepared to teach them, as we see in the Owens case. The Amschler case documents the process that an instructor at a college underwent after she was assigned to teach a health course that was new to her. Her experience is an example of how commitment grows over time. Teacher interest can also be developed through in-service education, as illustrated by the Drolet case.

WHAT SHOULD BE TAUGHT?

Much heat (but often not much light) has been generated in some communities in regard to what subjects should be taught. For example, whether sex education should be taught is often a topic for headlines in local papers. Ideally, curricula should be developed by school and community members working together so that community values are not likely to be violated. However, even this approach does not always work out. The Nybo case demonstrates a good attempt at cooperation between school and community on curriculum development. But even in this case, school and community values clashed in some communities.

WHY TEACH HEALTH IN THE SCHOOLS?

The best reason for teaching health in schools is given in the title of a kit produced by the American School Health Association: "A Healthy Child: The Key to Basics." This kit was designed to assist interested citizens in advocating for health education in their schools. The kit was issued in response to the current drive to get back to the basics. In its report dealing primarily with secondary schools, the National Commission on Excellence in Education (U.S. Department of Education 1983) recommends that five basic subjects be taught in the secondary schools: English, mathematics, science, social studies, and computer science.

Few would dispute the statement that a healthy child is the first requirement for learning the basics. The Surgeon General's Report on Health Promotion and Disease Prevention (U.S. DHEW 1979) indicates that all school-age children are not healthy. It addresses diseases and social problems that affect the health status of children of all ages. According to the report, the leading causes of death for children ages 1–14 are, in order of rank, all accidents except motor vehicle, motor vehicle accidents, cancer, birth defects, influenza, and homicide. For the 15–24 age group the leading causes of death are motor vehicle accidents, all other accidents, suicide, homicide, cancer, and heart disease. Whites have a significantly higher death rate from motor vehicle accidents than nonwhites, and nonwhites have a significantly higher rate for homicide than whites. These causes of death are preventable.

The social problems that affect the health status of children of all ages are issues society must tackle. But responsibility for doing something about these issues must be accepted by all institutions and all strata of society, including all age groups. Children need to learn how to maintain a healthy body and mind. Schools are one of society's institutions that must contribute to children's knowledge and skills in this regard (Fodor and Dalis 1981). But how does a mandate to teach health in the schools fit with the report of the National Commission on Excellence in Education (U.S. Department of Education 1983), with its call for instruction in the basics? The challenge to the school system committed to teaching health is to include health in the curriculum while strengthening the basics.

The commission's recommendations for curriculum development include a conceptual, problem-solving approach and instruction in the relationship and application of knowledge to everyday life. Early on, the School Health Education Study (1967) had devised a conceptual, problem-solving approach to teaching health in the schools.

The Education Commission of the States (1982) points out that the purposes of health education are similar to those of education in general—that is, to equip the student with the knowledge and skills needed to make informed decisions about choices in life. The commission recognizes the importance of teacher preparation and of developing students' ability to think critically and to assume responsibility. These issues are also noted by the Commission on Excellence in Education.

Some school administrators may cry poverty and lack of time as arguments against including health in the curriculum. The response to their argument is quite straightforward: It just depends on how you want to spend your resources. There is plenty of money—the total school budget. There is a great deal of time—the entire school day.

REFERENCES

Education Commission of the States. 1982. *Recommendations for School Health Education: A Handbook for State Policymakers*. Denver.

Fodor, J. T., and Dalis, G. T. 1981. *Health Instruction: Theory and Application*. Philadelphia: Lea & Febiger.

Kime, R. E.; Schlaadt, R. G.; and Tritsch, L. E. 1977. *Health Instruction: An Action Approach*. Englewood Cliffs, N.J.: Prentice-Hall.

Rash, J. K., and Pigg, R. M. 1979. *The Health Education Curriculum: A Guide for Curriculum Development in Health Education*. New York: Wiley.

U.S. Department of Education. National Commission on Excellence in Education. 1983. *A Nation at Risk: The Imperative for Educational Reform*. Washington, D.C.: Government Printing Office.

U.S. Department of Health, Education, and Welfare. 1978. *The School Health Curriculum Project*. DHEW Publication no. (CDC) 78–8359. Washington, D.C.: Government Printing Office.

U.S. Department of Health, Education, and Welfare. Office of the Assistant Secretary for Health and Surgeon General. 1979. *Healthy People: Surgeon General's Report on Health Promotion and Disease Prevention*. DHEW Publication no. (PHS) 79–55071. Washington, D.C.: Government Printing Office.

Elementary School Health Education

Charlotte Owens, B.S.

No person is better suited to teach health than the classroom teacher, simply because he or she sees the child more often than anyone else except, possibly, the parents.

In the schools of Baltimore County Maryland, health is taught by the method of "fitting it in whenever you can." As a separate curriculum it is nonexistent, at least on the elementary level. Health is primarily incorporated into the science curriculum. However, the county encourages that it be taught whenever it is deemed appropriate.

MY INITIATION INTO HEALTH TEACHING

After graduating with a B.S. degree in elementary education in June 1980, I immediately obtained an interview with the county's school personnel office, my first and roughest interview. In August I accepted an offer to teach fifth grade in an area called Middle River. Although I was declared excess personnel after two years, I was, luckily, able to keep my position as a result of another teacher's transfer. As I was interested in child health, I began working toward a master's degree in health education. My first few classes in this program alerted me to how limited health teaching was in elementary schools in my county. Looking back on my teacher preparation experience, I couldn't recall any specific content courses related to teaching health. I began to realize that the only way health

---

Charlotte Owens is a fifth-grade teacher at Sandalwood Elementary School in Baltimore, Maryland. She is currently working toward a master's degree in health education.

was going to be taught in Middle River schools was to take the initiative myself.

Throughout the school year, as I taught the fifth-grade curriculum in science, I extended the units to include more than the county required. It was hard to decide what part of the unit to delete so as to replace it with something that might not otherwise have been taught. Reorganizing the time for this extension was also difficult.

The fifth-grade units most closely related to health are "All Systems Go" (circulatory, respiratory, and digestive systems), "Plant and Animal Cells" (if you stretched some of the concepts), and "The Use and Abuse of Nonfood Substances" (drug unit).

I was particularly impressed with the drug unit and the objectives the county designed for it. The curriculum emphasizes good decision-making skills. Students were presented with facts about drugs, given specific skills to enable them to make important decisions, and encouraged to decide for themselves what choices they wanted to make in life. This kind of unit lends itself well to class discussion and role-playing techniques, which I use in many areas of the curriculum.

I was interested in the unit also because it provided essential preparation for students to enter middle school and high school. Aside from the obvious drug abuse problem existing in those schools, I was concerned that the students be socially and emotionally ready. I perceived good decision-making skills to be most effective in preparing them.

The students come to the school from a variety of backgrounds. The Middle River area was originally a community based on heavy industry. Many of the old houses and trailers are still in use today, and the people tend to be middle-class, blue-collar workers. But new developments are springing up to house higher-income people.

The school is situated right in the middle of the community and pulls students from both sides of the track. Regardless of which side the students live on, both populations share similar problems. Many of the children are living with one parent as a result of separation, divorce, or runaway spouses. Some students are living with grandparents and don't even know their parents. Many are physically and verbally abused. Those whose parents work long and inconsistent hours are strongly influenced by older brothers and sisters. As a result of these circumstances, many of the students are forced to grow up faster and become more independent than they might normally. They are in desperate need of good decision-making skills.

IMPLEMENTING THE DRUG PROGRAM

The drug unit is scheduled for approximately four weeks. It covers the effects of drugs on the systems of the body and the use and abuse of tobacco, alcohol, and narcotics and other hard drugs.

My goals for the unit are (1) to initiate discussion; (2) to enable the children to feel comfortable about expressing their feelings, to respect each others' opinions, and to realize what's right for one person isn't always right for another; and (3) to increase the students' awareness about drugs so they can make informed decisions.

The students participate in various activities to help reinforce these goals. During one part of the unit, the students bring in empty containers of prescription and over-the-counter drugs. They practice reading labels and comparing them to determine similarities. Role playing is used to mimic consumers entering a drug store to purchase over-the-counter drugs or get prescriptions filled. We discuss the kinds of questions consumers should be asking about their drugs.

Tracing time lines seems to be an equally enjoyable activity. The students use adding-machine tape to plot the history of drugs from caveman days to the present.

The students also make contracts to break a bad habit. Popular targets for reform are chewing their fingernails, eating junk food, and not getting enough sleep. The contracts are signed by the student, teacher, and parent(s). Often the students will persuade their parents to devise a similar contract, usually about drinking or smoking. Discussions are held on ways to help parents cut back on alcohol and tobacco.

Community agencies are involved in the course, too. Representatives of the American Lung Association visit the school to demonstrate "Smoking Sam," a mannequin that smokes a cigarette and allows the students to see the effects of cigarettes on the lungs. Another community organization offers a "Kool Kat" presentation, which stresses values and peer pressure among students.

Decision-making skills are taught in the following sequence (Bailey 1981):

1. Defining the problem
2. Considering and listing alternative solutions
3. Gathering facts and opinions
4. Weighing the facts and opinions to decide on a solution
5. Being prepared to accept the consequences for a decision

I read to the class from a book of open-ended stories related to drugs (Velder and Cohen 1973). The students work through the five steps just listed to decide how they would have ended each story. For similar situations, I use role playing and ask the children to put themselves in the enacted position. Sometimes they read newspapers or magazine articles and identify the decision-making process used by a particular person in an article. They are permitted to interject their own feelings in deciding what they would have done in the situation described (Greenberg 1978).

Students are evaluated through tests to see whether they have obtained the factual knowledge. However, it's hard to measure their values and beliefs. One can only hope that they've acquired the skills to make rational decisions and that, when confronted with situations like those they've studied, they will select the best choices for themselves.

I believe the need for drug education in this geographic area and particularly with this age level is critical. The students are susceptible to peer pressure and vulnerable to unfamiliar situations. The drug education curriculum is, I think, essential and very appropriate for the grade level.

CONCLUSION

Involvement is needed by students, parents, community organizations, teachers, staff, and administrators to promote health education in the schools. Although the ultimate goal is to develop health education as an integral part of the curriculum at every grade level, it is possible to incorporate it into other subject areas until we can reach that goal. The need is obvious, the students want to learn, and as responsible adults we have an obligation to help them.

REFERENCES

Bailey, J. 1981. *Drug Use in American Society: An Epidemiologic Analysis of Risks.* Minneapolis: Burgess.

Greenberg, J. S. 1978. *Student-Centered Health Instruction: A Humanistic Approach.* Reading, Mass.: Addison-Wesley.

Velder, M., and Cohen, E. 1973. *Open-Ended Stories.* New York: Globe Book Co.

Analysis

At first reading, this case telling of the solitary efforts of an elementary-classroom teacher appears inconsequential. However, it is representative of many individual efforts to initiate health instruction in the schools and illustrates the integrative method of health instruction noted in the introduction to Part 1.

Owens was interested in the health of her students but had received no training, in her teacher preparation program, to teach health. She used good educational procedure by conducting a needs assessment to select topics for her curriculum. She learned about the community and the changing social and economic conditions and related these factors to the students' immediate and future needs for health instruction. Because of the social conditions and type of family life, she gave the drug unit priority and emphasized decision-making skills.

Owens used a variety of teaching methods, a basic principle of good teaching. John Dewey's "learning to do by doing" philosophy was implemented by using methods that required the students to be active rather than passive (Dewey 1938). Owens also involved community resources. This is a useful procedure, for it brings up-to-date information into the classroom, helps build support for the program, and serves as a means of communicating with the community.

The elementary teacher is in daily contact with the children. Most elementary teachers keep weight/height/age records on their students, and many assist in vision and hearing tests. The teacher's involvement with these measures of health status allows the teacher to make health instruction relevant and to weave it into many aspects of the curriculum (Schaller 1981). The integrative method of teaching health at the elementary level can be effective. But it can be even more so if the school system has a health education coordinator who can assist teachers in developing health units, in identifying appropriate materials, and in incorporating health instruction into the general curriculum. An additional function of the coordinator is to provide in-service education on health topics and issues for the elementary teachers.

This case illustrates that individual effort can make an impact. Owens worked within the structure to add health education to the existing curriculum and obtained administrative support for the extra health instruction. She was willing to do the extra work, deal with the administration, and get acquainted with the community to meet a need of her students. This case raises the issue of how health should be taught at the elementary level. If a school system is not yet committed to teaching health, the individual teacher may be able to teach it if interested. In this case, the administration allowed the teacher to do as she wished. Many other administrations would do the same. But the burden is then on the teacher to take the initiative and spend the time and energy needed to develop health units. That asks a great deal of the individual teacher, although there are many like Owens in our school systems.

References/Select Resources

Burke, A.; Olsen, L. K.; and Redican, K. J. 1982. "Analysis of the Long Range Effects of the Science Health Curriculum Project: Grade 5. *Health Values: Achieving High Level Wellness* 6 (July–August):26–32.

The School Health Curriculum Project (SHCP) is an example of a comprehensive health education curriculum that shares many of the components of the concept of high-level wellness. The purpose of this study was to analyze the long-range affective and cognitive effects of the fifth-grade unit of the SHCP. This article provides information on the pre- and posttests that revealed a cognitive retention of above 80 percent.

Cornacchia, H. H., and W. M. Staton. 1979. *Health in Elementary Schools*. St. Louis: Mosby.

Describes the total school health program: instruction, services, safety, guidance, and other environmental needs. This book provides the daily information wanted by teachers to improve their skills and to enhance their contribution to the health of the school-aged child. It can serve as a resource for principals and supervisors as well as for classroom teachers.

Dewey, J. 1938. *Experience and Education*. New York: Macmillan.

This volume is must reading for anyone who chooses education as a career. Dewey articulates here many of the principles inherent in the practice of health education. Among these are the role of the environment in "teaching," the involvement of the learner in planning learning experiences, and the influence of past experience on future learning. Understanding the source of these principles will enrich the health educator's professional life. A close reading of this volume will be of value to anyone concerned with contemporary issues in education. Interestingly, the basic issues have not changed much during the past 50 years.

Ensor, P., and Means, R. K. 1985. *Instructor's Resources and Methods Handbook for Health Education*. 3d ed. New York: Wiley.

A concise reference for the beginning or experienced teacher. This handbook provides listings of teaching techniques, sample transparency masters, lecture and lesson plan outlines, bibliographies, and content outlines for a wide variety of topics.

Greenberg, J. S. 1978. *Student-Centered Health Instruction: A Humanistic Approach*. Reading, Mass.: Addison-Wesley.

This creative collection of approaches to motivate students for health offers a variety of teaching strategies, including value-clarification methods, useful from kindergarten through grade 12. The simple, easy-to-follow, adaptable lesson plans may be of value to both the beginning teacher and the experienced teacher.

Rash, J. K., and Pigg, R. M. 1979. *The Health Education Curriculum: A Guide for Curriculum Development in Health Education.* New York: Wiley.

A guide for developing curriculum for all levels of formal schooling and for the adult in the community. The authors emphasize the importance of developing a curriculum that is relevant for the community in which the school is located. Described here are the process of developing the curriculum with a school/community advisory committee; the teaching of health education through health services, related subjects, and as a separate subject; some useful methodologies; and the evaluation of school health programs. This book is a good introduction to curriculum development for all health educators.

Schaller, W. E. 1981. *The School Health Program.* New York: Saunders College Publishing.

This comprehensive text on school health includes, in addition to information about school health education, chapters on the organization and administration of a school health program and the requisite health services. Part 2 provides a survey of child health status and common problems that may be encountered. The appendix contains a resource listing of printed and audiovisual materials as well as sample school health records and forms.

Discussion Questions

1. Does an elementary school teacher need to consult with the principal or curriculum coordinator before deciding to give classroom health instruction?

2. Owens states that involvement by many different individuals and groups is needed to promote health instruction. Identify some of these important individuals and groups.

3. What are points pro and con for the integrated versus the separate discipline approach to health curriculum and teaching? Which approach might be most acceptable? When? Where? Why?

4. What might be the future of classroom health instruction in the 1980s and 1990s? Are there likely to be changes from now on? What factors might influence changes?

5. Design a workshop, including marketing strategies, for a statewide or system-wide teachers' workshop on health education for the purpose of helping elementary teachers teach health topics.

6. How would you go about identifying teachers like Owens who are enthusiastic about child health and about teaching health within the school curriculum?

Health Counseling: "I Think I'm . . ."

James F. McKenzie, Ph.D., and Roberta Ogletree, M.Ed.

The responsibility of health counseling will fall on the shoulders of every teacher sometime during his or her career, yet relatively few teachers feel qualified and comfortable in a health counseling situation. Knowing when, how, and to what extent to get involved are issues teachers must face in a health counseling situation. In dealing with these concerns, teachers must in addition weigh the impact of their professional, moral, ethical, and legal responsibilities on the students and on themselves.

The following case study is presented to provide all teachers with an opportunity to examine the teacher's role in a health counseling situation.

"Julie, has Dana Smith been in to see you today? She has been acting rather strangely lately—almost as though she has the weight of the world on her shoulders. Have you any idea what is bothering her?" Pam Page, the high school's physical education teacher, had stopped in to talk with the new part-time guidance counselor, Julie Newman, after school one Monday.

"As a matter of fact, Pam, Dana was in to see me ninth hour. Yes, I'm afraid something is bothering her. But I'm not really at liberty to say what it is."

Taken aback by Ms. Newman's reply, Pam Page did not know whether to drop the subject completely or to seek further information, even though Ms. Newman said she could not discuss it.

Her hesitation was relieved by the counselor, who continued, "Something has come up that may interfere with Dana's plans for going on to college next year. It is something personal and Dana is very worried and upset. She needs a great deal of understanding right now, and she needs to know that people care about her; her self-esteem is about shot and she really feels badly about herself.

"Dana has mentioned that you have asked her several times what was wrong, and she notices your concern. I feel that if you were to sit down with her, Pam, she would tell you her troubles and let you try to help her. She respects you and cares about what you think of her; that's why she hasn't approached you with her problem—she's afraid of how you would react to her situation."

Ms. Page was silent for a moment, then asked, "Do you think I should talk to her now? After all, she has come to you and confided in you; I don't want to interfere."

Ms. Newman rose from her desk and sat down in a chair next to Ms. Page. "Yes, I do, and I'll tell you why. Dana needs some mature guidance; she needs an adult to whom she can talk. She seems to trust me, yet I'm only here one day a week and certainly can't be of much help to her if I'm not here. But she sees you every day in your physical education class. You are available to her, and I'm sure she would be willing to talk to you if she just realized that you really want to help her."

"Do her parents know about this 'problem'?" Ms. Page queried.

"Dana doesn't live with her parents. They were divorced about five years ago, and now Dana and her two younger sisters live here in Taylorville with her aunt and uncle, who are the legal guardians. From what Dana has told me, her previous home life left a great deal to be desired and is probably in part responsible for the fact that she has such a poor self-concept." After a brief pause, Ms. New-

---

James F. McKenzie is Acting Assistant Dean for the College of Education at Bowling Green State University in Bowling Green, Ohio. Roberta Ogletree is an Instructor in the Department of Health and Physical Education at Lake Land College in Mattoon, Illinois.

man added, "Brenda Garrett is the only other person Dana has talked to about the situation. I don't know Brenda, so I can't judge just how much help she will be."

"Well, I guess I'll talk with Dana tomorrow and see what I can do," Ms. Page said. "I have no idea what this 'problem' is, but I'll do what I can to help her come to grips with it if she'll talk to me."

Ms. Page rose from the desk and thanked Ms. Newman for talking with her. The two women agreed to meet the following Monday when Ms. Newman made her next visit to the high school.

"By the way," Ms. Newman called out as Ms. Page was walking out the door, "I hope things aren't too rough and strenuous in your phys. ed. classes."

Ms. Page laughed. "They can take it!"

The next day, as her fourth-hour physical education class was dressing, Ms. Page asked Dana if she could stop in to see her after school. When Dana said that she had to catch the bus home, Ms. Page asked her to stop by her office after dressing.

When Dana came into her office, Ms. Page was seated behind her desk. She asked Dana to sit down.

"Well, Dana, I think you realize that I've been somewhat concerned about your recent change in behavior; you've seemed depressed and awfully quiet lately. I've asked several times if anything was wrong, but you've never given me a direct answer. Yesterday I went to see Ms. Newman to find out if you had talked to her and she told me that you had. However, she would not tell me what was wrong—she felt that would not be fair to you. She did suggest that I talk with you again.

"Dana, as your teacher I am concerned about your welfare and I would like you to know that if you feel you need to talk to someone, I'm ready and willing to listen and try to help if I can. I know that kids need help sometimes, and they don't always want to go to their folks even though they need to talk to an adult. So, I just want you to know that I'm willing to do what I can for you."

Dana shifted in her chair and asked, "Ms. Newman didn't tell you what the trouble is?"

"No, she didn't. You can trust her, Dana."

Dana nodded, seemed about to say something, but then stopped.

Ms. Page did not want to pressure her, so she said, "Dana, if you don't want to discuss the matter with me, that's fine. Ms. Newman felt, and I agreed, that you might need someone to talk to when she wasn't here. I am willing to be that someone if you'd like." At this point Ms. Page was ready to drop the matter, feeling that she had said all she could.

"But I do want to talk to you," came Dana's immediate reply, "It's just that I don't want you to think badly of me. I was going to talk to you in the first place, but Ms. Newman doesn't know me as well, and I really wasn't too concerned about what she thought."

("Okay, here it comes," Ms. Page thought to herself. "Just don't let yourself look shocked or upset by what she says.")

Dana shifted once again and took a deep breath before looking her teacher straight in the eye and saying, "I think I am . . ." another deep breath—"pregnant."

Registering no change of emotion on her face, Ms. Page continued to look Dana in the eye. She felt a surge of sympathy for what Dana must be going through.

"Are you sure?" Ms. page asked. "Have you been to a doctor yet?"

Dana replied that she had not, but her best friend, Brenda Garrett, was going to take her to the clinic in the nearby town of Carlton, where Dana's doctor was located, a week from Saturday.

"But why wait so long, Dana? The sooner you find out, the easier it will be on you. If you aren't pregnant, you can stop worrying; if you are, you can decide just what you are going to do."

"But I can't go any sooner. Brenda can't get her parents' car before then, and my boyfriend works until 5:00 every day, including Saturdays. My aunt and uncle only let me drive their car when one of them is with me, so I can't take their car. I really don't want my aunt to find out about this. They'd throw me out of the house."

Ms. Page interrupted, "But if you are pregnant, Dana, they are going to find out sooner or later."

"I know that, but if I'm not, I sure don't want them to know that I might have been. You see, they are doing my sisters and me a favor by keeping us—we could be living with my dad, but my aunt and uncle took us in. I'd really like to go on living with them."

Ms. Page nodded, "I understand, and I don't

suppose there's any need to get them all worked up until you know for certain. So how about Thursday after school?"

Dana frowned questioningly and asked, "What do you mean?"

Ms. Page rose and leaned against the edge of her desk. "I'll drive you over to the Carlton Clinic after school Thursday if you can go then."

After a moment's thought, Dana gratefully accepted the offer. She said that she would come up with some type of excuse to satisfy her aunt. Ms. Page told Dana to meet her in the gym lobby after school Thursday, and if she wished, she could take Brenda along as well.

Thursday afternoon, Ms. Page drove Dana and Brenda to Carlton, located 20 miles east of Taylorville. Once in Carlton, Ms. Page let the girls off at the clinic, telling them that she would return to pick them up in half an hour.

When Ms. Page returned to the clinic, she parked her car and waited for the girls to come out. After 15 minutes had passed and the girls had not shown up, Ms. Page decided to go inside. When she did not see Brenda or Dana in the front waiting room, she moved to the back hallway, where she found both girls waiting near the dispensary window. Ms. Page sat down next to Brenda and asked what was happening.

Dana, who was seated on the other side of Brenda, leaned over and announced that her test was negative and she was waiting for some medication the doctor had prescribed for her. At that point the clerk called Brenda to the window, gave her a package, and began writing out a receipt. On getting out her checkbook, Brenda discovered that she had already used her last check. She told the clerk that she had no checks left and had no cash with her.

Overhearing the conversation, Ms. Page went to the window and paid the bill herself. She was handed two receipts, one with Dana's name on it and the other with Brenda's. When she asked what the second receipt was for, the clerk said that it was for Brenda's birth control pills.

Surprised and angered, Ms. Page turned to Brenda. "I knew nothing about this! I brought you over here for the sole purpose of accompanying Dana—I had no idea that you had this trick up your sleeve."

No one spoke during the drive back to Taylorville. Ms. Page was unsuccessfully attempting to calm herself so that she could explain to the girls exactly why she was so angry.

After pulling into her driveway in Taylorville, Ms. Page broke the uncomfortable silence as she turned the motor off. "I hope you girls realize the position you have put me in. It is one thing to drive Dana to the doctor to find out if she is pregnant, but it is another thing entirely for Brenda to go to get herself put on the Pill. Had I known that you had intended to do that, I would not have offered to take you. And look at the predicament I am in now that I *paid for it!*"

Brenda interrupted to say that she would pay Ms. Page back as soon as she could.

"Of course you will, but those people at the clinic know me. I don't like the idea of any of them thinking that I took you over there just so you could get the Pill. I don't like that at all. Whether you go on the Pill or not is your own business, Brenda, but I want no part of it. Do you girls understand that if this should get out into the community I might get into serious trouble with the school board?"

For the first time since they had left the clinic, Dana spoke. "I guess we just weren't thinking, Ms. Page. But we didn't plan this. After I had my test, we decided to go back and ask the doctor about birth control pills; I decided not to get them, but Brenda wanted to go ahead. We really didn't know that you were going to come into the clinic, and we certainly didn't realize that Brenda was out of checks. We're sorry it happened the way it did and we'll never tell anyone what happened today."

Ms. Page relaxed somewhat. "Okay," she said wearily, "but I just hope that nobody over there tells anyone either."

The following Monday morning, Ms. Page met with Ms. Newman to discuss the events of Thursday afternoon. Ms. Newman revealed that Dana, quite upset about what Brenda had done, had already been in to see her.

"Julie," Ms. Page began, "I've been thinking about this situation all weekend and, quite frankly, I'm worried about what could happen if word about all this gets out into the community. I think that I should talk to Mr. Smith. If someone makes a complaint to the school board or to an administrator,

I think that Mr. Smith should be aware of the real story. What do you think?"

Ms. Newman agreed. "I think we should both go down and talk to him and let him know the entire situation so that he realizes we've been trying to help a girl through a crisis. Since I haven't talked with him about situations of this type before, it would be good for me to know just how he feels something like this should be handled from the school's point of view."

Mr. Smith, the principal, was free when the two women arrived at his office. He greeted them genially and asked them to sit down.

"Mr. Smith," Ms. Newman began, "Ms. Page and I are here to discuss a student counseling problem we've encountered. We have been counseling a girl who thought she might be pregnant, and in so doing, Ms. Page got involved in more than she bargained for."

At this point Ms. Page took over and revealed the entire chain of events. She then told Mr. Smith that they had come to him not only to let him know what had happened at the clinic, but also to ask his comments on handling a situation involving a pregnant student or one who thought she was pregnant.

Mr. Smith began by saying that he was glad that the students felt they could take their problems to Ms. Newman and Ms. Page, because students who need guidance and counseling often do not feel that they can talk with their parents about their problems. Most students talk to their peers, who are often an inadequate source of help and guidance.

"The fact that you took the one girl to the clinic to have the pregnancy test is not such a serious matter, Ms. Page, even though the girl's parents might object. I doubt that very much fuss would be made over it. However, the other girl is where the potential difficulty lies. Should her parents ever learn that you took her to the clinic and she got birth control pills while there, they'd be likely to object strongly. The fact that you were not aware that this was going to happen is in your favor. If the parents kick up a fuss, you have that to fall back on, provided the young lady is willing to be honest about the entire situation.

"If these girls do not spread this information around and if the people at the clinic don't start talking, I don't think that you will have anything to worry about."

"Well, that relieves me somewhat," said Ms. Page.

Mr. Smith rose as the women prepared to leave and made one last remark. "I'm very glad that you both are willing to take an active role in helping students with problems, but if this type of situation ever arises again, I would not recommend transporting the student to the clinic."

Ms. Page smiled and said, "Neither would I."

As Ms. Newman and Ms. Page walked down to the teacher's lounge for a cup of coffee, Ms. Newman asked, "Well, after all that has happened, are you glad that you got involved?"

Ms. Page contemplated that question momentarily, then replied, "You know, I think I am, but . . ."

Analysis

This case demonstrates an event frequently associated with health education instruction in schools. Students establish rapport with a health teacher so that the role of the teacher expands to include information and referral to outside agencies and individual health counseling.

Brammer's (1979) eight stages in the helping process provide a frame of reference for the case. Table 1 lists the eight stages and indicates the primary activities for each.

Table 1
Stages in a Helping Relationship

Stage 1: Entry	Lay groundwork of trust; enable the helpee to state request comfortably
Stage 2: Clarification	Clarify reasons for seeking help and get helpee's perception of problem
Stage 3: Structure	Formulate the contract, including conditions under which the relationship will work
Stage 4: Relationship	Build the helping relationship; increase depth and helpee commitment
Stage 5: Exploration	Explore changes needed and strategies likely to effect change
Stage 6: Consolidation	Explore alternatives, work through feelings, practice new skills
Stage 7: Planning	Develop a plan of action after deciding to terminate the relationship
Stage 8: Termination	Evaluate goals and terminate the relationship

Source: Brammer (1979:51–66).

The case focuses on a helping relationship between a classroom teacher and a student with a personal problem. A positive rapport was built up from classroom experiences that created trust. When the teacher asked the student about potential problems, the student felt she could share her concerns. This rapport was later threatened by the teacher's reaction to another student obtaining birth control pills. Some steps in the counseling process in Table 1 were followed by the teacher; other steps were violated. Although the teacher was well-intentioned, her understanding of the helping process and of appropriate responses for a helping person was somewhat limited.

The main issues raised by this case are the appropriateness of health counseling and the possible cognitive and value dissonance between the health professional and the community, including the school system. Given a particular community, options for an unwanted pregnancy may be limited.

If the teacher's personal philosophy and beliefs are different from those of the school system that hired him or her, the teacher has to decide whether to operate within these mores or outside of them and weigh the consequences. The eagerness and enthusiasm that many beginning teachers have to help students may place them at odds with the acceptable roles of a teacher or health counselor. Personal operating procedure may sometimes place a teacher's job in jeopardy. The beginning teacher needs to inquire beforehand whether there will be administrative support for counseling and what the acceptable counseling procedures are.

Sometimes being a "friend" or counselor to a student may meet the psychological needs of both the beginning teacher and the student. However, this mutual psychological meeting of needs is not an appropriate relationship for the professional.

Another issue the case raises is what "helping"/counseling really means. There are different kinds of counseling. As the case illustrates, it is important for the beginning teacher to fully understand these differences.

Following are brief definitions of different kinds of counseling.

Counseling is defined by Cottle and Downie (1970:1) as "the process by which a counselor assists a client to face, understand, and accept information about himself and his interactions with others, so that he can make effective decisions about various life choices. Counseling is conducted with clients whose behavior is within the normal range and this differs from therapy."

Crisis, or situational, counseling is a helping relationship in which a person is assisted in attempting to cope with a situation that cannot be readily solved by using coping mechanisms that have worked before. It is short-termed, brief, and directed specifically at improving the ability of the client to function at the same level as existed before the crisis period. The therapist or helping person assumes a more active role in such counseling but, by refraining from value judgments, maintains the client's integrity and positive regard (Aguilera and Messick 1978).

On the other hand, counseling may be a longer process, one known as psychotherapy, in which the primary goal is to assist "the person who wishes to relieve symptoms or resolve problems in living, or is seeking personal growth" (American Psychiatric Association 1980:116). Psychotherapeutic techniques differ in methodologies, goals, length of therapy, and indications for treatment. However, each type of psychotherapy strives to change behavior as a result of the relationship established between two (or more) people (Aguilera and Messick 1978).

This case presents a typical situation for the school health educator. Although students' problems may not always be as potentially controversial as this one, each will be considered serious by the student concerned. A health educator's knowledge of counseling procedures and mores acceptable to the community will help establish his or her reliability as a helping person and facilitator for problem solving.

References/Select Resources

Aguilera, D. C., and Messick, J. M. 1978. *Crisis Intervention: Theory and Method.* 3d ed. St. Louis: Mosby.

This text offers a concise, clear treatment of the basic theory and principles of crisis intervention. Different types of interventions for crisis are described and the functions of the therapist for each one defined. Group and individual therapy, barriers to therapy, manpower needs, and related issues are discussed.

American Psychiatric Association, ed. 1980. *A Psychiatric Glossary.* 5th ed. Boston: Little, Brown.

A useful glossary of psychiatric and related terms. Included is a table of research terms.

Brammer, L. M. 1979. *The Helping Relationship: Process and Skills.* 2d ed. Englewood Cliffs, N.J.: Prentice-Hall.

The author says this book is for people who want to help people. He provides clear descriptions of the helping process, helping skills, and different modalities for helping. He deals with both professional and nonprofessional helping. This is a good book for the part-time counselor like the schoolteacher in this case. Brammer provides appropriate caveats for the novice, as well as sufficient information on how to use counseling to help others.

Cottle, W. C., and Downie, N. M. 1970. *Preparation for Counseling.* Englewood Cliffs, N.J.: Prentice-Hall.

This book is for the professional counselor, the person who wishes to make counseling a career. It focuses on the information the counselor may need about a client and the variety of sources for this information. For example, the use of the case study, the sociogram, standardized tests, and observations are discussed. Although anyone interested in counseling would find this book useful, it is definitely geared to the full-time counselor.

Discussion Questions

1. Do you think Ms. Page should have approached Dana or waited until Dana came to her? Why?

2. Do you feel Ms. Page should have gotten involved? If so, how much and why? If not, why not?

3. Do school personnel have a responsibility to help students with personal problems? Why, or why not? If so, to what degree?

4. Was appropriate procedure followed in informing the principal of the incident?

5. Did the teacher follow appropriate health counseling principles and ethics in this strategy? At which steps in the process could the teacher have selected better approaches?

The Development and Implementation of a Women's Health Course

Denise Hope Amschler, Ph.D.

One of the realities that every health educator faces is having or wanting to assume professional responsibilites in a new area not covered in his/her professional training. In my case, teaching a course titled "Women and Health" was my challenge.

In 1975 a colleague, with tremendous foresight, initiated a course titled "Women and Health," but after several quarters moved to another college. The department chairman asked me if I would be willing to teach the course. After an initial reaction of being caught off guard, and a week of serious thought, I said yes.

During that week of deliberation my first big question was: "What *are* the unique health needs of women, and are there sufficient identifiable needs to warrant an entire women's health course?" It didn't take me long to determine that I, as a woman, had very specific health needs, including gynecological and nutritional considerations. Therefore surely other females must have the same concerns.

Assuming the course was eminently justifiable, where could I find resources for teaching such a class? My academic preparation proved to be very little help—only a smattering of sexuality courses from which to draw content information. I naively asked about a textbook, unaware that women's health courses were extremely rare and that textbook offerings were even more scarce. I purchased a copy of *Our Bodies, Ourselves*, published by the Boston Women's Health Book Collective. This classic book on women's health care gave me many ideas for building a new course. *Our Bodies, Ourselves*, presenting a women's health advocacy viewpoint, contains both traditional information and controversial presentations such as gynecological self-help concepts. I realized that I didn't have a sufficient background to always separate fact from rhetoric, so I then searched our university library for information that related to various women's health issues. Coming from a very conservative, Midwestern background, I knew that my level of awareness, as well as my level of knowledge, would have to increase.

Armed with as much information as I could collect within three weeks, I prepared a basic syllabus and a tentative course outline. I wasn't yet comfortable with my level of content preparation, but I was even more uneasy about the difficulty I'd had deciding philosophically just what approach I would take to teaching a women's health class.

At this point, "Women and Health" was being offered once in the fall and once in the spring quarter. The course had a "double listing," meaning that both undergraduate and graduate students could enroll. Typically, there were approximately 30 students per class.

All too soon came the time for my first class to meet. Had I known that first day of class what was in store for me that entire quarter, I probably would never have walked in the door! The first problem appeared almost immediately. While *I* had envisioned a somewhat more comprehensive, scientific treatment of various areas concerning women's health, a very pronounced faction of the class had been prepared to spend all quarter in discussion groups dealing with issues from what I considered to be a very narrow, pessimistic perspective. To me, these women were bitter, defensive, and ver-

---

Denise Hope Amschler is an Associate Professor of Health Science in the Department of Physiology and Health Science at Ball State University in Muncie, Indiana.

bally aggressive, and I must confess it was very intimidating. Most of the students in the all-female class resented being required to demonstrate increased knowledge levels about the medical aspects of women's health. It was obvious that they needed an avenue to vent their general feelings of frustration, and my class was it. A major dilemma for me was in interpreting this resentment and frustration. Was I, as an individual, the target? Was the structure of the course antagonizing these students by not giving them a needed forum to air their emotionally charged feelings? Did I miss a golden opportunity to undo the negativeness, to open the door for their and my learning and enrichment? Five years later, I still do not feel that I fully know the answers to these questions.

In retrospect, some of my mistakes are obvious. A very important aspect of teaching a new health education class is knowing where one stands philosophically, and I was very unclear in my own mind on this matter. Hence my goals, thoughts, policies, and so on were not strongly stated at the outset. Over the years I have discovered that knowing where one stands is more crucial in this course than in any other I have taught. Not only does one need to assess personal philosophy and needs, but it is very beneficial to assess, if possible, corresponding needs of the target group.

This philosophy must be shared with students from the very first day so that they know whether the course is likely to mesh with their motives for taking the class. I feel that being clear in one's own mind also enhances one's ability to be flexible about student needs. Having once established a basic philosophical premise, one is more comfortable with deviating from it within a certain range.

I also felt insecure during that first quarter. I was challenged on everything—my knowledge of the field, projects I assigned, attendance policies, and examinations. As a result, several students got the best of me psychologically. While trying to deal with this dissonance in my classroom, I found myself also dealing with it at home, in my sleep, in the grocery store, and when out with friends. There were some "good" days (when key troublemakers were absent or in more charitable moods!), but there were also some very dark days when the emotional climate in the classroom was so tense that it was difficult for learning to take place. While teaching, I often found myself concentrating on controlling my own anger, impatience, or insecurity, rather than on discussing the subject matter at hand. I had heard of "teacher burnout" and at this point felt it possible that I was yet another victim.

Although it was quite tempting to ask to be relieved of this course, I decided to give it another try, not wanting to admit defeat. Besides, whether or not I was consciously aware of it, I was becoming more personally involved in the women's health movement. My struggle with the class had forced me to examine my own values, beliefs, and convictions, many of which were starting to change. The next class of "Women and Health" proved to be a much more positive experience, and the start of many good classes that followed.

Why this turnaround? First of all, the mixture of students was different. It pays to bear in mind that individuals are by-products of their entire environmental interaction. Their attitudes and behaviors aren't created in a vacuum; therefore students' actions are not always focused on the classroom, but on life in general. (Incidentally, I later discovered that several of my key problem students from the previous quarter had been creating difficulties in other classes as well.)

Second, I had clarified my feelings about the class. I had decided that my goals for "Women and Health" would be as follows:

1. Determine what is unique about women to warrant the offering of such a course.
2. Identify changing problems and needs of women brought about by the changing cultural role of women.
3. Offer information and resources in sufficient amount to lay a foundation for decision making as it affects physical, mental, and social health.
4. Encourage each participant to discover her personal feelings about being a woman individually, and being women collectively.
5. To promote scholarly excellence in individual thought, study, research, written assignments, and performance on examinations.

I also knew that one goal would *not* be to *solely* promote an activist viewpoint, although there would indeed be times when such discussion would be appropriate, if not necessary. Politics, finance, law, and more, would need to enter our discussions. I was no longer afraid of creating dissonance for students; in fact, I wanted them to be sufficiently challenged on at least some issues to formulate their own opinions, because it is essential that women become intelligent consumers of health products, information, and services.

To communicate these decisions, I devised a little booklet about the course, describing my course philosophy, topics and assigned readings, objectives for the quarter, and major policies and requirements. This booklet was given to students on the first day of class and discussion was centered on it. I felt much more self-assured and was determined to make the quarter a success. To my great relief, this preparation, along with a fresh start with new students, marked the beginning of a positive evolution that is still in process.

For the last several years, "Women and Health" has emerged as my favorite course to teach, proving to me that first impressions aren't always the most accurate. The discussion that follows will attempt to identify and describe some of the specific factors that contribute to the ongoing process of educating women about their health in this course.

TYPES OF STUDENTS

There is a consistent diversity of students! Although 98 percent of the participants are female, they range from sophomores to graduate students. There is no prerequisite for this elective course; therefore some students have had no previous health courses, whereas others have taken three or four related health courses. Typically, very few of the students are health education majors, and it is not unusual to have students representing 15 major fields in one class. Personal motives and word-of-mouth recommendation are the two most common reasons cited for electing the course. Most students are white, but there is usually a smaller number of Black females enrolled as well as an occasional student of Spanish or Asian descent. Handicapped students enroll, as do students with chronic health problems, both emotional and physical. Philosophical differences abound, ranging from ultraconservative to ultraliberal. Generally, there are several "predictable" groups of students, as is typical in a women's health class.

Each class contains a faction of "women's movement activists" who generally take other courses in women's studies and often participate in local activist groups such as the National Organization for Women or in agencies that offer specialized services to women. The direction in which the women's health movement has traveled in recent years has no doubt been a partial reflection of the growth and maturation of those most actively involved with it. Changes in political structure, economics, technology, and medicine have also contributed their influences. The women's movement has opened up a tremendous opportunity for increasing health awareness. Receptivity levels for women's health education are wonderfully high, yet how many professionals are aware?

Another major group comprises students representing white, middle- or upper-class America. These young women often have a sorority affiliation, look and dress very nicely, and are quite cordial on a daily basis. They typically are more interested in health issues that concern them immediately on a personal level than the more global matters that confront women as a population. These students tend to be liberal about some of their own behaviors, but often demonstrate judgmental standards toward those who belong to different socioeconomic classes and cultures.

There is also a smaller, but yet pronounced, group of conservatives in each class. Very often these women have been raised in an environment that has offered them very limited exposure to issues involving women. They generally know only and have accepted only what they have been told and find the class to be both intriguing and upsetting. For instance, there might easily be several students in each class who feel that a woman's rightful role, no matter how well educated she may be, is at home, caring solely for her husband and children. An occasional student will feel that she is being exposed to an indecent film when observing a demonstration on the self-speculum examination. When I catch myself being surprised at these attitudes, I quickly recall my own conservative upbringing and try to express more empathy. Some of the more conservative students struggle and grow in the process of dealing with exposure to new ideas even though they may retain their original personal value system.

The last major identifiable group is composed of the "nontraditional" students—those who are typically in their late twenties or older and who are returning to school after years of being away. Very often these women have children or grandchildren, have had some outside work experience, and may be widowed or divorced. They are highly motivated, are appreciative of the work I do as their teacher, and have more of a personal attachment to many of the issues discussed. Perfect or good attendance is standard for these women, and they have a measure of security that only age and experience seem to bring.

Each quarter there may be two or three brave male students who sign up for the class and stay with it. Some are there out of curiosity, and some at the request of their girlfriends or wives, but usually they do not markedly influence the tone of the class. In five years, I have had only one experience with an antagonistic male.

In summary, the "Women and Health" class, now filling three sections per quarter, can be a potentially volatile group. The potpourri of backgrounds, attitudes, and knowledge levels can be as exciting as it is emotionally draining.

CONTENT AND PRIMARY METHODOLOGY

One of the major problems I have encountered in teaching "Women and Health" is how to effectively cover a wide range of topics in one brief quarter. As a minimum, students may expect to receive exposure to the following areas: anatomy and physiology of the female reproductive system; normal sexual functioning as well as sexual dysfunction; the gynecological exam; fertility and infertility; gynecological health problems (mild to severe); structure and function of the breast; benign and malignant breast disorders; special nutritional needs of women; health implications of working in and outside the home; alcohol and tobacco abuse; rape; wife abuse; women as consumers of health products, information and services; and female aging.

To achieve maximum use of the time allowed for the course, I have tried several different strategies with varying levels of success. At times, I have deleted entire units in order to cover the remaining ones more thoroughly. I did so reluctantly, because it seemed that important material was being sacrificed. At other times, I have given out an inordinate amount of supplemental reading material in addition to lecture and discussion. This approach seems to work as long as the readings are carefully chosen and not in excess.

For several quarters, I prepared and handed out fact sheets for many of the units. In outline form, each fact sheet on a particular topic contained key points, spellings, and statistics. Unfortunately, my bright idea backfired in a way I hadn't counted on: A noticeable number of students began to rely on the availability of these fact sheets, thereby generating a false sense of security about their own decreasing need to prepare for class. As a result, I now give out these fact sheets only occasionally, and extra copies are not available after they are handed out in class.

Finding the ideal textbook for "Women and Health" would certainly contribute to solving the time dilemma. There are a number of gynecological health books on the market, many of which are good, but when I use these, I must add several other books to provide enough information for the course. I have used several different leading textbooks over the past years, and though each has major strengths, I still must supplement heavily with other materials. Activist-type books turn many students off and may contain a greater number of inaccuracies. I prefer to use a textbook that speaks to its readers in a challenging, noncondescending way, and this has also posed problems for the students with a limited health background.

OTHER METHODOLOGIES

Films have been very well received by women and health students. There are many excellent films available, and it is always a difficult decision to choose five or six of the best ones to show each quarter. I generally choose some films that represent the more open-ended type story, while the remaining films are more factual or scientific in nature.

I purposely show one film each quarter that will expose students to the activist side of women's health movement. The film depicts the problems many women face with the health care system. Those women portrayed are generally the uneducated, the poor, and the minorities, who speak and dress in ways that do not conform to those of the general college population. This film, in particular, evokes compassion from some, contempt from others. Students who have had problems receiving good health care find it believable, whereas an occasional physician's wife taking the course may become defensive and even hostile, feeling that the film presents a distorted picture. Open-ended films dealing with topics such as sex roles, childbearing decisions, and alcohol abuse likewise evoke varied reactions from the class. Several very factual films often used in class offer amazing demonstrations and photography that would otherwise be unavailable. I utilize these films in the areas of nutrition, fertility problems, and cigarette smoking, and have been very pleased with their overall quality and effectiveness in conveying information.

Having access to models, charts, instruments, slides, and transparencies has been helpful, especially in the teaching areas of sexuality and gynecology. During discussions about reproductive anatomy and pelvic exams, students can much better gauge the actual size of an organ and its proximity to another when life-size models are used. Likewise, I bring both a plastic and a surgical steel speculum to class. After I explain their features and how they operate, each student has the chance to open and close them and make comparisons. A common reaction is "This is the first time I've ever seen a real speculum, much less handled one!" It is interesting to note that well over 50 percent of students in the classes have never had a gynecological exam. Two very common reasons for not doing so are "I didn't know why I needed one" and "I was afraid of what the doctor would do!" Many students make their first appointment as a result of this class.

A complete assortment of currently available contraceptive devices is a very necessary part of teaching a unit on birth control. Though many students are familiar with the oral contraceptive and perhaps the condom, a significant number have never had an opportunity to examine and compare different types of diaphragms, spermicides, and intrauterine devices. The majority have never seen a diaphragm introducer or even heard of the cervical cap.

Occasionally I've had a few problems obtaining needed teaching aids. Procurement of several types of contraceptive devices and pills understandably requires physicians' prescriptions, but these can generally be obtained without too much trouble. The local medical supply company required a physician's prescription to obtain a speculum. The apparent rationale: owning a speculum would make a self-induced abortion easier for a woman to accomplish. I wonder, though, just how many females in such a desperate situation would seek out a medical supply company to purchase a speculum? Or might it be possible that requiring a prescription is a ploy to discourage self-exams?

The use of guest speakers in my women's health class has been a bittersweet experience. Local agencies, serving battered wives and women with other emotional problems, have been most helpful. There has also been positive response from other faculty members to speak on topics such as women's fitness and the changing sex roles of women.

However, other experiences with guest speakers have been less than ideal. Unfortunately, it has proven very difficult to bring in a physician to answer medical questions from the class. On several occasions I have invited physicians to come to class, and in each case, the physician declined on the grounds of being unable or unwilling to take time away from the office. As a result, the actual physician-client encounter for many of my students must be delayed until the female actually enters the physician's office.

Another valuable lesson was learned when a guest speaker did consent to come and speak about rape crisis and prevention. One quarter, I invited the director of public education from the local police department to speak about current legal aspects of rape, rape prevention, what to do in case of rape, and the status of the crime on the national and local level. The officer assured me that there would be no problem and that he felt comfortable dealing with this sensitive topic in the classroom. On the appointed day, the officer (late 40s, lined face, conservatively dressed) walked into my classroom, large legal code book in hand. After introducing him to the class, I took a seat in the back of the room, prepared to take a few notes on the presentation.

The officer opened his large code book on the lectern and proceeded to read from the legal statutes for the remaining 45 minutes. He never varied his presentation. He did answer our questions, but he did so by reading more quotes from his book!

He provided much information, but the students just weren't receptive to this style of delivery. He didn't win any votes, either, when he concluded his presentation by assuring us that our town and campus really didn't have a rape problem!

EVALUATION

Though I usually conduct what might be termed a "hard evaluation" of the course through rigorous examinations and assignments, my assessment of the total impact of the course on individuals comes about mainly through reflection.

The very nature of the "Women and Health" course seems to provoke conflict within students. The dissonance experienced by some may remain solely internal or it may be openly shared in reaction papers, in class discussions, or in private conversations with me. Having spent most of their lives in a conservative state, nearly all the students are amazed at how little they had previously learned about their own bodies. In Indiana public schools, most had never received sex education, even though some may have been sexually active. Although most sexually active students on campus do use some form of contraception, they are likely to be uninformed about contraindications and risk factors associated with a particular method.

In spite of the students' access through class to fairly up-to-date research about the use of certain methods, there are yet many cases where this information is openly rejected. A case in point was Ms. C, a young married graduate student, who one day submitted a reaction paper saying, "How dare you upset me so badly? How dare you tell me that I should go off the Pill for three to six months before trying to conceive?" Feeling that I was somehow directly speaking to her, she was personally offended when information disseminated to the class contradicted her own beliefs. I have found that some aspects of contraceptive use are akin to cigarette smoking—that is, there is a coveted behavior that is unsafe yet very hard to change, despite the facts.

There have been countless cases of young women entering the class with an existing emotional conflict, hoping to find the answers they need to bring about a solution. At times, students are simply seeking out an environment in which others are likely to understand the situation they face and demonstrate to them that theirs is not a unique problem.

When the trust level is high enough, some students will spontaneously share information about current or past conflicts. They generally volunteer this information at appropriate times, when related material is being discussed. It is not unusual for females to reveal that they have personally experienced an eating disorder, such as anorexia nervosa or bulimia. In addition, there have been several cases where middle-aged women in class have shared past histories of having agoraphobia (also known as "housewives' disease"). It is no longer a great surprise when these very personal comments are shared; in fact, when students hear their peers describing a condition in the first-person tense, a greater degree of reality and authenticity is lent to the discussion.

Generally, persons who openly comment on their present or past condition give their own clues about how much they want to say. Sometimes classmates will ask questions such as these: "What was it like?" "How did you know something was wrong?" "How did you solve the problem?" And they will receive very candid replies. At other times, there is a definite message conveyed that the student herself wants information only and doesn't want to reveal too much at that point.

Victims of rape, wife abuse, and sexual harassment have also shared particular aspects of their ordeals. Very occasionally there have been tears or bursts of anger as these experiences are described. When this happens, the rest of the class generally reacts in a quiet and compassionate way. We all—the students and I—often develop a greater level of sensitivity by the end of the quarter.

Though these examples do not represent daily or even quarterly occurrences, such episodes are nevertheless frequent enough to merit consideration when planning curriculums and methods of presentation.

A role that many women's health teachers are asked to play is that of medical and psychological consultant. Sometimes counseling students is very comfortable and gratifying to me; at other times I have the distinct feeling of being out of my league. Although I hold no medical degree, it seems that

I still represent some students' closest link to someone who has needed information. Unplanned pregnancies, problems with contraception, symptoms of a reproductive tract disturbance, and problems with friends are all concerns brought to my office. Often the situation can be easily resolved, but for more serious cases I became more familiar with area gynecologists, voluntary agencies, and social services in order to make the needed referral.

POSTSCRIPT: PERSONAL REFLECTIONS ON MY ROLE

My bookshelves now groan with an ever increasing volume of reference books, ranging from gynecological and obstetrical texts to books by Betty Friedan and Germaine Greer. *Ms* and *Savvy* subscriptions were added several years ago, along with a membership in the National Women's Health Network in Washington, D.C. So many more outside resources are now available to provide current information than existed five years ago.

Many women's health issues are gaining increased coverage, and as the public's awareness grows, its needs for resources likewise expands. I routinely speak to civic groups about specific topics such as breast cancer, cigarette smoking, and the consumer aspects of women's products, as well as the broader topics of working women and the women's health movement. There is a large demand from area newspapers, radio, and television for information and interviews, providing a wonderful opportunity to reach a much larger audience. It is truly exciting to be a part of these many forms of community health education. It must be noted that part of the growing concern among women's groups is increasingly related to the curtailment of social services provided by all levels of government. Many of these services directly affect the lives of women in the areas of family planning, wife abuse, pregnancy alternatives, and nutrition.

In conclusion, my teaching the "Women and Health" class represented just the beginning of a commitment that soon led to a much broader involvement with the surrounding local and state community. I am willingly and enthusiastically committed to improving the health status of women and now feel very fortunate to be in a position enabling me to do this.

I heartily endorse the concept of women's health classes at the university level. My only reservation is that anyone undertaking such a course assignment be prepared to experience (1) a challenge regarding your traditional concepts about teaching health education, and (2) a personal challenge regarding your own new involvement and understanding of women's health issues.

Analysis

At least once in their career, most health educators are faced with assuming new tasks or responsibilities for which they have had little or no training or preparation. In this case the challenge for Amschler was to teach a course whose subject matter she knew very little about. In addition to raising her own level of knowledge, she had to plan the curriculum.

To boost her knowledge, Amschler examined what the previous course instructor had done, did library research, and reviewed textbooks and resource material. Researching a health/disease topic is a basic skill that all health educators should master. Amschler knew, of course, how to teach; she just did not have enough background to teach a course in women's health issues. But she made up for this lack because she knew how to research the topic and knew what questions to ask.

The possible topics health educators can work with are so numerous it is impossible for one person to be informed in depth on all of them. Health educators tend to have in-depth knowledge about health/disease areas with which they have worked or in which they are interested. When they encounter a topic that is unfamiliar to them, they do what Amschler did—they learn about it. Health educators bring to every project knowledge and skill in helping people learn/change regardless of the subject; and they know what questions to ask about any health/disease topic and are able to evaluate the answers.

It is important to note that there are some basic differences between developing courses at the college level and doing so at lower levels. To a great extent these differences stem from the changing nature of students from the lower levels to the college level. The typical college student either has made the transition or is in the process of becoming an adult learner. Knowles's (1978) theory of adult learning, labeled andragogy, is based on four assumptions that are different from pedagogical (child learning) theories. These assumptions are concerned with (1) changes in self-concept, (2) the role of life experiences, (3) readiness to learn, and (4) orientation to learning.

As Knowles states, the adult learner is characterized by possessing a deep need to be perceived as self-directing. And as the person gets older, he or she accumulates more experiences and thus becomes a rich resource for learning. "Accordingly, in the technology of andragogy there is decreasing emphasis on the transmittal techniques of traditional teaching and increasing emphasis on experiential techniques which tap the experience of the learners and involved them in analyzing their experience" (p. 56). The adult's readiness to learn is less a product of biological development and academic pressure than it is a matter of relating to the tasks required to perform social roles. The adult "comes into an educational activity largely because he is experiencing some inadequacy in coping with current life problems. He wants to apply tomorrow what he learns today, so his time perspective is one of immediacy of application" (p. 58). Finally, according to Knowles, although individual differences are important in dealing with children, they become more pronounced in adults because of differential experiences.

As we noted earlier, some college students have made the transition to adult learners while others may be only in the process of changing; a few have not even begun the transition. Instructors faced with this mix of students indeed have a difficult task in planning learning experiences. The logical way to overcome this problem is to perform a needs assessment. However, the health educator in a school setting generally has less opportunity to adequately assess needs before a course begins than the health educator in the community who is responsible for planning a program. As we saw in this case, the needs assessment was more of an ongoing activity once Amschler began teaching the course.

This ongoing assessment resulted in the development of philosophical premises, clarification of goals and objectives, and a more self-assured instructor, as was reflected in the booklet describing the course that Amschler distributed to students.

In addition to the content-process issue, the role of the health educator as counselor is also important to consider (see the case by McKenzie and Ogletree, p. 25). As both Gapinski (1979) and Brammer (1979) indicate, basic counseling and helping techniques can be readily mastered by most who find themselves in a position that requires these skills on occasion. But it is important for the health educator as counselor to recognize, as Amschler did, when the counseling situation necessitates the intervention of other professionals and to be able to make referrals.

Finally, although this case is set in a classroom, a health educator working in any setting could be faced with tasks similar to those Amschler describes. Health educators in all settings have to deal with the challenge of researching a topic with which they are not familiar. They also have to create an environment conducive to learning, use group process skills, and understand the target population and the larger community to which it relates.

There are, of course, differences among settings. The target population in this case has many characteristics different from those of target populations in other settings, for the structure of a college or school system differs from the structure of a hospital or a business. But our point is that the basic knowledge and skills needed are the same in all settings; only the application is sometimes different.

References/Select Resources

Brammer, L. M. 1979. *The Helping Relationship: Process and Skills.* Englewood Cliffs, N.J.: Prentice-Hall.

This book is must reading for anyone who is routinely thrust into a counseling or helping situation, as was Amschler, but has had no formal training. As Brammer notes in his introduction, the book is not on psychotherapy or on the pathology of human interaction—that is, situations in which a specialist is required. Rather the book is intended to assist the helper to become a more aware and effective person and acquire the basic skills needed to achieve a satisfactory conclusion in a helping situation.

Gapinski, P. A. 1979. "The Winking, Blinking and Nod of Health Counseling." *Journal of School Health* 49:509–513.

This paper provides a model for basic health counseling skills based on the following three communication skills: (1) reflective listening, (2) assertiveness training, (3) and problem solving and conflict resolution. Gapinski includes a list of guidelines for use in determining when to end a health counseling session.

Knowles, M. 1978. *The Adult Learner: A Neglected Species.* Houston: Gulf.

Knowles was the first to popularize the term *andragogy* to distinguish adult learning theory from child learning theory. For the most part Knowles's work has been applied to the human resource development field, that is, training programs in industry. But his theory of adult learning is very useful to anyone who has responsibility for educating adults. The assumptions underlying his theory, such as the importance of self-direction and the learner's experience, will be very familiar to health educators.

Discussion Questions

1. Should the instructor have asked the argumentative students to drop the course, especially after she found that they were disruptive in other courses as well?

2. How does an instructor or health educator go about assessing the situation when he or she intuitively senses conflict, "bad vibes" that are not conducive to a good working atmosphere?

3. Were the adjustments in teaching methodologies justified by this instructor?

Might she need to change methodologies in the future, even though she currently seems to have things organized for the best way to teach?

4. Is it appropriate for a health educator to play an "advocate" or "activist" role within the classroom? How should controversial issues be handled? Is it appropriate for the health educator to state his or her views?

5. If a male instructor were to teach the course, would it be appropriate for him to assume counseling as part of the course, as the female instructor did in this case? What special problems might the male instructor as counselor encounter?

6. Should the course include various consciousness-raising activities or be limited to factual health and medical matters?

Curriculum Development with the Pima Indians of Arizona

Kerry J. Redican, Ph.D., Larry K. Olsen, Dr.P.H., Charles R. Baffi, Ph.D., and Thomas L. Dezelsky, H.S.D.

The Gila River Indian Reservation lies in the desert approximately 35 miles southwest of Phoenix and is the home for the majority of Pima Indians. The major health problem affecting the Pimas is Type II diabetes mellitus, or noninsulin-dependent diabetes. Since 1965 researchers have observed the Pimas to determine the prevalence and incidence of diabetes as well as its association to factors such as obesity.

Knowles and co-workers (1978) reported that the diabetic prevalence and incidence rates of the Pimas far surpassed those of the general population. The age-sex adjusted prevalence rate was 12.7 times that in Rochester, Minnesota, the community used as a comparison group for the study. This high prevalence rate is approached only by that of the people of the small Pacific island of Nauru. The Pima incidence rate of 26.5 cases per 1,000 person-years, with a peak incidence in early adulthood, is the highest diabetes incidence rate known in the world.

According to the Southwestern Field Studies Section of the National Institute of Arthritis, Metabolism and Digestive Diseases, diabetes appears in over 50 percent of all obese Pimas 35 years of age and older (Howard 1984).

Kerry J. Redican is an Associate Professor and Charles R. Baffi is an Assistant Professor of Community Health at Virginia Polytechnical Institute and State University in Blacksburg. Larry K. Olsen is a Professor and Thomas L. Dezelsky is an Associate Professor of Health Science in the Department of Health and Physical Education at Arizona State University in Tempe.

THE NEED

A need was seen by both reservation personnel and outside agencies for a school curriculum focusing on diabetes prevention. To secure money for the development of the Diabetes Prevention Curriculum, funds were transferred from various Bureau of Indian Affairs sources to the Pima tribal council.

The reservation school personnel felt that they lacked the skills necessary to develop such a curriculum for elementary school children. Since several members of the health science faculty at Arizona State University had worked previously with the Gila River Indian Reservation community on health-related projects, they were asked to be consultants in the development of this curriculum.

GETTING STARTED

Four preliminary meetings were held at various sites on the reservation with State Department of Health Services personnel, various tribal leaders, tribal elders, school personnel, and the consultant team. At these preliminary meetings, the following issues were discussed:

- The importance of the project
- The relation of this project to the Tribal Health Plan
- Demographic characteristics of the population
- Sociocultural issues
- Previous curricula in the health field and the impact of those curricula

- Approaches to the development of the curriculum
- Grade-level placement
- Teacher training
- Student academic ability
- Availability of various health education materials for the schools
- Time constraints for the curriculum
- Coordination of the entire project
- Evaluation strategies

These meetings gave the consultant team a chance to travel throughout the reservation to observe conditions and visit with residents, school personnel, and other personnel who would be involved in the project. The meetings with the tribal elders were particularly critical. They provided a forum for explaining to the consultant team the key cultural elements that should be woven into the fabric of the curriculum. These preliminary meetings also provided the opportunity to ensure that there was community support for involvement in the curriculum that would result from the development efforts.

TRIBAL HEALTH PLAN

The goal of the Tribal Health Plan was the development of a comprehensive school health program. It was critical that the project's curriculum model be flexible enough, although specific to diabetes, to be used when more comprehensive health curriculum development occurred.

THE SCHOOL SYSTEM

The school system presented other problems. The system on the reservation was, in fact, a conglomerate of reservation schools, parochial schools, and a community school. With such diversity of schools and administrative patterns, community support and curriculum flexibility were critical. To address these issues, the consultants met with the school officials on numerous occasions throughout the development process.

These discussions resulted in the selection of grades 1, 3, and 5 for the pilot testing of the curriculum. It was felt that emphasis on prevention at lower grade levels would produce the most positive results. A series of health curriculum models was presented to district supervisors, principals, and teachers of grades 1, 3, and 5 who might be involved in the pilot testing.

SPECIAL CONSIDERATIONS

It was important that the curriculum be filled with hands-on health activities, make optimal use of currently available materials within the schools, and include free and/or inexpensive instructional materials that would be available to all the schools. Further, it seemed necessary to utilize the services of various community health-related personnel as resources for the teachers.

As a result of all these discussions and concerns, an eclectic curriculum model was developed, embodying key elements included in the School Health Education Study (1967), the School Health Curriculum Project (U.S. DHEW 1978), Hoyman's Spiral Approach (1947), and selected traditional unit approaches.

THE CURRICULUM MODEL

We will briefly discuss here each of the models that provided the basis for the eclectic curriculum.

SCHOOL HEALTH EDUCATION STUDY (SHES)

The conceptual orientation of the SHES model was retained for the Diabetes Awareness Project. It was felt that the entire effort would thereby be more amenable to incorporation with any subsequent development of comprehensive health education curricula.

SCHOOL HEALTH CURRICULUM PROJECT (SHCP)

The SHCP is a multimedia, hands-on approach to health education. Moreover, a rather detailed teacher training component is embodied in its overall philosophy. This project also draws widely upon community resources as an adjunct to material purchased for use in the curriculum.

The Diabetes Awareness Curriculum adapted the SHCP's concept of intensive teacher training to acquaint teachers and other personnel with the philosophy, methods, materials, and use of the curriculum. This concept was retained because extensive literature about the SHCP indicates that teacher training is an integral aspect of the success of that project.

The SHCP intersperses the resources of large and small groups. Similarly, the new curriculum used materials from the reservation school as well as materials from health agencies such as the American Diabetes Association, the American Heart Association, the Arizona Department of Health Services, and the Maricopa and Pinal County Health Departments. These free materials were supplemented with materials from commercial companies. The consultants could thus incorporate sociocultural issues considered important by the tribal elders.

HOYMAN SPIRAL APPROACH

Hoyman's proposal for health education is based on a spiral approach to learning. He begins by finding out what the children's knowledge and interests are and then builds on these to broaden their base of knowledge. He introduced the concept of the developmental level of the child as one of the foundations for the introduction of new material. Thus maturational level and differential intellectual capacity, as well as student needs and interests as seen both by the child and by the health professional, became organizing elements for the curriculum.

TRADITIONAL UNIT APPROACH

The traditional approach to curriculum development has been to base content in specific units of instruction. The consultant team started by securing copies of previously developed diabetes content units. These units were then organized into a traditional unit framework. By doing this, the team was able to ensure fairly comprehensive coverage of the content as it fit into the project framework.

CONTENT AND ACTIVITY CONSIDERATIONS

In developing the curriculum, the consultant team discussed the interests and life-styles of Pima children and learned a great deal about their basic interests. What became quite noticeable was the apparent lack of interest in engaging in much physical activity. Because of the tribal elders' wish to make the children proud of their heritage as outstanding runners, an effort was made to integrate various movement activities into the curriculum. Beginning with rather simple movements, these activities then progressed to more vigorous ones. Careful attention was paid to ensure that they were not extraneous to curricular goals and that they required only enough initial skill for a child to experience success.

In meetings with tribal elders, several traditional games were suggested that could be integrated into the curriculum. Evolved from the basic material from the elders, these games were incorporated into the various learning activities in such a manner as to gradually increase physical activity and content as the curriculum progressed.

Commercial materials were examined by the consultants as well as by the tribal school personnel. The criteria for inclusion of an item in the currriculum were that it was not culturally or sexually biased; it fell within the basic skill level of the students who would be using it; and it furthered the development of a relevant concept. In most cases, material had to be adapted to stress cultural points that the tribal elders wanted to preserve. In addition, Pima vocabulary, games, and foods were incorporated into the unit where applicable.

TIME CONSIDERATIONS

Too often a curriculum is developed by three or four persons over a summer. In the fall, the "guide" they produce is distributed to teachers, along with the standard office memo suggesting that teachers examine the new curriculum and incorporate it into their schedule. The ideas have generally not been tried in the classroom, so it is largely unknown if they will work for the students for whom they are intended. Further, teachers may not be familiar with the background or philosophy that led to the development of the guide.

In an attempt to overcome such problems, it was decided that moving slowly while keeping the teachers well informed of the process would probably yield the best results. Therefore about four months were allotted to develop the curriculum guide for pilot testing. During this phase, a conceptual framework would be constructed and discussed with school administrators and the pilot teachers to ensure their understanding of the underlying philosophy. This timing also allowed teachers and others to provide suggestions for the curriculum.

It was also decided that the curriculum would cover approximately 20 days of regular classroom time and that each day would be the equivalent of one regular class period (approximately 30 minutes per grade per day).

TEACHER TRAINING

Following agreement on the conceptual framework and total classroom guidelines, it was decided to conduct an intense one-day workshop. In the workshop the consultants would distribute the guide and instruct the reservation teachers and administrators on how to use it. Further, each person would be provided with the materials necessary to implement the curriculum. After the pilot program began, the consultants planned to meet with teachers and tribal elders to discuss and evaluate the curriculum. At these meetings, suggestions for revisions of the guide would be made. The guide would then be revised and a final copy printed. It was to be distributed to the other teachers in the district when each of them attended a workshop. The purpose of the second workshop was to train at least one teacher at each grade level within each school in the use of the guide. This procedure would also allow training for teachers who would be new to the school district. Pilot teachers were to have an opportunity to work with the consultants in conducting the teacher training. Thus a built-in source of teacher training could be developed.

The teacher training component was modeled after that used in the SHCP. The Arizona Department of Health Services made initial contacts with the school district's central administration and then with the various schools. In this way the local people were kept informed of what was happening and the teachers were more motivated to become involved with the training.

It was decided that each school would pilot a different grade-level unit but that every pilot teacher would be familiar with the contents of each of the three units of instruction, not with just the one he or she would be teaching.

TEAM APPROACH

A team approach was used for the teacher training. School nurses, the principal, at least one specific grade-level teacher (1, 3, or 5) and one support person (usually a librarian or the person who had library responsibilities) attended the teacher training workshop. The team approach has been shown to maximize interaction between persons who play different roles within a school. Further, their differing perceptions of the curriculum and their suggestions for improving the guide could be incorporated into revisions. This approach also facilitates reinforcement for teachers who are trying something innovative in their classrooms and provides them some psychological support. Having more than one teacher trained in an innovative program is always a good idea anyway in case the one teacher leaves.

Although the time was short, during the training workshop the consultant team discussed every activity included in the guide. Obviously, it would have been better to have had the teachers experience all the activities. However, time and economics dictated that one day was the maximum time a school's personnel could be absent from school. To compensate for the lack of teacher training, the consultants made themselves accessible by telephone or appointment and spent a great deal of time talking about the guide to the people who would be using it. With the telephone the teachers felt they had a hotline they could use if they did not understand something in the guide or did not remember what was done in the workshop. The nature of each call to the consultants, was recorded so that the questions could be addressed in the revised unit.

The first group of trainees piloted the curriculum in their respective classrooms. The teachers were asked to keep detailed notes on specific activities they used, how the children received them, and their own overall perception of them. By having several key activities available, the guide became considerably more flexible and allowed each teacher to consider student differences when selecting classroom activities. A wider range of activities could thus be included in the final draft before training other teachers.

The project took about four months to complete the developmental and initial teacher training. At each grade level, there were enough activities correlated to specific behavioral objectives to last for approximately 40 classroom periods, each 40 minutes in length. Most implementations would be for only 20 classroom periods. However, enough activities were included so that a teacher would have options as to which activities he/she wished to use.

THE FIRST DRAFT

The first draft of the guide was presented to tribal administrators and was well received because of its flexibility, individualization, and cultural responsiveness. The one-day workshop was conducted during early spring. All the schools implemented the program during the spring semester and were ready to discuss revisions by late spring.

DIABETES: INFORMATION AND AWARENESS PROGRAM

The final curriculum unit(s) developed for the reservation schools was entitled "Diabetes: Information and Awareness Program for Grades 1, 3, and 5." The overall goal, as developed by the consultants and tribal leaders, was to provide students with decision-making opportunities to reduce their personal risk factors associated with the development of diabetes. Six major concepts were developed, each relating to a particular aspect of diabetes. From these six concepts, long-range goals in the cognitive, affective, and psychomotor domains were developed. Finally, grade-specific behavioral objectives and suggestions for content, learning activities, materials, and evaluation activities were incorporated. The conceptual model for this process was patterned after that used in the SHES (Figure 1).

CONTENT AREAS

When dealing with risk factors of a disease such as diabetes, several content areas must be addressed. The guide addresses mental health, chronic diseases, nutrition, personal health practices, community health, and exercise. Basically, each concept stresses a different content area, thus making the curriculum somewhat global in scope.

RECONVENING SESSION

A debriefing was held between the pilot teams and the consultants. During this meeting, the teachers presented their anecdotal records of the activities they used in their classrooms. On the basis of these sessions, the curriculum was revised and final copies were sent to the pilot teachers, administrators, and project coordination personnel.

Interestingly, the Native American teachers were reticent in criticizing the curriculum. The prevailing impression was that they did not want to hurt anyone's feelings. This cultural element apparently overrode the need to constructively criticize a curriculum in order to better it.

The Anglo teachers were more likely to offer criticism. Using the initial comments of the Anglo teachers, the consultant team was able to elicit comments from the Native American teachers by showing them that they were interested, wanted their comments, and were not hurt when the comments were made.

Native American teachers spoke in a soft voice and tended to avoid direct eye contact. The consultants realized that this was not apathy, but rather a cultural element related to difference in communication patterns and to a history of years of exploitation by the majority society. Reactions to this exploitation were demonstrated in the underlying questions: "How long will this one be here?" and "We really are not ready to talk with too many people, so why do you want to talk with us?" The consultants tried to follow the Pima cultural pattern of nonverbal communication to maximize the interaction between them and the teachers.

CULTURAL AND ORGANIZATIONAL INFLUENCES ON DECISION MAKING

Staff turnover is a problem experienced on many reservations. This turnover is not confined just to teachers, but extends to all reservation personnel. Further, the salary level for teaching staff is below that of nonreservation school districts. The result

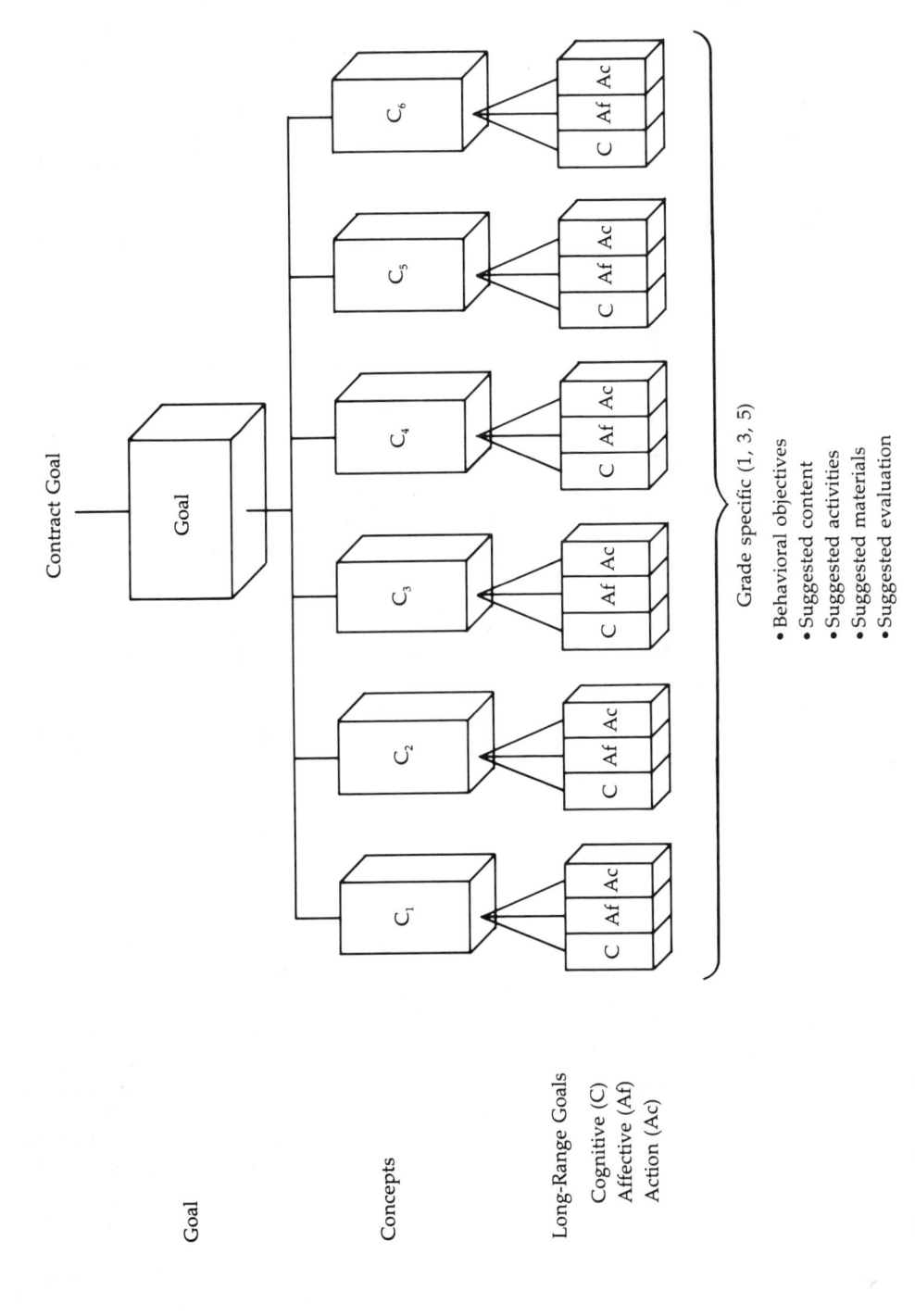

Figure 1
Curriculum Development

is that teachers who have to stay, or want to stay, in the greater Phoenix area to teach will accept a position on the reservation until they can obtain employment elsewhere. The major exception is the Catholic Sisters who teach in the parochial school. But even they may be reassigned on very short notice. Thus continuation of any innovative program becomes quite difficult.

To combat the problem of losing a program as a result of staff turnover, the consultant team stressed the need for a mechanism whereby an ongoing program of in-service education could be assured. A concept included in the teacher training component was to train the pilot teachers to the extent that they could form a cadre of teachers who could train new teachers in the district. Additionally, since two or three teachers in each building had been trained in each grade-level unit of the curriculum, it would be unlikely that all trained teachers would leave the district simultaneously. This situation, to a degree, helped ensure a continuing training program within both the school and the district.

Unfortunately, the central project staff, as part of the Arizona Department of Health Services, was also rather mobile. In the course of this project, the consultant team dealt with four different project officers. Each project officer had varying degrees of expertise in the control of diabetes and in the concept of curriculum development. Fortunately, the consultant team kept exact records of its agreements with the project officers, so that although there were personnel changes, the project could proceed with a sense of continuity. It is strongly suggested that, regardless of the project or the group with whom one might work, every decision be put in writing and signed by all parties involved. At the very least, the decisions should be put into memo form and copies sent to everyone concerned. This procedure will help avoid any hard feelings in case a consultant tells a new project officer that the prior project officer did things differently. Any alterations can then become points of negotiation between the project officer and the consultants.

Tribal elders pride themselves that their word is their bond. They feel that once their word is given, the matter is closed. Consultants need to be quite careful about the wording of follow-up letters, because these letters could be construed by the elders as mistrust of them. It is invaluable for the consultant team to keep a careful record.

The reservation leaders would not initiate memos to the consultants, so the consultants had to alter their usual work style and initiate very carefully worded memos. In general, these memos placed all responsibility on the consultant. For instance, by wording the memos, "We want to be sure that we have not misunderstood what you would like in regard to . . . ," the consultant was saying that the elder knew what was wanted but that the consultant was not quite sure that he understood the elder's message.

RISK REDUCTION FUNDS RELEASED

Shortly after the completion of the Diabetes Awareness Project, the Gila River Indian Reservation received a federal Risk Reduction Grant that allowed it to implement a variety of health programs, including the Diabetes Information and Awareness Program. One of the key elements was to develop a school-based curriculum that dealt with smoking, alcohol, and drug use. Thanks to the success of the Diabetes Awareness Project, the consultant team was asked to help develop this curriculum using the project as the model for the Risk Reduction Curriculum. As a result of the risk reduction contract, school health education became a viable part of the Department of Human Resources of the Arizona State Department of Health Services and was reflected in the development of Project Health Promotion, the Gila River Reservation Health Risk Reduction Project.

POSTSCRIPT

Several major problems confronted the consultants not only in the construction of the Diabetes Awareness Project but also in its implementation. These problems included continual staff turnover, long waits for approval of various materials from tribal elders, and the school district's lack of appropriate materials for the activities recommended in the guide.

It is a good idea to remember, too, that the Native American population tends to make decisions more slowly than a consultant might like. The key here is to present a well-documented case and allow for rather lengthy delays as decisions are made. This delay factor can be advantageous in that it gives the consultant a chance to learn about the culture and how it may affect, positively or negatively, any project proposed. Decisions within this culture are made by a tribal council, and everyone must be given an opportunity to react to the proposal. Often counterproposals will have to be negotiated, and the consultant should be prepared for that process.

In this case therefore each decision was reached by using the tribal political avenues, a procedure that, to the consultants, seemed rather slow. For this reason even rather simple projects could not be done in a short period.

The tribal elders had been deceived on many occasions by prior consultants and were thus rather suspicious of any outsider trying to develop and implement a program. This overall attitude tended to slow the decision-making process even further.

The suspicion with which outsiders are viewed creates potential problems for consultants who are not cognizant of, or do not take into account, the long history of deceit foisted upon the Native American population. This suspicion, coupled with the cultural elements of passivity, lack of eye contact, and reticence to criticize work presented to them, can cause outsiders to take a negative attitude.

The Native American population here, as elsewhere, has experienced much frustration over time. They have not been given the same opportunity to adjust to a fast-moving society as have other ethnic groups. Rather, they have become almost a forgotten people, pushed to a few square miles of desert and left, to a great extent, to fend for themselves. The result has been the development of numerous health problems. Many of these problems can be prevented through a well-developed program combining health education and preventive medicine.

Professionals working in this type of situation must be prepared for frustration. They must be extremely organized and sensitive to human needs. Fast-paced movement will not work in this culture. One must take care to learn about tribal and community politics. If one does not recognize the various political factions at work in the community, and how to work with them, any project will fail. It must also be realized that it is better to be successful with one small part of a program than to attempt a major effort and do a sloppy job, or fail. Failure, in the minds of these people, means one more way they have been exploited.

The Gila River Indian Reservation has a serious diabetes problem. Education is a key component in the prevention of diabetes or at least in limiting its effects. The education component for this reservation was developed and successfully implemented.

A formal evaluation of the curriculum has not been and may never be conducted. This situation is partially due to economic considerations because the true impact of the program will not be evident for many years. Some evaluation efforts have occurred, but things move slowly. Several of the teachers who were in the pilot study have written to the consultants about their activities. This gesture, of itself, is significant because the Native American teachers are usually not willing to talk about their concerns, lest they hurt someone's feelings. For health educators who are eager to follow elaborate models and professional procedures, transcultural experiences can be frustrating and humbling. Perhaps the key lesson from this project is the awareness of the chasm between life at the grass-roots level and professional life in a fast-paced techno-society. This contrast does not discount the value of theoretical models, but emphasizes the need to incorporate them into everyday human experience. Change requires time and it requires consideration for the human element of a program.

REFERENCES

Howard, B. (Phoenix Clinical Research Section, National Institutes of Health). 1984. Telephone conversation, January.

Hoyman, H. S. 1947. "Oregon's Four Cycle Health Curriculum." *Journal of Health, Physical Education and Recreation* 18:486.

Knowles, W. C.; Bennett, P.H.; Hamman, R.F.; Miller, M. 1978. "Diabetes Incidence and Prevalence in Pima Indians: A 19-fold Greater Incidence Than in Rochester, Minnesota." *American Journal of Epidemiology* 108:(6):144–156.

School Health Education Study. 1967. *Health Education: A Conceptual Approach to Curriculum Design.* St. Paul: 3M Education Press.

U.S. Department of Health, Education, and Welfare. 1978. *The School Health Curriculum Project.* DHEW Publication no. (CDC) 78-8359. Washington, D.C.: Government Printing Office.

Analysis

This case presents a unique glimpse of a planning project for a health education curriculum aimed at a special target population. The authors served as curriculum planners, facilitators, trainers, and outside consultants. In addition to needing the skills of educational planning, the authors were required to work transculturally to provide a service that was not available within the resources of the reservation.

As presented by the authors, the main theories in this case involve curriculum planning for a school system. Knowing the ultimate goal of the reservation schools was to have a comprehensive health education program, the authors adapted several known curriculum models and approaches. The three approaches to curriculum planning are well described by Kime, Schlaadt, and Tritsch (1977).

At the base of their planning was the concept of involving as many school district adminstrators and pilot teachers as possible from the very beginning. This approach served to involve these people in the planning as well as to ensure their later use of the materials. The teachers thus had more interest in the curriculum because it contained their ideas, but the time-consuming work of putting the curriculum together was handled by the consultants.

Some components of organizational development are present in this case. Not only were the consultants preparing a curriculum for school health instruction, they were attempting to create the structure to support the implementation and continuation of the curriculum. In addition, they were setting the foundation for development of a more comprehensive curriculum. Therefore attention had to be given to all groups in the organization, that is, the total reservation. In organizational development theory, the case could be interpreted as managed change (Huse 1980). The initiation of the change came from within the organization as a request for help in preparing a curriculum for teaching about what it considered a serious health problem. The three basic requirements of the intervention theory and method as developed by Argyris (1970) are present in the case:

1. The intervenor must help the client system generate valid information about the system.
2. The client system must have free choice among alternatives after the generation of valid information has provided the system with a cognitive map or outline.
3. The client system must have a high degree of ownership of the course of action or choice available.

Another, more elaborated model of planned change that can apply to the implementation of a schoolwide curriculum is the model developed by Lippitt, Watson, and Westley (1958). Basic to this model are two features:

1. All information must be freely and openly shared *between* the client and the change agent.
2. The change agent and the information are helpful only when and if the information can be directly translated into action.

Since events for most health education efforts occur within some type of organizational structure, concepts and models of organizational change have value for health educators. In addition to their expertise in education for health, health educators must have an understanding of organizational structure and decision making and of organizational change to deal with the reinforcing and enabling factors that prevent or support the educational activity. By making samples of existing curricula available for review, the consultants in this case accelerated the process of selecting the content and activities. As an educational theory and as a tool, hands-on experiential learning activities predominated within each grade-level unit.

Throughout this case principles of participatory planning were used as much as possible. One of the goals of the consultants was to build the curriculum with supporting factors so that it would continue to be used after they left. Frequently a project will fold when the consultants leave or the original monies are exhausted. By including several levels of school administrators and teachers in the planning and early stages of the curriculum, there was a greater chance that the curriculum would continue. Few people like to abandon projects on which they have spent much time and hard work.

The consultants were constantly aware of the need to create a climate of cooperation and communication. The tool of the confirming memoranda helped them not only to keep records but to keep the momentum going after a certain stage or decision had been reached.

Respect for local customs and different ways of working enabled the consultants to learn from their clients as well as to provide expertise. It seems strange that respect needs to be mentioned under a principle of practice. Yet, it does, to call attention to the gap that frequently occurs between provider and client. The provider often becomes caught up in the details of the work and forgets that he or she is working with people—that the work is still a social interaction.

An underlying issue that cannot be overlooked in this case is the cultural and social relationship between the clients and the consultants. Social and political issues were present. They did not need to be addressed directly, but recognition of their importance and pervasiveness in all facets of the client relationship had to be considered.

The issue of the traditional unit approach to curriculum and health teaching had to be addressed. The conceptual approach had come to be the primary accepted approach to school health in the past 20 years, but old ways die slowly and in some cases they may be the best ways. In this case the unit approach, in addition to the conceptual approach and activities from well-known health education projects (the School Health Education Study and the School Health Curriculum Project), was incorporated, thus providing a firm philosophic base upon which to build a more comprehensive curriculum in the future.

This case required the health educators to have considerable knowledge and skill. Perhaps the most significant professional skill was the ability to establish trust between the health educators and the clients. This ability illustrates the translating of a professional code of ethics into practice. And with any minority group or subtarget group, that is fundamental.

References/Select Resources

Argyris, C. 1970. *Intervention Theory and Method.* Reading, Mass.: Addison-Wesley.
Chris Argyris presents here his theory of intervention as applied to organizational development. Health educators will see clear parallels with their own work, particularly in regard

to planning and needs assessment. Beyond this, however, the health educator who assumes the role of consultant will gain much from this book. The second part of the book presents a number of cases that illustrate the theory developed in the first part.

Huse, E. F. 1980. *Organizational Development and Change.* 2d ed. New York: West Publishing.

This well-organized text explains principles of organizational development to assist organizations in improving productivity and the quality of work life. Using a systems approach, Huse describes underlying concepts, principles, and assumptions of organizational development. This is an excellent reference for health educators responsible for supervision or those who are building a health education department, section, or team.

Kime, R. D.; Schlaadt, R. G.; and Tritsch, L. E. 1977. *Health Instruction: An Action Approach.* Englewood Cliffs, N.J.: Prentice-Hall.

This book is an excellent reference for teachers who are responsible for curriculum planning at both the elementary and the secondary levels. Three approaches to curriculum planning are discussed: unit approach, the conceptual approach, and the competency-based instruction approach. As the authors indicate, the trend is now toward the latter two approaches.

Klein, N., ed. 1979. *Culture, Curers, and Contagion.* Novato, Calif.: Chandler & Sharp.

Many classic medical anthropology articles are presented here. Of particular interest is the selection of articles on health belief systems. Several articles deal specifically with the health care systems and health belief systems of Native Americans.

Lippitt R.; Watson, J.; and Westley, B. 1958. *The Dynamics of Planned Change.* New York: Harcourt Brace Jovanovich.

This early text on planned change is intentionally content-free in that it doesn't describe what the result of the change should be. The emphasis is on the change process itself. The authors also discuss the effect of change on subparts of a system. They note how change in one subpart can affect other parts intentionally or unintentionally. They also note the danger of selecting a subpart for change that is too small and thus unable to resist forces outside the subpart.

Spector, R. 1981. *Cultural Diversity in Health and Disease.* New York: Appleton-Century-Crofts.

The focus here is on the health care system and health-related issues affecting a variety of ethnic groups. The cultural issues of health and illness are explored in several major areas: for example, provider awareness; consumer-oriented issues surrounding the provision and acceptance of health care; broad issues such as poverty; and traditional health beliefs and practices among selected populations, including Native Americans.

Discussion Questions

1. How was an educational needs assessment conducted in this case?

2. Would it have been appropriate to have conducted an organizational diagnosis—that is, an assessment of the resources and attitudes of the various groups within the reservation (school system, public health system, tribal elders, etc.)—before beginning to write the curriculum?

3. Do you think only one curriculum approach should have been selected rather than combining elements of several?

4. Could there have been any way of speeding up the process of curriculum development in this case? Is it acceptable for things to move slowly at times? Why or why not?
5. Was there enough opportunity for the classroom teachers to contribute to the curriculum? Could other approaches have been used?
6. Did the consultants devise any ways to save time while moving according to the pace of the clients?
7. What was the decision-making process for this project? Were there various levels of approval? If so, how was this discovered by the outside consultants?

Organizational Dissonance

Valorie E. Nybo, Ed.D.

This case is about the Better Health for Students Project (BHSP). The BHSP began in 1977 and is still operating. For the first three years it was administratively responsible to the Community Outreach Program (COP). The COP, located on the campus of the state university, was funded by a private foundation. The school project was funded by the State Department of Public Health. For accounting purposes, the department chose to have the program administered by the COP.

The BHSP has facilitated the development of a school health education curriculum in a number of communities in the state. The BHSP operated for the first three years despite major barriers: constant turnover of administrative staff in both the BHSP and the COP, disastrous problems with evaluation, and administrative styles that were not consonant with the goals of the BHSP.

This case study will describe the process by which the COP and BHSP staffs assisted coordinators in local communities to carry out the task of developing and implementing school health education curricula. The story of how the coordinators worked in the communities is another story and requires a different case study.

Figures 1 and 2 will help you follow the chronology of events and identify the cast of characters. Figure 1 gives the organizational structure of the university campus when the BHSP contract was signed by the COP in 1977; and Figure 2 shows a reorganization in 1978 that created a School of Human Resources with the COP director as the dean. This reorganization had considerable influence on subsequent events.

In addition to the BHSP, the COP was responsible for three other grant projects. The BHSP shared common services such as office space, secretarial services, and evaluation services with these projects. The directors of each of these projects made up the COP management team.

This case describes the first three turbulent yet productive years of the BHSP. An overview of the project will be presented first, and then the three major barriers just referred to will be discussed in detail. The nature of these barriers, the way in which they affected the BHSP, and how they were dealt with will provide the substance of the case.

You should keep in mind that all three barriers operated simultaneously. For purposes of analysis, each is treated separately. Therefore there will be repetition of some events as each barrier is discussed.

OVERVIEW

The BHSP resulted from discussions among a number of public health leaders in the state regarding the lack of good health practices among students and the long-term value of "good" school health education. The State Department of Public Health gave the COP one and a half million dollars for four years' support of the BHSP. The originally stated purposes were as follows:

1. Distribute the funds on a competitive basis to local school districts for the implementation of comprehensive K–12 (kindergarten to grade 12) health education curricula models.
2. Identify 16 pilot school districts that will implement the process of developing and implementing school health education programs, a process to be extended to 96 school systems in the three years of the project.

Valorie E. Nybo is the Executive Director of Health Programming, Inc., in Augusta, Maine.

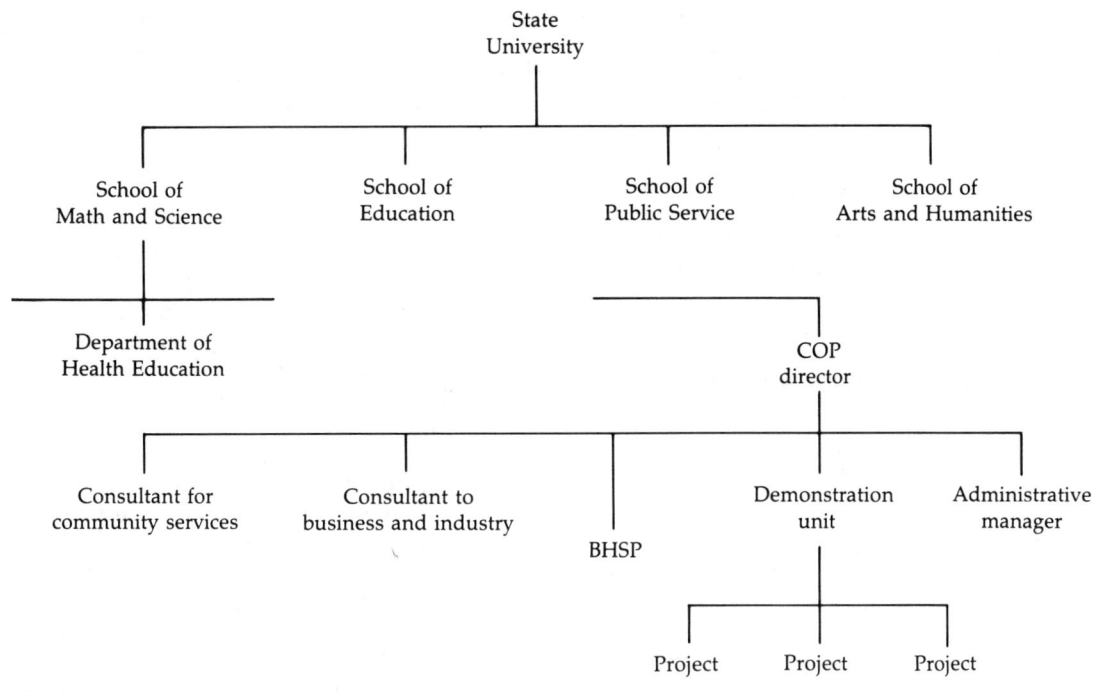

Figure 1
Organizational Structure of the State University, July 1977

*Funded by private foundation
**Funded by State Department of Public Health

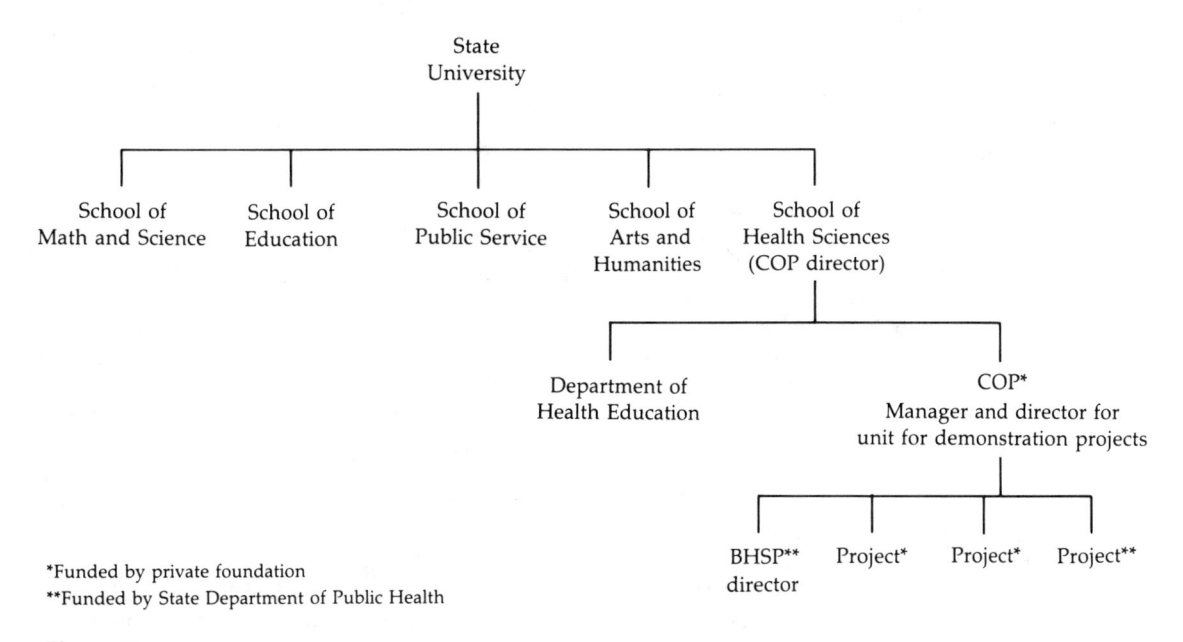

Figure 2
Organizational Structure of the State University, September 1978

3. Train curriculum coordinators within those districts in such areas as resource development, curriculum goal setting, techniques of staff and community development, and related skills required to design comprehensive community-based curriculum programming in health education.

Since most rural communities tend to have a strong sense of autonomy, additional specific objectives required that a model of community involvement be followed in developing the curriculum in each community. The most important quality for community coordinators was seen to be the ability to work with local people and local schools.

When the school project was funded, the following chronology of events occurred, beginning in August 1977:

1. The first BHSP director was hired; he had been associated with the successful curriculum development project in one community in the state but had no formal training in health education.
2. Through a request for proposal process, 16 communities were funded for the 1977–1978 school year to develop a K–12 health education curriculum.
3. A training session was held for the 16 coordinators hired by the local districts. This was a week-long live-in program. Few of the coordinators had professional training in health education or any academic background in health.
4. The training program was designed to give the coordinators usable skills to fulfill their functions. These functions were defined in the BHSP contract with the State Department of Public Health as follows:
   a. Coordinate and supervise the development and implementation of a comprehensive, K–12 health education curriculum.
   b. Develop a process for involving the school staff and the community in the design of a K–12 health education curriculum.
   c. Work with the various community-based agencies and resources to ensure optimum utilization of their services and expertise.
   d. Interpret the curriculum to the community and the various publics.
   e. Serve as a clearinghouse for materials related to health education.
   f. Provide and coordinate in-service training for the teaching staff.
   g. Assist with ongoing evaluation of the curriculum.
   h. Serve as a consultant to neighboring school systems during the second, third, and fourth years of the grant period, assisting them through the same process of curriculum development.
5. The coordinators began work, set up community advisory committees, and did community needs assessments for school health education. The advisory committees reviewed the survey results and existing curricula, and all but one community decided to write their curriculum rather than adopt an existing one. Even though some of these curricula were "square wheels," they belonged to the communities. The sense of ownership was high. Most communities eventually discovered that the square wheels rolled better when they rounded off the corners and set about revising them.
6. Since the community was seen as playing an important role in the health education of children, the coordinator and advisory committee often conducted community open forums, effective living workshops, nutrition workshops, health fairs, and the like.
7. As the first year of curriculum development activities progressed, there began to appear in the local papers articles and letters to the editors condemning the school health education effort as subversive. One article read: "The health education program . . . is the use of psychological and psychiatric techniques used on normal healthy students in order to change their values and attitudes (behavior) [sic] in political, social and moral areas; in other words brainwashing."
8. In the spring 1978, the BHSP issued a second request for proposals and funded 16 additional school districts for the 1978–1979 school year. The original notion of

extending the project to 96 school districts in the third year was abandoned as impractical.
9. The budget for the BHSP did not include funds for adding staff to assist the additional site coordinators. The BHSP director would now have 32 school districts with which to work.
10. In contrast to the first-year coordinators, all but three of those hired for the second year had academic training in health education.
11. Separate training programs were held for first-year (1977–1978) coordinators and second-year (1978–1979) coordinators in the late summer of 1978.
12. In the first 15 months of the BHSP, in addition to the difficulties of their tasks and the abuse to which their programs were subjected in the media, coordinators had to deal with three different COP executive directors, three different BHSP directors (between July 1977 and October 1978), and repeated shifts in approach, emphasis, and philosophy.

BARRIER 1: TURNOVER OF ADMINISTRATIVE STAFF

In August 1978, the BHSP had funded 32 sites and one staff person to help site coordinators. The COP was persuaded by the funding agency, the State Department of Public Health, to hire an assistant coordinator for curriculum development to give the BHSP director some help with the 32 sites. One of the original 16 site coordinators was given this position. Around this time, the following events occurred: (1) In September the third COP director was appointed; (2) in October the first BHSP director resigned with two week's notice; and (3) in October the president of the University unilaterally reorganized the university structure, removing the Department of Health Education from the Liberal Arts College and creating a new School of Human Resources, headed by the COP director, who then had responsibility for the COP projects and the academic program in health education.

With the resignation of the BHSP director, the new staff member (of three months) was appointed interim-director (BHSP director 2). The funding agency objected on the grounds that the two jobs were too much for one person and asked that the COP appoint someone else. The chairman of the Health Education Department was appointed interim-director (BHSP director 3). This switch in directors occurred during the second-year training program for the original (1977–1978) site coordinators who were aware of what was going on and were not happy about it. They like BHSP director 1 and were unhappy about his resignation; felt BHSP director 2, "one of them," had been unfairly treated by removing her after two days; and felt BHSP director 3 was a flunky of the new COP director, who was seen as an "outsider." (It did not help that the new COP director worked one day a week for the first three months of his appointment while commuting from his other job out of state.)

At the beginning of the second year (1978–1979) of the project, BHSP had (1) 30 unhappy site coordinators (two sites had dropped the project partly because of the bad publicity); (2) COP director 3, who was viewed with suspicion; and (3) one staff member, with limited experience, available to consult with the 14 first-year coordinators and the 16 new coordinators.

Two promises had been made to coordinators by the COP and BHSP staffs: (1) assistance in analyzing their community's needs assessment and (2) the provision of morbidity and mortality data for their community. Neither promise was kept the first year because there was no staff to carry out these responsibilities. In an effort to keep this promise, two data and research coordinators, trained health educators, were hired in October and November 1978. They discovered they had to write 16 different computer programs to analyze the needs assessments. The 16 new communities had developed 16 different surveys, with no consideration for computer analysis. Getting to the computer required a three-hour trip, one way, which only multiplied the coordinators' frustrations. Finally, they discovered the morbidity and mortality data were the property of the state hospital association, which would not release them. Appeals to higher authorities for these data proved fruitless.

Meanwhile, the one assistant curriculum coordinator neccessarily spent most of her time with new sites just as the data coordinators did. The 14 original sites received few direct services and weren't happy about it.

In January 1979 the interim BHSP director was replaced by director 4, and a second assistant curriculum coordinator was hired to work with the sites. The BHSP staff now included a director, two assistant curriculum coordinators, and two research and data coordinators (Figure 3). Four of these persons had been on the job less than six months. Three of the four were the first trained health educators hired for the BHSP.

These new staff members encountered considerable hostility in the field. They got questions such as "What are you people doing with those millions of dollars you have over there?" and "Why did you come here?" One staff member had moved several thousand miles from a much more urban area. This made no sense to the natives. The assumption was that she was a flunky of the COP director. With regard to the budget question, the site coordinators knew that COP director 1 had bought rugs and carpets of various sizes (the size of the rug in your office indicated your status on the staff). This incident raised questions among coordinators about the fiscal responsibility of the COP.

The new BHSP staff members shared a common goal. Each had taken the job with the project because they believed in the philosophy—that is, community involvement in school health education—and they wanted it to work. Therefore they agreed as a group to work together, to support one another and the site coordinator by doing the following:

1. Answer all incoming requests, even if the answer was "We don't know." (Incoming requests from the sites had too frequently gone unanswered—part of the reason for the anger of the site coordinators.)
2. Make all decisions pertaining to policy or staff activity by consensus. This was agreed on despite philosophical disagreements among some staff members, such as the need for training in health education (about which a couple of staff members were known to have had shouting matches.)
3. Refer to themselves in the field as the BHSP staff, not the COP staff, and explain that the BHSP was state-funded and the COP was a foundation-funded university activity to which the school project was related administratively. (The staff had noted that the anger of the site coordinators was directed more at the COP than at the BHSP.)

The BHSP staff carried out these agreements faithfully and greatly improved relationships in the field. But it was the beginning of serious trouble back home with the COP director.

While the BHSP staff was trying to get its act together, a Technical Review Committee, originally organized by the COP for evaluation activities, became an advisory committee to the COP on paper, but in fact was advisory to the State Department of Public Health about the BHSP. This committee, mindful of the frustration and anger of the site coordinators, requested that they meet to identify their problems with the COP administration of the BHSP and make recommendations to the committee about renewing the contract with the COP for the student project. As a result of the site coordinators' recommendations, the committee recommended to the State Department of Public Health that the contract not be renewed with the COP but be transferred to another campus of the state university.

BHSP staff members were not allowed to attend these meetings, nor to have any input in this decision. This lack of communications created a "them against us" atmosphere. The staff members felt the Technical Review Committee's decision was punitive to them because of prior problems over which they had no control. Paranoia was the order of the day. They were convinced that they would all be fired if the BHSP was moved. Rumors to that effect were rampant.

Although staff members expected they could get other jobs, they had just come to the state, believed in the program, and thought that as a team they could make the project go, if allowed to. Per order of the COP director or university president, their only line of communications to the State Department of Public Health and the Technical Review Committee was through the university chain of command, that is, the COP director, university vice-president, and university president.

The staff had begun to build a constituency among site coordinators by keeping their promise to provide services. They called coordinators to ask that they write the State Department of Public Health to support keeping the project with the COP. Their point was they were blamed for activ-

August 1977	September 1978	October 1978	October 1978
Director 1	Director 1	Interim director (director 2)	Interim director (director 3)
	Curriculum coordinator 1		Curriculum coordinator 1
			Data coordinator 1
			Date coordinator 2

January 1979	July 1979	September 1979
Director 4	Director 5	Director 5
Curriculum coordinator 1	Data coordinator 1	Curriculum coordinator 3
Curriculum coordinator 2	Data coordinator 2	Curriculum coordinator 4
Data coordinator 1		Data coordinator 1
Data coordinator 2		Data coordinator 2

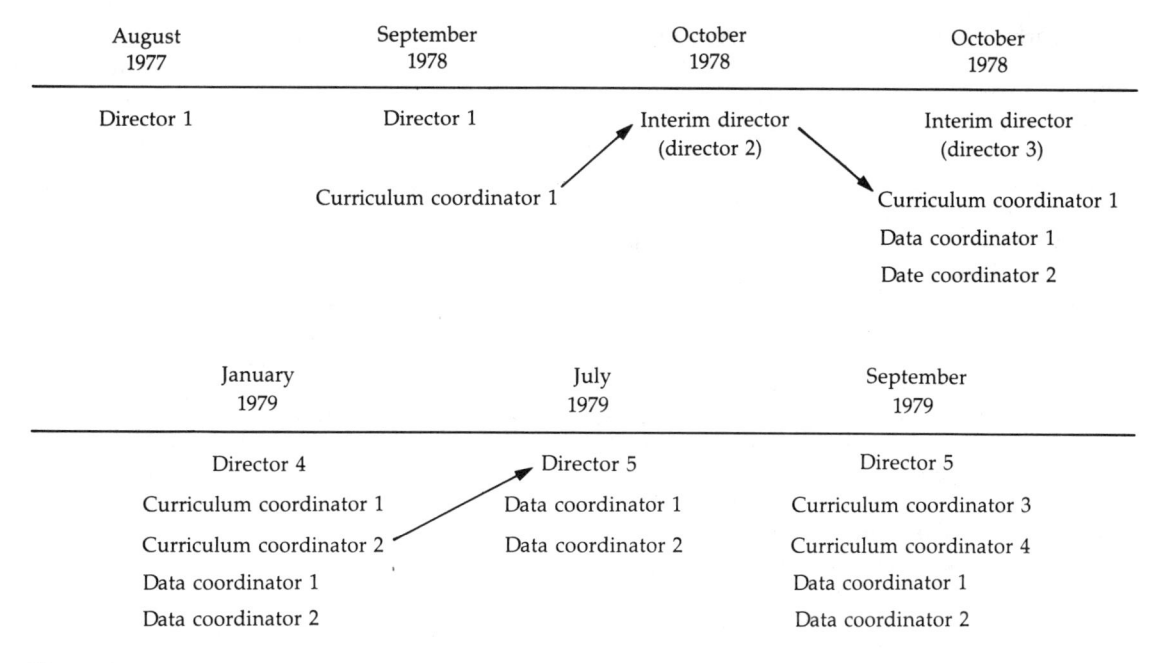

Figure 3
SHEP Staff Changes, August 1977–September 1979

ities that occurred before they arrived; they were trying and were making improvements. Fifteen coordinators wrote letters of support. The president of the university solicited similar letters from school superintendents. Several were received.

A new governor was elected in January 1979 and the deputy commissioner of public health, a political appointee, with whom the COP and the BHSP had been working, was replaced on April 1. In reviewing the recommendation of the Technical Review Committee, which had met March 27, the new deputy commissioner called in the BHSP staff for their perspective. He asked them as well about complaints from some of the first-year coordinators that they were not receiving services from BHSP staff. The staff was able to document that services were being provided. The deputy commissioner decided not to accept the recommendation of the Technical Review Committee and left the BHSP with the COP.

Just as things began to settle down after this trauma, BHSP director 4 resigned in the spring of 1979, the end of the second year of the project.

One of the assistant curriculum coordinators was offered the position. Even though the staff had "saved the project" (or so they thought) in the last crisis, evidence that the COP director was not happy with staff members identifying themselves as the BHSP, not the COP, was mounting. He set up administrative procedures and reporting mechanisms that were cumbersome. The university president, who had a strong interest in the COP and the BHSP, was reaching further and further into the day-to-day operations of the school project.

The assistant curriculum coordinator decided to take the position of BHSP director, basing the decision on commitment to the concept, a belief in the competence and support of the project staff, the sincerity of the State Department of Public Health, and the ability of the site coordinators to get the job done, given half a chance.

On July 1, 1979, the BHSP had director 5. Hope was high among the staff that things would improve. In September a successful, positive, enjoyable resident-training program was held for the second-year (1978–1979) coordinators. The training program for the first-year (1977–1978) coordinators was not so pleasant; it was hostile. The site coordinators' anger toward and frustration with the COP and the BHSP staff were rampant. For the first four days of the five-day workshop, the workshop staff could not reach the site coordinators. They were prepared to believe nothing that was said nor accept anything offered. The workshop staff (the BHSP staff for the most part) with the aid of a consultant pulled all the tricks out of the hat. Nothing worked. Finally, on the fifth day, the BHSP staff responded to anger with anger. They were not responsible for the gripes of this group of coordinators. They were trying to right the wrongs of the past and to give service; every problem the coordinators raised, the staff answered. For example, the project staff said: "You wanted the opportunity to share problems and achievements with one another, but in a session conducted the day before yesterday you were given precisely that opportunity and refused to participate." And, "You want a network for sharing information about the quality of audiovisual materials available, but you refuse to provide evaluation of materials you use through the network that we developed with your input last spring."

When the BHSP staff shared their feelings of anger and frustration with the coordinators in this way, one coordinator said, "Let's let bygones be bygones and start again," and a fresh though tenuous beginning was made.

From October 1979 to June 1980, progress in BHSP sites improved; morale among site coordinators was up 100 percent. The sense of a common purpose between the staff and the site coordinators was strong. When a negative article about the BHSP appeared in the papers in spring 1980, 12 letters to the editor in defense of the program were sent from the sites. For the first time since it began, the school project was in good shape.

However, the survival of the BHSP at the COP again became an issue during the 1979–1980 school year; it looked as though the new BHSP director's worst fears about the issues she identified when she took the job would be realized.

Several factors affected the BHSP's relationship with the COP and the university:

1. The COP and BHSP staffs and the staff of the Department of Health Sciences at the university were all housed in the same building. All these staffs were younger than the majority of the university staff and, unlike most of the latter, were unmarried and female. Further, most of their salaries were higher than those of the university faculty. These factors again created a "them and us" environment.
2. There were fundamental differences of opinion between the BHSP director and the university president and between the BHSP staff and the COP director.
3. The issue of evaluation was boiling. Despite considerable funds provided for evaluation of the school project, no agreement was reached between the State Department of Public Health, the COP, and the BHSP as to how this project was to be evaluated. Evaluation contracts were left to experts. Extensive surveys were sent to hundreds of school personnel statewide. Tons of data were gathered. But contracts with evaluators consistently terminated before data analysis was completed, and analysis that was completed was too late to be of great use.

BARRIER 2: EVALUATION DISASTER

Evaluation had begun to be an issue for the BHSP fairly early. The overall goal of the project—"to reduce the incidence of preventable health problems among children in the state"—was recognized as one that could not be evaluated in either the short or long term. Some persons proposed changes in student health behavior and status as the only appropriate level of evaluation. Others felt the effectiveness of provision of services to sites should be the primary level of evaluation. Still others proposed evaluating the achievement of contractual objectives in individual sites. In any case, one thing was certain, the parties involved—that is, the funding agency (State Department of Public Health), the COP, the university, and site personnel—had not agreed on what was to be evaluated, the method of evaluation, or who was going to conduct the evaluation.

The BHSP grant proposal required that the locally developed curricula be evaluated by a panel of nationally recognized experts, COP director 1 had contacted several nationally recognized school health education experts and asked if they would be willing to serve on an evaluation panel. The majority responded that the evaluation of the curricula would more appropriately be done by people from the state who could evaluate in light of local circumstances. As a result, in fall 1978, a Technical Review Committee was formed by the COP and charged with evaluating the curricula. The evaluation was to assess the following:

1. Accuracy of information presented
2. Practicality of implementation
3. Focus of the curriculum on significant health problems in the community
4. Quality of content from an educational point of view
5. Identification of criteria for successful completion of the objectives

The Technical Review Committee held its first meeting in August 1978. During the next few months numerous things went wrong. A team of evaluators was sent to one school district without the district's being informed they were coming. One team was given the wrong curriculum; an error discovered only after the team arrived to do on-site interviews. Results of four initial site evaluations were reported in technical Review Committee minutes without sharing them with the communities evaluated. One community, in registering a formal complaint that negative remarks were made about its curriculum and implementation plan, pointed out that it had not been asked for complete information or given the criteria upon which it was evaluated. Excerpts from a letter received by BHSP director 3 from one superintendent suggest the degree of concern about evaluation and the extent of the commitment to the project at the grass roots:

> It is a great concern to me that the technical review committee is "floundering" . . . because it . . . has had little guidance in determining the purpose of the review. The idea of a group . . . evaluating a program on criteria drawn up in isolation with little, if any, understanding of the job being done . . . is outrageous.
> It is not surprising that coordinators who have been hurt personally and professionally by the completed reviews, and those coordinators who have yet to be reviewed, are concerned when they are told to place the "new approach" on the back burner while the technical review is still taking place, and even more puzzling is the fact that the technical review is evaluating programs developed on a program-centered base.
> My initial reaction was to withdraw from COP after this year as we had done the task as originally planned. However, after considering the possibilities, I felt I could not allow what I considered a valuable project to be terminated so easily without seeing it through to its completion.

The superintendent also referred to the "new rules of the ball game," reflecting that the sites' perception of the basis for the curriculum was different from the COPS's, which was again different from the State Department of Public Health's perception. The Technical Review Committee's teams were asked to evaluate whether the curriculum was focused on the significant health problems of the state or area. Sites being evaluated had developed their curriculum from what they perceived to be a wellness orientation and were upset that criteria were "being changed."

It is likely that the sites' perception of a change in expectations was facilitated by poor communications. The deputy commissioner of public health spoke to the director for health education (state project officer), who transferred the message to the COP director, who informed the BHSP director, who interpreted it to the sites. Under the best of circumstances this method of communication is like playing "Gossip." Each person in line probably interpreted the messages to the next in a manner that was perceived to make the message as acceptable as possible.

It also appears that semantics was an issue. Site contracts required that the curriculum address health problems such as obesity, dental disease, and accidental injuries. Site personnel tended to translate that requirement into wellness- or prevention-oriented objectives. The State Department of Public Health expected objectives that measured improvement in health status: for example, students will lose ten pounds; students will have fewer cavities. Excerpts from a March 1978 letter from the director of health education in the State Department of Public Health to BHSP director 1 illustrate this dilemma.

> While some of the content areas can be easily linked to specific health problems or conditions, we are somewhat confused by such topics as Body Awareness, Education for Survival,

Personal Health, Physical Health, You and Your Body, and Health and Daily Living. We are sure that a number of interesting topics will be included in these areas but we are unclear about health problems that they will attempt to address. . . .

As an example, our concept of an objective under a topic area called Emergency Care would state "all graduating seniors will be able to adequately perform mouth-to-mouth resuscitation when appropriate." We find these objectives to be quite different from statements such as "students will be aware of dangers around the home." The problems to which these two examples might relate could be heart attacks, electrical accidents or drownings. Not only are objective statements like the latter non-measurable, but if we are talking of an integrated curriculum I have trouble determining who is accountable for the instruction. We felt that we must make our feelings clear at this point in the curriculum development process.

When COP director 3 arrived in September 1978, there was a strong need to fill the full-time position of evaluator. Evaluation problems were common to all COP projects, not only to the BHSP. The same evaluator was to be involved in all projects at any given time.

Two issues were critical to evaluation:

1. The major actors had different perceptions, as noted earlier, of the goals of the school health education curriculum.
2. A full-time staff position for evaluation of all COP projects had been budgeted but not filled. (A consultant was hired for the position in February 1979.)

The first consultant came to the state for several weeks to plan the evaluation and returned to his home base (3,000 miles away) to write surveys. The BHSP staff began distribution of survey forms to coordinators in April 1979. Each site coordinator was asked to distribute surveys to principals, teachers, school board members, community committee members, and students.

Most of the groups that were asked to complete the forms received more than one from different sources (i.e., the COP, BHSP staff, and the coordinators) within a short time. For example, the coordinators received the following:

1. One-page curriculum committee survey from the BHSP staff at coordinators' meetings
2. Two-page "Participant Expectations of BHSP, Part 1" at a coordinators' meeting
3. Two-page "Participation Expectations of BHSP, Part II" at a coordinators' meeting
4. Six-page "Satisfaction with COP Related Activities" survey mailed by the COP director
5. Sixteen-page "Coordinator's Round 1 Survey" mailed by the BHSP staff

Thousands of surveys were printed, numbered consecutively, distributed, and collected. Sites were not adequately forewarned of the extent of the evaluation activities. The contracts required that sites participate in the COP evaluation, and most did, but grudgingly. A few sites refused to allow the surveys to be distributed in their districts. BHSP staff members were no happier with the surveys than were site personnel. They were asked to complete more surveys than any other group.

In December 1979 the contract with the evaluator ended without completion of the data analysis for BHSP surveys. A second group of consultants/external evaluators was hired in March 1980 to complete the data analysis and conduct follow-up surveys. The BHSP staff voiced their concern about inappropriateness of some of the surveys used the previous year and worked with the new consultants to construct the surveys for spring 1980. The questionnaires were shortened dramatically in an attempt to include only those questions that provided data directly related to the BHSP.

Meanwhile BHSP director 5 held a series of meetings with superintendents of participating districts in September and October 1979. In particular, the superintendents expressed confusion about the purpose and necessity of student surveys. Discussions resulted in agreement on the purpose and the method of assessing students as follows:

1. Student assessments will directly measure, over time, changes in students' health knowledge, attitudes, and behaviors, giving a direct measure of the impact of health education programs being implemented in the schools.
2. Student assessments will provide school districts with a measure of student change over time and should help identify areas of the curriculum needing further revisions to meet student needs.
3. Over time, student assessments should show the desired changes in students' knowledge,

attitudes, and behaviors that will justify the expenditure of time and money on school health education.

BHSP sites were to participate in a student assessment program through one of the following options:

1. Sites will participate in a pre- and posttest of students provided by COP. The pretest is to be conducted during the fall of 1979 and the posttest is to be completed during the spring of 1981; or
2. Sites will develop their own pre- and posttests to be given on the same schedule. Sites choosing this option will work with the BHSP staff during the development stages of the instruments in order to (a) assist in developing a format which will enable the staff to provide the site with computer analysis of their data and (b) enable the establishment of a core group of topics or questions which will provide COP for some comparison of groups of sites over time.

In addition, it was suggested that some mechanism be developed to identify the products of participation in the BHSP that were not measured by student assessments: for example, community education efforts, changes in school smoking policies, and establishment of health related projects. Generally, it was felt that these products, which were readily identifiable, should be as important in the justification for continuing the programs as documentable changes in students, which were much more difficult to measure over a short period.

The final insult in the evaluation process occurred when the evaluators claimed that the data yet to be analyzed for the previous year had been stored on tapes that were illegible by the computers to which they had access. Attempts to have these tapes "translated" proved fruitless. Completed data from hundreds of student assessments gathered dust. The sites would never receive a report of the data they had supplied to the evaluators by all those surveys.

BARRIER 3: ADMINISTRATIVE STYLE

The third major issue influencing the progress of the BHSP was the difference in administrative style of the university, COP director 3, and the BHSP director. This has been alluded to previously. The COP director's style had the most direct influence on the BHSP staff and therefore on BHSP activities. His decision-making style was individual, not collateral or participatory. This style conflicted with the way the project was structured. COP staff committees (a personnel committee and a program committee) were organized to advise the COP director. Because of this structure, the staff expected to have effective input in decision making. But apparently they were too optimistic.

Input would be solicited from these committees, but the COP director would proceed on the basis of decisions made before asking for that input. Program directors were expected to stay within a budget but had no fiscal authority. The COP director could and did transfer funds within and between various project budgets without consulting or informing program directors.

This kind of conflict between the staff and the COP director was perceived by staff members of all COP projects as interfering with the accomplishment of their project goals. It resulted in a strong letter from the management team (all COP project directors) to the COP director in February 1980 outlining staff concerns and requesting a change in the way in which the COP was administered. Since the director did not respond to this letter, the staff sent it through the university chain of command.

For the next two months, a member of the management team periodically asked the university administration about actions on the issues they had raised. The administration, having apparently taken no action, offered no substantive replies.

There was little time for the staff to feel disappointed or defeated. Two events occurred on the heels of the staff's complaints, galvanizing its members into action. First, the COP director was offered a second contract by the administration. Although he did not accept the contract, the offer made it very clear to the staff that the administration approved his administrative style and gave no credibility to the staff's complaints. Second, the COP director recommended to the university administration that a staff member's pay be docked for three days for alleged failure to fulfill job responsibilities. The action was approved by the administration without informing or discussing the allegation with the staff member involved.

The staff member documented that the charges were false and resigned from the COP. Demoralization among staff was the order of the day.

In May 1980, BHSP director 5 and the COP staff member who had resigned went to the State Department of Public Health, the funding agency, to express their belief in the value of the COP projects and their concern that it would be difficult to operate viable programs under the current COP and university administrative style. They asked whether the projects could be moved to an organization that offered a style consonant with the project goals. The department agreed.

POSTSCRIPT

Two major projects were removed from the COP and were subsequently administered by other organizations. The staffs of both projects moved with them. One of the projects has since run its course and ended. The BHSP is still thriving in its new environment. Though several staff changes occurred in the two years following the move, all were agreeable and constructive for the staff and the project. The statewide support for the BHSP and school health education in general continue to grow and thrive.

Analysis

This case focuses on a group of health educators as trainers and consultants for a special project designed to develop a comprehensive health education curriculum in the school districts of a rural state. The case presents administrative issues: rapid turnover of administrative staff, evaluation, and administrative styles that were not consonant with project goals.

The health educator coordinators who provided direct service to the communities found these issues to be serious barriers to the goal of the project, that is, developing a comprehensive curriculum for school health education. The case describes how the health educator trainers and consultants dealt with these barriers.

Concepts about conflict resolution explain the actions taken by the health educators in this case. Ross and Mico (1980) identify five general conditions under which conflict occurs. Two of these are relevant to this case: (1) Conflict occurs when value differences are not mutually understood or mutually accepted, and (2) conflict occurs where there is a major imbalance in the power and influence held and exercised by interdependent parties. The desire to achieve power is invariably countered by the defense to hold it, and the resulting struggle frequently results in a win-lose interaction.

Zaltman and Duncan (1977:269) state that the strategies for conflict resolution range "from avoidance, smoothing-playing down differences, confronting the conflict, to forcing resolution through some coercive means."

Confrontation was chosen by the health educators as their method of dealing with the issues. The barrier that most directly affected staff was administrative style. This barrier made it difficult to deal with the other two, the evaluation disaster and staff turnover.

Staff went about their task of confronting this barrier systematically. They met, agreed on, and wrote down their major concerns; they expressed these in a letter to the administrator of the agency to which they were administratively responsible. Receiving no response, they took the letter up the chain of command. Periodic contact over a two-month period with the higher authority's office brought no reply. At the end of two months, the administration responded indirectly in ways that made it clear to staff that their grievances had not been and would not be heard.

Staff then moved from confrontation to "forcing resolution through some coercive means." They took their complaints to the funding agency and "forced" a physical move of the project to the site and administrative control of another agency. The school project is still thriving in that setting.

This case raises a number of interesting issues. Among these is commitment of staff. We assume that all professionals are committed to the goals of their profession and, of course, to the goals of professional activities in which they engage. But few of us have that assumption tested. The health educators working on the project described in this case did; they performed well under fire.

It would have been easy to resign, and under the circumstances totally justifiable. But they chose to confront a situation they believed would eventually destroy a health education program of potential benefit to the children and adults in the communities they served. They could have lost their battle to save the project and probably would have if the funding agency had not agreed with them.

Social support is a second issue this case identifies (Gottlieb 1981). It is clear in reading the case that there were multiple problems contributing to the untenable climate at the COP for the school project: for example, the "them and us" issue that surfaced more than once under different guises; and the communication problem that plagued the project in every conceivable way—misinterpretation of words and/or concepts, verbal messages garbled in delivery from one person to another, inflammatory newspaper publicity, and rumors.

The staff members could easily have been sidetracked by any one of these issues. They were not. They put things in perspective and analyzed problems objectively. This allowed them to focus on major not minor concerns. Once major concerns were identified, they did something about them.

It was possible to live through the trauma, keep their heads, analyze objectively, and develop constructive solutions because they supported one another. One person could not have managed this; but a group with a common goal, commitment, and good leadership could and did.

Administrative support is considered absolutely necessary for the practice of health education (Mathews 1982). This case raises questions about the level of support required. The objective of the BHSP was the development of a relevant curriculum in the school districts. Despite chaos at the COP, this process was going on. The local coordinators had support from their communities and superintendent. What they needed now was training and technical assistance from the BHSP, but lack of appropriate administrative support at the COP interfered with that.

This case demonstrates that it is possible to defy the barriers, to confront difficult issues and develop a constructive solution. The stakes for which the staff were fighting were high. Over time, a well-developed and well-taught school health curriculum should contribute to improved adult health—a goal worth the trauma and work that such a confrontation demands.

Although this case deals with organizational issues, the raison d'être for the case, the development of a curriculum for health education in school districts, offers an excellent example of the involvement of the community in school health education.

Financial support for the school districts was minimal, but community interest maximized the potential of each dollar, and communities eventually provided support for the program.

Understanding the structure of organizations, the decision-making processes in organizations, and organizational politics is critical for the health educator. Even the beginner must understand the relationship between these processes and what the health educator can accomplish in an organization. Health educators functioning in administrative or supervisory positions must be able to analyze these processes to promote, develop, and maintain health education programs in the organization. This case illustrates that the task is not easy.

References/Select Resources

Gottlieb, B. H., ed. 1981. *Social Networks and Social Support.* Beverly Hills: Sage Publications.

This book of readings is directed at mental health workers who are interested in social support issues as they relate to clients. However, a close reading (particularly of Part 2, on social network analysis and social support) will provide insight into the necessity for and use of the health educator's own professional support networks. In the final analysis these readings emphasize the need for social supports if we are to function effectively as individuals and professionals.

Katz, D., and Kahn, R. L. 1978. *The Social Psychology of Organizations.* 2d ed. New York: Wiley.

The authors describe social psychological principles that can be applied to all forms of work organizations. Chapter 10, "Power and Authority: Rule Enforcement," as well as other chapters on conflict, management, and organizational change are particularly pertinent to this case, which involved so much conflict. The effect of conflict on the interdependent behavior of a total system is applicable to any organization.

Mathews, B. P. 1982. "Administrative Climate: Its Implications for Health Educators." In *SOPHE Heritage Collection of Health Education Monographs,* vol. 1: *The Philosophical, Behavioral, and Professional Bases for Health Education,* edited by S. K. Simonds. Oakland, Calif.: Third Party Publishing.

The questions posed and the issues developed in this article are as important today as they were when first published in 1962. Mathews correctly points out that the administrative climate of the organization that employs the health educator is a major determinant of the health educator's effectiveness. "The most effective health educators," as Mathews notes, "are likely to be those who take into consideration not only the concerns and motivations of the learners but the practical reality of the administrative climate and the pressures it imposes." Hence it is necessary for the health educator to systematically diagnose the administrative climate to determine what effect it will have on programming and on the health educator as a professional. The task then may be for the health educator to try to change a less than supportive climate. However, this task can be very difficult and generally should not be undertaken by the new professional who has not developed significant credibility within an organization.

Ross, H. S., and Mico, P. R. 1980. *Theory and Practice in Health Education.* Palo Alto, Calif.: Mayfield.

This is a useful volume for the beginner and a good reference for the seasoned practitioner. It offers a comprehensive listing of theories, models, strategies, and issues for the practicing health educator. The authors' treatment of conflict and the resolution of conflict, an issue relevant to this case, illustrates their brief but adequate description of all concepts and issues in the practice of health education.

Zaltman, G. 1973. *Processes and Phenomena of Social Change.* New York: Wiley.

A collection of views on social change and theories of forces for and against change. The factors that precede and result from change are presented. Value systems and change strategies are discussed. This is a useful volume for helping health educators to understand macrosocietal issues and to gain a perspective on general social change in the valuing of health and on the meaning of change in health habits, hospital utilization, doctor-patient relationships, and health service organizations.

Zaltman, G., and Duncan, R. 1977. *Strategies for Planned Change.* New York: Wiley.

This volume offers a clear and comprehensive treatment of the change process. The authors identify four factors that facilitate the capacity of an organization to adapt its structure to deal with change. Dealing with conflict is one of these factors. The other three are effective intrapersonal relations, the ability to switch the rules as needed, and the willingness to institutionalize a structure that allows for change.

Discussion Questions

1. What are the pros and cons of the stand the staff took? Was there another way in which they could have handled this situation other than resigning?

2. What are some of the techniques you would have used in handling the uncooperative first-year coordinators at the week-long workshop?

3. Develop an outline for a training program for new coordinators, given their job description in this project.

4. Assume you are the health educator on this project. You have gone to one of the communities at the request of the school health curriculum coordinator. You find that he is having a problem with his community committee, for it wants to institute a curriculum that he feels is not adequate. The committee wants to avoid any reference to sexuality in the program but especially in the high school. A major problem in that community is teenage pregnancy. How would you advise the coordinator to deal with this problem?

5. What do you think might have been done to improve relationships between the COP staff, the BHSP staff, and the faculty members of the university?

Health Education Required for High School Graduation: From Resolution and Action to Law

Mabel Crenshaw Robinson, Ed.D.

This case study will describe the process by which comprehensive health education was recognized as an integral part of quality education in the high schools of Alabama. In 1978, Act 853, mandating comprehensive health education, was passed by the Alabama legislature. The bill required that all students entering the tenth grade during the school year 1982–1983 and thereafter successfully complete a full semester's course in health education. Course content, credit for the course, and the qualifications of the instructors also were set forth in the bill.

Ten years of activity preceded the passage of this bill. We will report in detail on the last three years of this activity. During that time, the author was the health education consultant for the State Department of Education and was intimately involved with the process. We will describe briefly events from 1968 to 1974, give a chronology of events from 1975 to 1978, and end with a description of the role of the health educator in the passage of Act 853.

BACKGROUND

A State Planning Committee for Curriculum Development was organized in 1968 to prepare a Health Education Curriculum Guide for grades K–12. The committee held two workshops on curriculum development in health education and published a draft of a guide in 1969. The Huntsville school system used the guide in 1970–1971. On the basis of the experience of this school system, a revision and rewriting team was organized. This group gave the final draft to the printer in January 1972, and it was distributed to all public school districts in the state.

Despite the availability of the guide, including an endorsement from the state superintendent of education, there was no apparent increase in the teaching of health education in the public schools over the next four years.

CHRONOLOGY 1975–1978

JANUARY 1975

The state superintendent of education appointed me health education consultant to the State Department of Education. This position had been vacant for eight years. Although a curriculum was developed and distributed, there was no other contact with the school systems relative to health education. An Advisory Committee to the health education consultant was appointed. Eight individuals knowledgeable both in health education and in the state system were invited to serve on this committee by the state superintendent of schools. The Advisory Committee, together with the consultant, identified areas of need such as (1) information on what was being taught in the schools in health education, (2) professional preparation, (3) legislation, (4) public relations (5) finances, and (6) program implementation. The first priority, however, was to get some kind of official recognition for a health education curriculum in the schools.

Mabel Crenshaw Robinson is a Professor of Health Education and Assistant Dean in the School of Education at the University of Alabama in Birmingham.

1975–1978

The State Board of Education required that all teacher certification criteria be reviewed and new standards set. At that time there was one certification for both health and physical education teachers. The state health education consultant negotiated with the physical education consultant to separate the certification for these two groups. The law requires that teachers of health education must have the same qualifications as teachers of any other subject. Physical education majors had only one course in health education; therefore they could not be certified as teachers of health. In this instance logic prevailed. Certification for teachers of health education was established.

1976

The health education consultant and members of the Advisory Committee developed a booklet entitled *Health Education in Alabama Schools: Planning for Action;* The American Lung Association and the University of Alabama in Birmingham printed the booklet. The content included a definition of comprehensive health education, a list of members of the Advisory Committee, task force membership, and the health education coordinators for each district. The material was distributed widely throughout the state and was an excellent resource for local school personnel.

SUMMER 1976

A committee was appointed to revise the 1972 Health Education Curriculum Guide. The consultant assumed major responsibility for this task.

JUNE 17, 1976

A resolution in support of a comprehensive health education curriculum in the schools developed by the Advisory Committee was passed by the State Board of Education. A commendation for this action was subsequently passed by the Alabama House of Representatives. The resolution was distributed to all school superintendents and principals and to deans of education and health education professionals in the colleges and universities. The resolution "urged" that health education be taught in the schools.

JULY 14, 1976

An orientation meeting for the 100 members of the State Health Education Coordinating Committee was held at the State Capitol, and 75 attended. Many members of this committee were serving on task forces, chaired by members of the Advisory Committee. The task forces were set up for the specific needs identified by the health education consultant and the Advisory Committee. Members of the coordinating committee included the state superintendent of education, the state director of public health, legislators, members of the radio and press, physicians, PTA members, members of the Auxiliary of the Alabama Medical Society, judges, representatives from the Governor's Committee on Physical Fitness, presidents of universities, and administrators of public and private schools—in fact, anyone remotely concerned with health education. This orientation meeting was the first time the superintendent of public education and the director of public health sat on the same platform and both advocated comprehensive school health education.

1977

Five regional workshops to assist schools in planning a health education curriculum were held at Athens College, the University of Alabama–Tuscaloosa, Auburn University, the University of Alabama–Birmingham, and the Mobile city schools. These workshops were staffed by members of the State Department of Education, Governor's Physical Fitness Commission, State Department of Public Health, Arthritis Foundation, American Lung Association, American Heart Association, American Cancer Society, and other organizations.

MAY 25, 1977

The State Board of Education passed a resolution recommending the inclusion of cardiopulmonary resuscitation (CPR) training in the school curriculum. Twenty-four workshops were held to train instructors in CPR. The state superintendent of education recommended that every member of the Division of Instruction and others in the State Department of Education take the basic CPR course; 700 did so.

SUMMER 1977

The state superintendent of education recommended to each of the 127 school districts that a health education coordinator be appointed. Notices of meetings and workshops of interest to teachers and principals often got lost on the superintendent's desk. There was a need for someone in each local school district to be the link between that district and the state consultant's office. Most of these coordinators were not health educators, because there were few in the schools at that time. But many did perform a useful function in keeping teachers and others informed about workshops, in-service programs, and available resource materials.

A survey of health instructional practices in the state at the elementary and secondary levels was conducted. One thousand of 1,310 questionnaires distributed were returned (76 percent). Ninety-six percent of the schools surveyed said they had a comprehensive health education program. Survey data suggested that superintendents and principals did not know the meaning of health education. Some thought that health and physical education were the same, others that health and science were the same. It was clear we had to define what we meant by comprehensive health education. The need for this survey was identified by the Advisory Committee and further defined by the Needed Information Task Force. The consultant developed and implemented the survey and analyzed survey data.

The Professional Preparation Task Force developed a survey for college and university professional preparation programs in health education. The data showed that only three institutions (out of 27) offered an undergraduate major in health education. Clearly, one pressing need was to prepare more teachers of health education.

AUGUST 1977

The state PTA organized a Health Education Committee and invited a representative of the State Department of Education to be a member. It sponsored a one-day workshop on health education and invited the state superintendent of education to give the keynote address. The program focused on implementing a health education curriculum in the schools.

The auxiliary of the Alabama Medical Society devoted its fall conference to "Health through Education" and chose as its project for the year a public relations campaign to inform the state about the importance of health education. It developed television spots shown in January. At about the same time, a brochure it had put together—"What in Health Do Our Schools Teach?"—was distributed to all school districts, every doctor's office, and other appropriate locations.

FALL 1977

Workshops for principals and health education coordinators were held in eight sections of the state at one of the state colleges and universities. The purpose of the workshops was to define the meaning of comprehensive health education, that is, what should be included in a school health education curriculum and how to promote the concept of comprehensive school health. The workshops were conducted by health education specialists from the State Department of Education and members of the Advisory Committee. Both voluntary and public agencies offering material for school health education were invited to participate. Faculty from local universities hosted the workshops.

1977–1978

Conferences and workshops were held throughout the state, sponsored by a number of different groups, to acquaint people with the meaning of comprehensive school health education and to promote curriculum development in local school districts. The chairman of the Senate Health Education Committee of the Alabama legislature participated in several of these meetings to garner support for a bill on health education he was planning to introduce.

1978

The Committee of a Hundred was appointed by the State Board of Education so that the public would have some say in what was required for high school graduation. The state consultant nominated two health educators for this committee, and they were appointed. The committee held hearings throughout the state and deliberated over a two-year period. The consensus was to eliminate every subject except the "basics." All other subjects would be elective. The first to be attacked was health and/or physical education. The committee saw the two subjects as the same, but on being enlightened by the health educator members, recommended that health education be required for one semester.

The revised curriculum guide was published.

Legislative Act 853 passed. The act mandated that all students entering the tenth grade during the school year 1982–1983 successfully complete the approved courses in health education before graduation.

POSTSCRIPT

The passing of the legislation was, of course, the highlight of all the activities of the past ten years, but it was not the end of the battle to promote health education in the schools.

Following passage of legislation, there were a number of other activities, including the following:

1. We suggested to all school superintendents that the health education coordinator for the school district be a health educator or someone with a demonstrated interest in health education. This suggestion was well received and resulted in the appointment of new coordinators in many districts.
2. We continued to promote seminars and workshops throughout the state on all facets of school health education.
3. Since all institutions now had separate degrees in health education and physical education, to comply with the separate certification requirements, a passing score on a competency test was now needed for certification in health education. (All teachers are required to pass a minimal competency test.) Two members of the Advisory Committee were appointed to serve on a committee to develop minimal competencies for teachers of health education.
4. The State Board of Education now required that all undergraduates, regardless of their field of study, have a course in health education to receive professional teacher certification.
5. The State Health Education Coordinating Committee and its task forces were reorganized and set new goals.

The process never ends!

ROLE OF THE HEALTH EDUCATOR

In the chronology of events from 1975–1978, staff functions of the health education consultant have been mentioned. Developing survey instruments and analyzing data are functions common to the practice of health education and other professions as well. The "how to" of these functions is described in the literature. The major function I carried out, however, was the coordination of the political and educational process that led to the passage of Act 853.

It is clear from the case that hundreds of people were involved in and responsible for the passage of Act 853. Someone had to coordinate all these efforts and keep them focused on the goal. That was the job of the health educator.

Coordination of programs is one of the seven responsibilities of the health educator as defined by the Role Delineation Project. The description of the functions related to that responsibility, as defined in the verified role, fit very well the functions carried out in the passage of Act 853—with one addition: We were involved in a political as well as an educational effort. That part of our function could fit under Responsibility VI in the role, that is, "promotes organization and social development." Changes in policy and the development of new policies were an integral part of the total effort.

To briefly describe the role I played: Coordination required that the political and educational issues be identified; that progress by key target populations toward the goal of comprehensive school health education be tracked; and that the course of the issues related to the goal be monitored.

It is impossible to describe all the activities, but a few major ones will be illustrated to show how it is possible to coordinate a number of different efforts and track progress toward a goal.

First, though, you need to know that I have lived in Alabama all my life and my family has deep roots there. I know the political system. Further, I worked in the educational system, so I understood how it was structured and how it worked. I did not have to spend time learning about the environment in which I was to work. It would have taken a newcomer to the state much longer, simply because a newcomer would have had to learn his or her way around the system.

When I was appointed state school health education consultant and the superintendent of public instruction approved the idea of comprehensive school health education, I knew we had to move in two directions: (1) We had to do our homework; we had to know all there was to know about school health education; we couldn't afford not to have the answers when asked. (2) The idea of comprehensive school health education had to have backing from a number of publics: the powerful, the "little guys," and the people who were going to have to do the work—school teachers and principals.

To begin, I asked the superintendent to appoint the Advisory Committee: a group of professionals and lay people whose credibility and expertise was beyond question. This committee and I worked together to identify the issues and appoint task forces to begin to get necessary information on the issues, such as preparation of teachers to teach health education. We worked quietly and diligently for over a year before we asked the Board of Education for the resolution on comprehensive school health. We had gathered enough information at this time to warrant this request. The commendation from the legislature for this resolution was pro forma. But it had great publicity value. So when we surveyed school systems about current practice, asked them for a contact person for health education issues, and offered workshops to the teachers, we had something to point to that suggested health education was worth the attention of local school districts.

The School Health Education Coordinating Committee provided the opportunity to involve anyone interested in school health education at any level of activity they wished, from merely getting information about what was being done to active participation in one of the task forces. No one with an interest in school health could say they didn't have a chance to be part of the action. I played a major role with the Advisory Committee in identifying the 100 members of this committee. It was extremely important to include everyone with even a remote interest. We gave the formation of this committee a good deal of publicity in an effort to identify interested persons whom we did not know.

A critically important target population was the teachers and principals. In the final analysis, if they didn't accept the concept, there would be no school health education. Our workshops and conferences with this group were carefully developed. First we had to promote the idea, interest them in considering it, and then provide them with all the information they needed and all the resources we could muster to help them develop a school health education program.

My role was to identify potential contributors to the workshops at all levels of participation: publicity people, hosts and hostesses, panel members, program arrangers, and those who could maintain contact with participants. We involved as many teachers, principals, local superintendents, and academicians as possible. As often as we could, we applied the principle that one learns more by being involved than by sitting passively.

The entrance of the PTA and the auxiliary of the Alabama Medical Society on the scene was manna from heaven. We knew that the auxiliary was looking for a project. We urged its members to consider school health education. Their activities contributed a great deal to the general publicity but, more important, they helped us inform and get the support of two audiences critical to the development of school health education programs: parents and the medical profession. The support of the auxiliary gave credibility to the concept that we could not have gotten in any other way.

Paralleling all of our efforts to reach specific target audiences were our activities related to teacher preparation for health education. This was the issue on which we would easily have floundered badly. Everyone could agree that comprehensive school health education was a great idea, but if there were not enough teachers trained to teach it, we would have lost the ball game.

Persuading the Committee of a Hundred to leave health education in the curriculum was not easy. There was a strong lobby to cut back health and physical education. Our representatives to that committee had done their homework. They had convincing data about the value of health education. However, the data alone were not enough. Those representatives helped; they kept health education in the running. Health education *had to be a required course* somewhere in the 12 years of public school or our cause was lost. We asked for more than we thought we could get so that, when they cut back, we had something left. We did a good deal of informal lobbying on this issue. And that contributed greatly to our coming out of that committee with a one-semester requirement for health education.

It's appropriate to say a word about our informal activities in our push for comprehensive health education. I mentioned earlier that I've lived in Alabama all my life. I'm an active member of my community, so I know a great many people. I never lost an opportunity to mention the comprehensive school health issue to anyone I thought was interested or could help the cause along. It made no difference whether I saw them in the supermarket, at church, at a party, or walking downtown. I really believed in the importance of this issue. So did the members of the Advisory Committee; they too did informal lobbying. I truly believe it was the informal lobbying that won the day for us with the Committee of a Hundred.

Luck, however it might be defined, played a role in our success too. It was a stroke of luck that the State Board of Education required that all teacher certification criteria be reviewed and new standards set. This was a golden opportunity for us to separate from physical education so as to have separate standards for teachers of health education.

We were able to achieve this separation rather easily. It was a simple matter of reasoning: Physical educators were not qualified by state law to teach health education; that is, they didn't have a sufficient number of courses in health education. The physical education leadership saw this point and readily agreed to the separation.

Because I was coordinating all the activities related to comprehensive school health, I was able to see what was being done throughout the state. With statewide activities as a backdrop, the Advisory Committee and I worked together to orchestrate our plans to legislate school health education at whatever level we could. It was very clear to us that although some schools would institute a health education curriculum, many would not unless they were required to do so. The one positive assurance we could have that all schools would offer some type of health education course was legislation.

We were fortunate to have a state senator interested in school health education. He was instrumental in creating a Senate committee on health education; and it was he who introduced the legislation. We worked very closely with him, providing him with information, answering questions, introducing him to people knowledgable about school health education, and so on.

As you will note from the chronology, we kept up a steady stream of activity in the school districts. We involved universities and colleges as much as possible in this activity, thus introducing the academics to an issue with which they would have to be more involved if legislation for comprehensive health education passed. In 1975 there were only three schools offering a major in health education. Clearly, we needed many more.

As we worked with the schools, the PTA, the auxiliary of the Alabama Medical Society, and others, we identified persons with a strong interest in school health education. It was these persons, as well as the Advisory Committee and the Health Education Coordinating Committee, on whom we depended to muster support for the legislation when it was introduced.

The passage of the legislation was a coup. It happened because a number of different groups were keenly interested and sufficiently committed to support the legislation. The task was not easy. There was skepticism and opposition along the way. Our stance was to keep moving in the direction of the goal. We dealt with the opposition politely, but we did not let it stand in our way.

There was no budget for this project. Professionals who were involved either paid their own expenses or had them paid by their organization. All the volunteers paid their own expenses, and for some this was not a small amount. Many traveled hundreds of miles around the state, sometimes staying overnight and always having to pay for one or two meals. If people care enough to take money out of their own pockets to pay expenses, they have to believe in what they are doing. Such dedication was probably the greatest asset this effort for school health education had.

Analysis

This case focuses on two aspects of the role of the health educator: that of coordinator and that of facilitator for policy change and the development of new policy. The case describes a complex, long-term effort to make certain all graduates of Alabama public schools were exposed to a comprehensive course in health education before graduation. The staccato description of the events that culminated in the passage of the mandating legislation belies the extensive and intensive activity that occurred.

The health educator and the Advisory Committee were aware of the political reality: Though many school systems would express an interest in a health education curriculum, the only way to be absolutely sure that all school systems offered students a comprehensive course in health education prior to graduation would be to mandate the course. The leadership also understood that this could not be done unless there was sufficient public support for the concept of comprehensive school health education.

Lewin's concept of "imposed" learning/"learned" learning provides a theoretical base for the analysis of the process by which school districts would adopt a comprehensive school health curriculum. Lewin claimed that some people will not adopt or learn a new practice unless forced to do so. Learning is imposed in a variety of ways (e.g., reward or punishment, legal constraint). However, Lewin emphasized that no practice or new behavior could be imposed on a group or a culture unless there were enough members who wanted to see the new practice accepted (Lewin 1951). The health educator and the Advisory Committee in this case therefore planned activities to develop public support.

This theoretical perspective explains how the principal actors in the implementation of the law on comprehensive school health education—that is, teachers, principals, and superintendents—learned their role. One means of imposing learning is to use a step-by-step process. People will go along with something new although they are not sure where it is leading them. They take one step at a time, and each step has a potential for bringing them closer to "learned" learning. Diffusion of an innovation is an alternate theory (Rogers 1983). The principal actors gradually became aware of the issue, got interested in it, and pursued it through the process of evaluating it and trying it out. Finally, some adopted it because they believed in it, whereas others adopted it only because they were forced to comply with the law.

Both theories offer similar explanations. Diffusion of an innovation is perhaps more useful because it also suggests a strategy for proceeding. Specific methodologies can be attached to each step in the adoption process. This is helpful in program planning. A brief discussion of the strategies will throw further light on the application of this theory to practice.

Community organization was the main strategy used to organize the relevant publics to support both comprehensive school health education and the legislation for it. Many of the skills required for community organization are included under the health educator's role as coordinator (U.S. Department of Commerce 1982). All these skills have been well identified in the literature. Barry (1982:190–191) states that "understanding about and use of relationships is perhaps the greatest professional skill which the worker can bring to community organization practice." She goes on to say:

> In community organization practice, we work with many different organizations, groups and individuals. We bring representatives of these groups together. We work with persons at various levels on the socioeconomic scale, persons with different points of view, persons with various motivations, abilities, and field of competence. Part of our job is helping these community groups work together, each contributing his own competence towards a mutually acceptable solution to a problem.

The skills demonstrated in this case were not those of an amateur. It takes real skill to identify the strengths of individuals and groups and focus them on the desired goals.

Although community organization provided the strategy to organize enough support for the legislation to pass, diffusion of an innovation provided a strategy for helping the principal actors learn the meaning of comprehensive school health education and what was required to implement it in the school districts. Note how these activities were planned.

The resolution by the State Board of Education did not mandate school health education in 1976; it "urged" school systems to consider it. The school systems were thus alerted to the State Board of Education's interest but were not forced to take action before they were ready.

In the next couple of years a great variety of activities were carried out. All were planned to keep the issue of comprehensive school health education before the school districts. There was such a barrage of diverse activities that it was impossible for these target populations not to know what was going on. The need for multiple educational inputs to achieve complex and lasting changes in behavior has been identified by Green (1982:87).

Activities were then planned to gradually involve the target populations, both the schools and the public, in the issue of comprehensive school health education. In this way these activities also contributed to the development of support for the concept. The process is integrative.

Other activities paralleling the development of support included the separate certification for health education teachers and the development of a curriculum in universities to prepare teachers of health education.

The legislative activity by the health educator, members of the Advisory Committee, and others concerned with the issue of comprehensive school health education is not detailed in the case study, but it must have been extensive. Understanding the legislative process and knowing how to work with legislators and provide them with information—not too much, just enough—are important skills for the health educator.

This case illustrates the value of continuity of staff. Robinson was a member of the staff of the State Department of Education from 1965 to 1980. As in the Campbell/Williams case (p. 288), we have long-term continuity of staff and a credible, stable organization. When we compare the accomplishments of the people in these cases with those of people forced to operate on time-limited grants, we have to opt for funding community-based organizations that won't go away in three years, and for funding at a level that permits qualified staff to work with communities *over time*. Finally, the case raises the issue of the importance of a comprehensive analysis of the issues prior to beginning activity. There were many bases to cover to achieve the goal. Essential were the support for legislation from the target populations and from the superintendent of public instruction and the interest generated among and by community organizations. All this backing, together with the knowledge and skills of the coordinator and the Advisory Committee, contributed to the passage of legislation mandating the health education course. But it was the specificity of the legislation and the availability of the resources to implement it that made the legislation meaningful.

References/Select Resources

Barry, M. D. 1982. "A Theoretical Framework for Community Organization." In *SOPHE Heritage Collection of Health Education Monographs,* vol. 1: *The Philosophical, Behavioral, and Professional Bases for Health Education,* edited by S. K. Simonds. Oakland, Calif.: Third Party Publishing.

This article gives a clear picture of the major concepts in community organization, with examples of how these are applied. The role of the community organizer (i.e., the staff person, whether a health educator, a social worker, or a recreation worker) is described realistically and in detail. Although the use of community organization at the level discussed in this article is not a task for the novice, the beginner can nonetheless learn from Barry's thoughtful presentation of the issue. However, the beginner should function as a community organizer only under the supervision of an experienced health educator.

Green, L. W. 1982. "Determining the Impact and Effectiveness of Health Education as It Relates to Federal Policy." In *SOPHE Heritage Collection of Health Education Monographs,* vol. 2: The Practice of Health Education, edited by B. Mathews. Oakland, Calif: Third Party Publishing.

This major policy paper by one of the leaders in health education provides a systematic review of recent research in health education. Thirty-six specific recommendations based on this research offer the basis for future federal policy decisions. One of these recommendations identifies the need for multiple methods for effective programs, a principle applied in this case.

Iverson, D. C., guest ed. 1981. "Promoting Health through the Schools—A Challenge for the Eighties." *Health Education Quarterly* 8(1):1–117.

Iverson describes three major problems that must be overcome so that the efforts to promote the health of children and youth through the schools will be successful. He stresses the need for well-planned programs that can be adapted to meet local needs and points out that school health education and health services personnel must coordinate their efforts.

Lewin, K. 1951. *Field Theory in Social Science.* New York: Harper.

In chapter 4, Lewin describes the basic attributes of field theory and their relation to learning. He distinguishes between "learned" learning and "imposed" learning; the latter is often referred to as compliance. He identifies the conditions under which learning is imposed and the conditions under which individuals learn. People will allow learning to be imposed if the reward or punishment is great enough, if they perceive a choice as the lesser of two evils, if legal or social constraints are applied, if they don't feel they have a choice, or if they are "pushed into a situation which is not sufficiently different from the previous one to create great resistance." Lewin makes other useful distinctions in this chapter, such as the difference between cognitive and motivational learning.

Rogers, E. M. 1983. *Diffusion of Innovations.* 3d ed. New York: Free Press.

Rogers reviewed 3,085 studies on diffusion for this volume, an indication of the tremendous increase in diffusion research since his first publication in 1962, when he reported on 405 studies.

Here he extends diffusion theory to include factors that antecede and follow the adoption process, thus posing several questions. For example, Where did the diffusion come from? Which comes first, the need or the innovation? What kinds of problems are encountered, and how are they solved as the innovation is implemented?

In this case, the basic diffusion model was useful in planning strategy to involve teachers, principals, and superintendents. Knowledge was made available to them, learning experiences were planned, and opportunities were offered to simulate use of the curriculum, all of which helped them be persuaded to consider the health education curriculum.

Ross, M. G. 1955. *Community Organization.* New York: Harper.

This very influential book was one of the early efforts to define community organization and suggest methods of practice. According to Ross, community organization is "a process by which a community identifies its needs or objectives, orders (or ranks) these needs or objectives, develops the confidence and will to work at these needs or objectives, finds the resources (internal and/or external) to deal with these needs or objectives, takes action in respect to them, and in so doing extends and develops cooperative and collaborative attitudes and practice in the community." Although, as this definition implies, community organization cannot be imposed, there is a need for the community worker to take an active role in bringing about change. Values and problems need to be identified and methods selected. For Ross, community organization is based on the following assumptions: People can learn to deal with their own problems; people want change and can change; people should participate in and control change; self-change has a meaning and permanence that imposed changes do not have; a holistic approach is better than a fragmented approach; people often need to learn skills to make democracy work; and communities frequently need help in organizing to deal with their needs.

U.S. Department of Commerce. National Technical Information Service. 1982. *Role Refinement and Verification for Health Educators; Final Report.* Access no. (HRP) 09–04273. Springfield, Va.

This report describes the process by which the role of the health educator was verified. The data on the verified role support the hypothesis that there is a generic health educator at the entry level. The seven responsibilities of the generic, entry-level health educator and the functions included under these responsibilities are specified. The report should be on the bookshelf of every health educator.

Discussion Questions

1. Using the adoption process, plan a series of activities for the personnel of a school system to introduce them to the concept of comprehensive health education and to help them evaluate the concept and try it out. Specify the methodologies to be used at each step in the process.

2. Although adoption of an innovation provides both a theoretical base and a strategy for a part of the case, why doesn't diffusion of an innovation fit the case? (See Rogers 1983).

3. Consider the issue of "informal" lobbying. Identify instances in which it is ethical.

4. Prepare a draft of a statement of the superintendent of education to present to the State Board of Education relative to the resolution for comprehensive school health education. In preparing this statement, consider its length, the information to be included, and the format.

5. If you were the newly appointed school health education consultant in your state educational system, what steps would you take to get acquainted? Assume the superintendent of public instruction has made it clear that she wants to see all school systems include health education as a required course.

The Seaside Story

Judy Drolet, Ph.D.

INTRODUCTION

In the small coastal town of Seaside, Oregon, an annual week-long conference provides new directions for health education. Each June since 1977, representatives from school districts throughout Oregon have been spending five days living and learning the philosophy of wellness at the Seaside Health Education Conference (SHEC).

The SHEC serves primarily as teacher in-service for educators from varied disciplines (e.g., health education, physical education, home economics, science) who are involved with health education. However, participants also include administrators, food service personnel, school/district nurses, and counselors as well as parents and community members. Families of some school personnel have also been accommodated. Registration for the first conference in 1977 numbered 152 and increased to slightly over 500 in June 1982. Approximately 100 applications beyond the capacity were received for both Seaside V and VI. Participants frequently comment on the disappointment experienced by colleagues unable to attend.

A committee with representatives from the Oregon Department of Education (ODE), school districts and colleges, community agencies, and professional health organizations plans the SHEC each year. From 14 to 50 administrators, teachers, nurses, parents and community members offer suggestions on speakers, topics, and scheduling for each conference program.

As coordinating sponsor for the conferences, the ODE arranges housing in Seaside for those attending. In addition, through a cooperative effort, local proprietors prepare highly nutritious meals three times a day for the week.

Seaside I was a direct result of a two-year needs assessment conducted by Len Tritsch, health education specialist for the ODE. The assessment results indicated that health educators in Oregon six years ago lacked power to influence the future trends and status of their discipline. Thus participants in the SHEC of 1977 focused on "how to become a change agent" within their respective communities to follow the conference theme of "Health Education at the Crossroads."

The following year, Seaside II convened with the theme "Healthy Is In" and emphasized team participation (which we will discuss shortly). Seaside III was encouraging representatives from 67 school districts to pursue "Wellness as a Life-style," and in 1980 the Seaside IV theme was "I'm Promoting Health." "Come Alive: Seaside V" was the focus in 1981. Participants in Seaside VI were challenged to "Energize and Renew in '82."

Diverse sources offer financial support for the Seaside conferences. Funding for the first SHEC was provided by the Single State Agency housed in the Oregon Mental Health Division. Subsequent conference expenses were supplemented by the sponsoring agencies. Allocations from local school districts and volunteer agencies complemented Mental Health Division drug education grant money in covering 1978 conference costs and those of ensuing years. Partial funding was also acquired from portions of the Nutrition Education Training Programs. These expenditures, however, did not include the tuition fees for those wishing to receive college credit for attending the SHEC.

Judy Drolet is an Assistant Professor of Health Education at Southern Illinois University at Carbondale. She was formerly a Graduate Teaching Fellow in the Department of Health Education at the University of Oregon.

The initial Seaside workshop convened in 1977 with hopes of creating a solid health education network throughout the state of Oregon. Among other conference goals, participants were encouraged to (1) assess the effectiveness of health education in Oregon schools, (2) share successful health education techniques with others, (3) analyze their own daily eating, drinking, and exercise practices, and (4) take part in experiences designed to enhance positive feelings about themselves and their profession. The following year, to supplement the goals of Seaside I, participants were provided with opportunities to develop contracts for personal behavior change.

As the conference evolved, the initial goals were retained when the dimensions of wellness became the focal point. Health education teaching models were built on prevention coupled with self-appraisal of wellness. Course outlines and class activities related to nutrition, physical fitness, stress awareness, and management and environmental sensitivity were shared. The wellness dimension remains the core of the SHEC, along with sessions related to drug education, human sexuality, and innovative teaching techniques.

Two keys to the SHEC's success are the requirements of team participation and action plans. First, far greater positive impact is evident in districts where a group of administrators, teachers, staff, and community members participate. Second, each team is required to attend the entire conference and develop an action plan for improving or implementing a health education program. Thus the teams and action plans complement each other in helping those attending the SHEC achieve their conference goals. Team meetings are scheduled at the SHEC for evaluation, work on action plans, and sharing experiences of the day.

The SHEC offerings have evolved over the years. Seaside I presenters were from Oregon school districts and the ODE. By the second conference, nationally recognized experts were keynote speakers for both general and small-group sessions. The number and variety of topics offered in small-group sessions expanded each year. Seaside I offered 17 sessions; by 1980 and 1981, participants could select at least seven topics each morning and each afternoon of the conference. A sign-up procedure was used to allow manageable group sizes at each session.

A reorganization in format occurred in 1982, the result being 20 workshops and 53 sessions structured around *daily* themes. Monday's activities focused on physical fitness, Tuesday's on nutrition topics. Coping skills and other mental health sessions were scheduled for Wednesday. Longer workshops, lasting for either three or six hours, were offered on Thursday. These sessions provided in-depth hands-on training in skills for promoting wellness.

From the beginnning, representatives from a wide variety of community agencies concerned with school health education set up displays and provided materials throughout the conference. With the new format, community agency booths accented the daily theme.

Besides the professional development aspects, an observer of the Seaside conferences can immediately see that participants are having fun. Conference organizers try to create a supportive environment for work and play. Further, the coastal setting offers an ideal locale for social events and fitness activities. Exercise time is scheduled before breakfast and between sessions each day. T-shirts with the conference theme are sold each year. Participants are encouraged to become involved with planned activities (e.g., beach campfire picnics and sing-alongs, fun runs, talent shows, clogging and dancing, new games). Time is also allotted for relaxation, use of the city pool, and other recreational activities.

EVALUATION

In an evaluation of the 1977, 1978, and 1979 conferences (Seaside I, II, and III), survey results indicated substantial knowledge increases in five of six content areas. Attitude changes were also reported. Further, respondents described behavior changes resulting from conference participation (Dosch and Paxton 1981).

A five-year (1977–1981) evaluation was undertaken at the University of Oregon as a doctoral dissertation to assess whether participants in Seaside I through V perceived more health program changes within their schools than personnel not participating in these conferences. Specific details of the study design and the statistical analyses described next are given in Drolet (1982).

This follow-up study examined perceptions of how the current (1981) status of the following four components compared with that of 1977: (1) health-related curriculum, (2) specific indicators of overall support for health-related activities in the schools, (3) positive-health role models, and (4) personal behaviors.

In March 1982, 400 questionnaires on health-related topics were mailed to selected Oregon school personnel. SHEC participants received 200 surveys, and an additional 200 questionnaires were sent to a matched control group. The SHEC group returned 103 (51.5 percent) usable questionnaires, whereas the control group returned 69 (34.5 percent).

In addition, 74 individual interviews were conducted at Oregon school districts in March and April 1982 to triangulate with data collected through the mailed questionnaires. The interviewees represented (1) 13 school districts that participate in the SHEC, (2) 13 school districts that participated in the SHEC and also received funding for Nutrition Education Training Programs (NETP), and (3) 13 school districts that were not involved with either the SHEC or NETP.

The demographic characteristics of subjects in both the questionnaire groups and the interview groups were generally comparable. The majority of subjects were between ages 30 and 49, with equal representation of females and males. Nearly all respondents had bachelor's or master's degrees and were teachers or school administrators. Within the high school and community college subgroups, the largest proportions of teachers in the study were assigned to health education. This consistent representation of subjects allowed comparisons among the five study groups.

In response to questions about the health-related curriculum, both SHEC and control subjects indicated that in 1977 the health courses had focused on disease diagnosis and treatment. In the mailed questionnaire, both groups reported change toward the wellness model, but with greater change occurring in the Seaside group. SHEC participants had adopted the wellness model and concurrently achieved a more positive status for health education in the school curriculum.

Subjects in the interview groups also discussed changes in the health-related curriculum. Their responses were consistent with those obtained in the mailed questionnaire. Seaside interviewees (85 percent) reported "major" curriculum changes, whereas, three quarters of the control group perceived curriculum changes as "minimal." Over 95 percent of the SHEC subjects indicated that the changes involved adoption of the wellness model, whereas less than one-quarter of control group stated that the health curriculum in their schools focused on wellness.

Subjective comments were also recorded in the personal interviews. Refinement of the scope-and-sequence components and greater autonomy as a discipline were mentioned by the Seaside participants along with observations about the wellness orientation. Personal comments also indicated that, in some SHEC schools, health themes had extended to other disciplines, ranging from home economics and science to shop and theatre arts.

When participants return from the SHEC, they share materials, techniques, and new ideas with other school personnel to encourage support from administrators, staff, students, and parents for wellness concepts and health-related activities. Perceptions of past support for health-related activities (HRA) were not significantly different when the Seaside and control groups were compared. However, current support for HRA was significantly different between the Seaside and control groups. The following four indicators reflect the results of participation in the SHEC.

1. Fairly "extensive" efforts were made to encourage parental participation.
2. There was moderate subsequent parental involvement with HRA.
3. Somewhat "extensive" changes in the food services resulted from HRA at the SHEC-group schools.
4. Moderate financial support for HRA was maintained at a level equal to or beyond that at other school programs in SHEC-group schools.

When overall support for health-related activities became a topic of discussion in the interviews, responses supported the mailed questionnaire analyses on indicators of support for HRA. School administrators and teachers were perceived as being supportive of health-related activities by at least three-quarters of Seaside subject, whereas less than one-quarter of control-group members reported this support. Changes placing more emphasis on food service and expanding the food service activities have occurred at Seaside-group schools. In general, SHEC participants perceived that financial support for HRA was the maximum possible from the respective school budgets. The *proportion* of subjects in control-group schools reporting these changes was minimal. The differences between the study groups were found to be statistically significant.

Through subjective comments, specific examples of support for health-related activities were acquired. Several principals allowed teachers to use "prep" time for exercise, meditation, and other fitness activities. Athletic facilities in some schools are now available for use by teachers and staff. At least six districts are attempting to implement "WELLCHEC" insurance plans, whereby premium refunds are offered as incentives for reducing sick-day absenteeism. As you'll see shortly, the Pilot Rock School District is a prime example of SHEC-motivated changes.

The wellness model as well as the Seaside conferences operate under the assumption that role modeling exerts a strong influence on personal health habits. Consequently, the presence of positive role models is stressed at the conferences.

Seaside respondents to both the mailed questionnaires and the individual interviews placed more emphasis on the importance of role models than did the control-group subjects. Comparison of changes from past to present perceptions about role modeling revealed statistically significant differences between the two groups. The Seaside group tended to view everyone in the school district as necessary for positive role models. Likewise, a statistically significantly greater proportion of Seaside interviewees (75 percent) perceived "everyone" generally and the health teacher specifically as important role models, as compared to the control group (32 percent).

Subjective comments focused on the relationship of role modeling and effective teaching. Typical remarks were those of two high school teachers: "The only way to be a better teacher is to be a better person" and "Credibility as a health education teacher is acquired by role modeling." Numerous examples of how role modeling "creates a domino effect" were also offered.

As previously mentioned, one intent of the Seaside conferences was that those attending would influence the health habits of people at their schools. In the mailed questionnaire, changes in ten behaviors by four categories of school personnel were assessed. Twenty of 40 tests revealed statistically significant differences between the study groups in the proportion of respondents who observed the designated positive behavior changes in various categories of personnel. In each of the 20 cases, a larger proportion of SHEC subjects reported more positive behavior changes. The behaviors most frequently reported were related to exercise, nutrition, and weight control. Teachers exhibited the most changes.

Interview questionnaire results were once again consistent with those from the mailed questionnaire. Comparisons reflected statistically significant differences in seven of ten health habits. A larger proportion of Seaside participants observed positive behavior changes in other school personnel. Though specific categories of personnel were not delineated in the interviews, behavior changes in nutrition and exercise were again most frequently reported. Personal comments regarding changes predominantly described decreased smoking and increased exercise by personnel and students at the schools.

The Seaside conferences also strived to enhance the health status of each participant. An extremely important indicator of the success of the SHEC was personal application of the acquired knowledge and skills. Nine categories of behavior were assessed in the mailed questionnaire. Both study groups perceived their health-related behavior five years previously as positive. But further comparison revealed statistically significant differences: A higher percentage of Seaside participants than control-group subjects reported changes aimed at improving their already "positive" behaviors. Anecdotal remarks from the Seaside subjects related mainly to changes in smoking, exercise, and weight control.

The full potential impact of the SHEC is typified by the Pilot Rock School District in eastern Oregon (550 students and 39 teachers). According to the high school principal, Larry Wolfgram, it's hard not to be affected by wellness because everyone on the school staff is involved with health-related activities in some capacity.

Prior to Seaside I, the school district did not have a coordinated health program. Pilot Rock now has a total curriculum for grades K–12. The physical education program has also acquired a new orientation. A noncompetitive curriculum aimed at individualized fitness involved all students.

The food service personnel have made changes that improved district menus, offering more nutritious meals, including "waistliner" lunches. Ten-minute nutrition breaks are scheduled two hours before lunch. Juice, milk, whole wheat muffins, and other healthful foods prepared by the home economics classes are available.

Though the area is considered to be very conservative, the impact of wellness has extended further to include the local Pilot Rock community. A monthly "Heaven Can Wait" newsletter is distributed to the school board, classified staff, students, and community members. The district has organized a community fitness program highlighted by a community run that provokes a large turnout each year. Support from parents and community groups, such as the Lions Club, is strong and increasing.

The energy sparked at the Seaside conferences has spread throughout the Oregon school systems. What started as an attempt to bridge the communication gap perceived by Oregon's health educators has grown far beyond the expectations of those involved with its creation. The impact of the SHEC has extended from the classroom to the district and beyond to the local communities. The result is a strong and cohesive statewide effort for health promotion.

The story does not end at the Oregon borders. Conferences modeled after the SHEC are developing in several states, including Kansas, Texas, Virginia, Washington, and Wisconsin. This growth enhances the possibility of having a national network for promotion of wellness.

REFERENCES

Dosch, P., and Paxton, C. 1981. "Recharging Professionally." *Health Education* 12(6):34–35.

Drolet, J. 1982. "Evaluation of the Seaside Health Education Conference and Nutrition Education Training Program in Oregon School Systems." Ph.D. diss., University of Oregon.

Analysis

The role of the writer of this case is not revealed until the last part. She was the evaluator of the follow-up study conducted after the program had reached its five-year point. The specialized skills needed by Drolet centered on evaluation design and the ability to direct a major evaluation project through its design, data collection, statistical analysis, interpretation, and report writing.

A then/post design was used to conduct the follow-up evaluation. In a then/post design, data on conditions (knowledge, attitudes, and practice) before and after the program are collected concurrently after the program is completed. As Howard (1980:94) notes, the then/post design can eliminate the response-shift bias that can occur in the pre/post designs. In training programs, "one specific objective is to change a subject's awareness or understanding of a particular variable. One might contend that to the extent that an intervention meets this goal, it will alter subjects' perspectives in evaluating themselves on that dimension. In such a case, conventional pretest and posttest ratings would relate to different scales and hence would fail to adequately reflect change due to treatment."

In the evaluation of this case, we can use the question of how well a curriculum has adopted a wellness perspective as an example of how the then/post design can eliminate response-shift bias. *Wellness* is a term that has both a colloquial and a specialized meaning. In the latter sense, a wellness-oriented program or curriculum has a particular philosophical base that focuses primarily on skill development for health maintenance. It does not focus on disease or disease processes. Persons who are asked to rate on a pretest whether their curriculum focuses on wellness may indeed not understand what the concept really means unless they have had some training. Without this understanding, their responses may not be valid.

Next it is important to consider the use of a comparison group in the design. We don't know whether there was something special about the Seaside participants before they attended. Drolet states the participants and the comparison group were matched. However, what we don't know is whether there were any initial differences in the participants' school systems. Indeed, perhaps the motivating factor for sending the participants to Seaside originally was the school or school system's prior commitment to change. Such a commitment might have made for an important difference between participants and the comparison group.

A particular strength of the design in this cases was the use of both written questionnaires and interviews. These permitted the evaluator to triangulate, or verify, data to strengthen conclusions drawn from the study (Patton 1980).

In addition to the evaluation design, this study is of interest because of the impact the Seaside program had on the planning for comprehensive school health education in Oregon.

The formal and informal activities during the week of SHEC were designed with the intention of eventually effecting change in the school districts represented at the conference. Conferees were exposed to practices that if adopted could result in improved health. They were also provided with information and materials for teaching health in the schools and with methods for effecting change in their school system.

Skills in knowing how to go about making changes in a school system are frequently overlooked in the preparation of school health educators. They need skill in group process and community organization to promote their programs. Enthusiasm and mere appeal to reason are often not sufficient to do so.

At the SHEC there was no pressure on participants to do anything when they got back home. The conference was organized so as to motivate conferees to *want* to effect change back home.

Three motivational elements focused on this goal:

1. The effect created by a sense of common purpose, that is, the promotion of school health education.
2. The fun philosophy, the underlying philosophy of the conference that "these things aren't just good for you, they are fun too."
3. The requirement that only teams from school districts could attend; the team had to include a teacher and an administrator; the latter could be a principal or superintendent; community members, school committee members, and other school personnel were also eligible to attend and were welcomed.

The sense of common purpose, or "group belongingness," as described by Kurt Lewin (Lewin and Grabbe 1945), was created and/or enhanced by the conference planners. They depended on this feeling as a motivator for involving participants in the informal social and fitness activities. Many of the participants may not have gotten up in the morning at home to run or swim or do other physical activities.

But because they were part of a group interested in school health education, whose members had come together for a week to work and live together, they went along with the crowd. Many probably assumed that they would not continue these activities. Lewin explains that participation results from a sense of group belongingness, a "we feeling."

As a result of participating, many were sold on the usefulness of these activities to their life-style. They liked how they felt after a week of exercise, good nutrition, and fun. Further, their feelings of good health were reinforced by what they heard in the classroom and what they saw in the displays and films that were part of the program.

The term *peer pressure* is common in the literature, especially in reference to the behavior of adolescents. As it is used, it suggests that individuals are pressured into doing something they don't really want to do in order to be acceptable to the group. This concept has negative connotations. The "we feeling" is the positive expression of the same concept.

Robinson (1977) discusses the use of fun in health services and in education. She cites giants in the field of literature and psychology, such as Marshall McLuhan and Carl Rogers, as noting that laughter is a great aid to learning. If one is having a good time, one is relaxed and remembers the experience with pleasure. Empirically, we know we remember more of the good times than the bad times in life. There is little research on the role of fun in education, but we can hypothesize that one retains more of what is learned in a happy, relaxed atmosphere than in a grim, stress-filled environment. This was the premise on which the organizers of the SHEC operated. Their results suggest that they may be correct.

During the SHEC week the "we feeling" and the fun philosophy motivated conference participants to *learn about* improving both their own health status and the health education programs in their schools.

The requirement that a team rather than individuals be present from school districts fulfilled functions that differed from those of the "we feeling" and the fun philosophy in effecting change in the school districts. It is a fundamental principle of all training that trainees must have support back home to practice the new knowledge and skills obtained in the training program; otherwise they cannot apply them. (Lynton and Pareek 1978). The team members attending the SHEC provided support for one another in carrying out changes in their personal behavior or in the school district. The requirement that an administrator be present gave teachers the support they needed to effect change in their classroom instruction. Teachers and community members supported school administrators who wished to effect changes in the system. Change must occur at all levels to be worthwhile. Thus the team requirement placed an advocate for change at all levels in the structure of the school district.

Modeling (Bandura 1977) was a major strategy used by conferees back home to promote a healthy life-style. They practiced the behaviors they had learned at the SHEC conference. Their colleagues observed that they looked better, felt better, and were enjoying life. Therefore their colleagues tried out the behaviors and many of them decided to adopt them. This is a classic application of the modeling principle.

The importance of a philosophy of health education is clear in this case (Taba 1962). The director of school health education for the state of Oregon and the planning committee for the Seaside conference believed in wellness. They defined it, described it, and focused all the resources of the conference on it. A defined philosophy gave the conference direction and allowed for a cohesive, comprehensive approach to the issues. All the elements of the conference reinforced one another, thereby enhancing the learning potential.

This case describes an innovative way in which to interest and involve teachers in teaching health in the schools. It illustrates that many of the stated barriers to school health education, such as a lack of time and lack of money, are myths. The creative use of *available* time and money can overcome these assumed barriers.

References/Select Resources

Bandura, A. 1977. *Social Learning Theory.* Englewood Cliffs, N.J.: Prentice Hall.

Bandura's theory holds that human behavior is motivated in part by forces outside the individual. In its simplest form this theory deals with the concept of modeling, one familiar to most educators: People learn from what they see and feel in their environment. Hall called this informal learning. Social learning theory does not hold that people automatically respond to external stimuli, but rather that they are influenced by them and that "they select, organize and transform the stimuli that impinge upon them." This behavior is readily apparent in training programs such as Seaside, where participants process what takes place and then apply it to their work environment. Bandura runs a middle course in defining the causes of human behavior. According to him, it is neither totally within the power of the individual to do as he or she pleases, nor is it totally within the power of the environment to influence the individual. There is a continuous interaction between the two. He says, "Both people and their environment are reciprocal determinants of each other." The material in this book is presented clearly and concisely.

Howard, G. S. 1980. "Response-Shift Bias." *Evaluation Review* 4(1):93–106.

In this important paper, Howard describes a heretofore unrecognized threat to internal validity—the response-shift bias. Howard shows how it can invalidate pre/post designs. To get around this difficulty, he suggests the use of a then/post design. An example of this threat to validity is its occurrence in an assertiveness training program. On a pretest, individuals may rate themselves as moderately assertive. After the program, they may still rate themselves as moderately assertive; hence it would appear the program had no effect. However, with a then/post design the same individuals, when asked to rate how assertive they were both before and after the program, may report being more assertive after the program because the program changed how they viewed assertiveness.

Lewin, K., and Grabbe, P. 1945. "Conduct, Knowledge and Acceptance of New Values." *Journal of Social Issues* 1(1):53–64.

In this paper, Lewin discusses the reeducation process. He identifies ten principles basic to the process of reeducation that he equates with the acceptance of a new value system because he sees reeducation as similar to the process of acculturation. In this case, the participants in SHEC did develop a new value system for health.

Lynton, R. P., and Pareek, W. 1978. *Training for Development* West Hartford, Conn.: Kumarian Press.

This book was written for those preparing to work in 3rd world countries in the process of development. However, the principles of and strategies for training are so well presented that we recommend it for anyone involved in training.

What is especially useful is the section in the book that looks at the trainee "back home." For example, after the training program how useful were the knowledges and skills learned?

Patton, M. Q. 1980. *Qualitative Evaluation Methods*. Beverly Hills: Sage Publications.

Among the many important issues in this book, Patton describes the need for triangulation, a process by which one sees whether data collected by two or more methods provide similar findings. This process is one way to assess the validity of methods that are employed.

Robinson, V. M. 1977. *Humor and the Health Professions*. Thorofare, N.J.: Charles B. Slack.

This book defines and describes different styles of humor. Robinson discusses how humor can be used in education and in curing illness and how health professionals can learn to introduce humor into their role.

Taba, H. 1962. *Curriculum Development Theory and Practice*. New York: Harcourt Brace Jovanovich.

This classic on the subject of curriculum development is *must* reading for all health educators regardless of the setting in which they work. For example, in the first part of the book, Taba discusses many issues relevant to program planning such as the function of the school, the culture of the community, the educational implications of this culture, and the theoretical foundation for curriculum development (program planning).

Discussion Questions

1. Using the PRECEDE model, outline a plan for introducing and implementing health/wellness education into the school systems of your state. You may use ideas from this case for your diagnosis and your implementation plan.

2. Should the term *wellness education* replace the term *health education* in the curriculum of the school system? What might the implications and ramifications of this change in terminology be?

3. Was it an advantage or disadvantage that the program evaluator at the five-year mark had been uninvolved in the previous activities?

4. How would you have designed the evaluation if you had been involved in the program during the planning phase?

5. Using Rogers's adoption-diffusion theory/method, outline a plan to change institutional attitudes toward wellness/health promotion programs in a medical setting, school system, or work site. Identify the barriers you might encounter in each setting.

PART TWO

Case Studies in Medical Care Settings

MEDICAL CARE SETTING

Health education has always been a traditional part of medical care; it is integral to the role of the provider. The employment of the professional health educator by medical care organizations, however, is relatively new. The Public Health Service promoted studies and demonstrations in the late 1940s and early 1950s. The Veterans Administration (VA) and the National Tuberculosis Association, now the American Lung Association, joined forces in the 1950s to demonstrate the value of health education by employing health educators in two VA tuberculosis hospitals. It was not until the late 1960s and early 1970s that medical care institutions began to hire health educators in sufficient numbers to make the medical care setting a viable source of employment for them. The "patient's right to know" movement, emerging emphasis on quality assurance, cost control, Health Maintenance Organization (HMO) legislation, and the increased interest in education by the consumer and the provider alike, all helped to contribute to this growing need for health educators (Richards and Kalmer 1974).

The eight cases describing the practice of health education occur in a variety of medical care settings: acute and chronic care hospitals (Biel and Skiff); ambulatory clinics (Bartlett and Schwartz/Morris); HMOs (Davis, Estabrook, Miller, and Zapka). Although the project described by Zapka occurred in HMOs, the substance of the case study, management issues, is applicable to any setting in which a health educator practices. The issues raised by the remaining seven cases are specific to medical care settings and will be discussed here in more detail.

These seven cases all raise one critical issue: the need for health educators to understand the philosophical and organizational barriers the medical care system presents to any health education effort that makes demands on the system. These demands require changes in the behavior of the medical care staff or changes in organizational behavior or policy.

Kouzes and Mico's (1979) description of the structure of human service organizations, including medical care, helps us understand the reasons for some of these barriers. They refer to the three domains in human service organizations: policy, management, and service. They state (p. 450) that each domain "functions by a separate set of governing principles, success measures, structural arrangments, and work modes . . . [each of which] is incongruent with the others, and . . . each domain gives rise to its own legitimating norms which contrast with the norms of the others."

The policy domain espouses participatory decision making, the management domain uses a hierarchical mode of decision making and the members of the service domain make individual, autonomous decisions. These decision-making modes also pertain to all other aspects of each of the three domains.

Most health educators would identify with the norms of the policy domain, yet they must work within the management and/or the service domain. Although the interaction among the domains influences everything within the system, health education activities are more directly influenced by the service and management domains. The influence of the management domain may appear less obvious than that of the service domain because it is often exerted by default. Notable exceptions are the Skiff and Estabrook cases. Biel does appear to have management support, but because she has not challenged the system, the extent of this support remains undetermined. The cases in this section, with the exception of the studies by Biel and Estabrook, clearly illustrate the direct effect of the service domain on the health educator's work.

THE ROLE OF THE HEALTH EDUCATOR IN MEDICAL CARE SETTINGS

A number of different roles are played by the health educator in medical care settings. Each role is appropriate, but a comprehensive approach allowing all roles to be carried out simultaneously is clearly preferred. Many HMOs with a staff of health educators do offer such a comprehensive approach.

It is our position that the role of one-to-one counseling for the health educator in a medical care setting is appropriate only if the health educator functions as an extension of the educational arm of the provider of medical care. The health educator cannot replace the provider's educational role; he or she can amplify it. Although this role provides excellent experience for the beginner, great care must be taken that providers do not see the health educator as someone to do "education" because they themselves do not have the time.

The number of possible roles for the health educator in a medical care setting can be arranged on a continuum of simple to complex. The complexity of the role depends on the degree to which it makes demands on the system of the three "domains." The Estabrook and Schwartz case studies discuss roles that were prescribed by the administration. All the other cases had health educators who selected roles that were directly related to their training and experience. The beginner chose a task such as organizing classes for patients, while the more experienced health educators chose more complex roles.

The Biel case illustrates the way in which it is possible to work successfully in a medical care setting, provide a service of value to consumers, and not make demands on that system. Davis offers a glimpse of the transition from that type of role to the more complex role of integrating health education into patient care. Skiff and Bartlett both demonstrate that, to do this, you must make demands on the system. Davis discusses the need to earn personal and professional credibility before venturing into the lion's den.

Skiff was able to plunge directly into the issue of integrating educational concepts into patient care. This was an appropriate role for her, because she brought with her the experience to cope with the intricacies of planning and implementing this type of program, and she had the maturity to deal with the frustrations bound to be created by this approach.

Bartlett encountered double trouble because he not only wanted to integrate educational concepts into patient care, but also wanted to integrate the concept of prevention of disease. His analysis of why this innovation was ultimately unacceptable identifies the characteristics of the system that work against the acceptance of an innovation at the implementation stage: that is, complexity of the innovation, lack of both formalization and emphasis on following specific rules or procedures, and decentralized decision making. Bartlett also identifies resident and faculty attitudes about prevention and analyzes the power of the health educator to work effectively with residents and faculty.

If the health educator has the experience, the training, and the stamina, the roles played by Skiff, Bartlett, and Davis should be enacted. These roles are theoretically sound and, in the long range, offer the greatest potential for ensuring that patient education will be integral to patient care.

EDUCATIONAL COMPONENT OF THE ROLE OF THE MEDICAL CARE PROVIDER

Skiff's perspective that the providers of medical care are the first-line educators of patients is theoretically sound. Role theory holds that the occupation of a position in a social system is a role that carries with it expectations from those who interact with it (Merton 1957). Thus patients have expectations of doctors, nurses, dietitians, physical therapists, and other providers of medical care. One of these expectations is that the provider will help them learn to cope with their illness. The provider fulfills this expectation either positively or negatively in every encounter with a patient, by what is said and done and by what is unsaid and not done. There is no way a provider can avoid this expectation.

The second theory that supports Skiff's Perspective is the concept of informal learning (Hall 1973). Informal learning, commonly referred to as modeling, is a major concept of Bandura's (1977) social learning theory. Modeling, or social learning, means that individuals learn from their environment through what they see being done, what they hear, and what they feel. The application of this informal learning to the provider's role in patient education is clear. Learning occurs during the patient/doctor interaction—that is, history taking, physical examination, and the diagnostic process.

The physician, the nurse, and other providers tell the patient whether they care and give the patient clues about the seriousness of the condition through their body language and what they do or do not say to the patient (Redman 1976:10).

The expectations attached to the role of the provider and the fact that learning occurs informally will not change. This theoretical perspective also reinforces our position that health educators providing one-to-one counseling cannot replace, but can merely extend, the provider's educational role. Patient education, therefore, cannot be considered an appendage to medical care; it is an integral part of that care.

The two major differences between the provider's educational function and the health educator's function in medical care settings are their role identification and job responsibilities. The physician's primary professional identity is in the area of medicine, the nurse's is nursing, the dietitian's is nutrition, and the health educator's is in the area of education. The primary responsibility of physicians, nurses, dietitians, and other providers is to provide medical care for the patient. In carrying out their specific patient-care role, they are all responsible for educating the patients with whom they come in contact. The health educator's primary responsibility is the overall planning, implementation, and evaluation of education programs for a variety of patient needs. The difference between these roles seems obvious. Most providers of medical care usually do one-to-one patient counseling, although nurses and dietitians sometimes do work with groups of patients. Their concern usually centers on the needs of individual patients rather than on program planning for groups of patients. Exceptions here are those providers who have switched roles and chosen to function as educators in medical care settings.

ADMINISTRATION'S PERCEPTION OF HEALTH EDUCATION

The fact that five of seven health educators in these case studies chose the role they would play rather than having that role defined by the administration raises questions about the perception and understanding of administrators in medical care institutions regarding the role of health educators. The one instance (Estabrook) in which the administrators knew specifically what they wanted occurred in a well-established health education department. In the Schwartz case, the administrators knew they wanted to evaluate a health education program and did hire a health educator and an evaluator to accomplish this. But the administrators did not fully understand the educational process, as demonstrated by the fact that they were unaware that the physicians and nurses in the ambulatory clinics were not doing—and indeed did not even know how to do—patient education. That no attempt was made to gather baseline data on the status of patient education suggests that the administrators were totally unacquainted with the basic facts about program planning and implementation.

This situation suggests that an important task for the profession of health education is to begin to educate administrators. The Skiff and Miller case studies offer examples of two different approaches. Both systems were in the position of having fewer resources than needed and so were able to offer services only to those who expressed interest in having them. They marketed their services well, worked with those who were ready to learn, and allowed the diffusion process to work with others. Although this process helps, a broader effort is needed. The profession of health education must market its services on a scale that is larger than that of individual health educators in specific settings.

THE CULTURE OF MEDICINE

A primary responsibility of health educators is to help the providers of medical care, the first-line patient educators, to maximize their educational potential. Skiff, Bartlett, and Davis all indicate that this is not an easy task and progress is slow, yet they all met with some success. Possibly greater progress would be possible if the health educator better understood the norms and values of the physician, who seems to be the provider who is most difficult to reach.

Several factors inherent in the culture of medicine contraindicate involvement in patient education. Skiff says the "most difficult task was to get [physicians] to understand what is involved in planning and implementing educational programs." The Davis case raises a similar issue. Physicians' perceptions of education/learning derive from their experience with the educational system. Most physicians, as well as other professionals, assume that "to tell is to teach." In medical schools the faculty member who gives a "good" lecture is rewarded. Rewarding the good lecturer reinforces the physicians' misconceptions of the learning process. This is one reason why they emphasize their need to give the patients information about their illnesses. The health educator who attempts to broaden the concept of education to include the affective component and the environmental issues that influence a patient's illness deals with issues with which most physicians have had no experience and often do not fully understand.

There is a difference between the physician's and health educator's orientation to their work. The physician is task-oriented, the health educator process-oriented. Physicians are trained to do "for" the patient. In some instances the nature of their work requires just that (e.g., setting a broken leg, removing a gallbladder). But effective patient education requires that the provider work "with" the patient.

The physicians' need to "have the answers" sets up other barriers. As Skiff noted in a personal communication in 1982, "In order to practice medicine, the physicians need to pursue some course of treatment and be able to defend it; they need to resolve the ambiguities inherent in the diagnostic process; and, related to outcome issues, they need to satisfy patients'/families' expectations (often unrealistic). In other words, physicians must have answers." Health educators must be more flexible because they are working with human behavior rather than with disease and do not always have "answers" for patient education. The "solution" to the educational problem depends on the patient and on his/her family and environment.

Finally, the reward system in medicine creates another barrier. Skiff expresses disappointment because she was unable to gain entrée to graduate medical education. Her hope was to reach interns and residents so as to enable them to integrate principles of patient education early in their career. This was a reasonable goal, but it was not realized. Why? The reasons are threefold: (1) In medicine, patient education is not rewarded by peers, mentors, or third-party payers; (2) modeling is an important methodology for teaching clinical medicine, yet there are few physician models doing patient education whom the intern or resident can copy; and (3) although a course in medical school may introduce humanistic issues, the concepts are rarely reinforced in clinical clerkships.

We should not underestimate how important it is that the physician understand and implement the educational component of his or her role. The physician is, and will continue to be, the primary source of medical care for most people. Haynes, Taylor, and Sackett (1979:19) report that about 50 percent of those who see a physician do not follow a long-term prescribed medication regimen. Even if we assume that a certain percentage of these regimens would not definitely help the patient, there are still a large number of people who suffer ill health needlessly because they have not learned to follow a prescribed regimen.

Health educators need to recognize that physicians have values and norms that differ from theirs. They need to understand what those values and norms are and how they can use educational interventions in that culture. At the same time, it is hoped that physicians will make the effort to understand the norms and values of health educators. Both professions are working toward the same goal, that is, the good of the patient/consumer. Each profession needs to try to heighten its understanding of the other.

CONCLUSION

In the past ten years, more and more health educators have found positions in the medical care setting. Most of these positions have been in hospitals, although some have been in HMOs. In some sections of the country, these positions have replaced those formerly found in health departments.

The obstacles to the optimum practice of health education in this setting are very real. The health educator has a great deal of responsibility, but very little authority. The system functions in an environment that is not conducive to coordination or cooperative planning or joint decision making. Cooperation and support are necessary tools of the trade in health education.

REFERENCES

Bandura, A. 1977. *Social Learning Theory.* Englewood Cliffs, N.J.: Prentice-Hall.

Hall, E. T. 1973. *The Silent Language.* Garden City, N.Y.: Doubleday (Anchor Books).

Haynes, R. B.; Taylor, D. W.; and Sackett, D. L. 1979. *Compliance in Health Care.* Baltimore: Johns Hopkins University Press.

Kouzes, M., and Mico, P. 1979. "Domain Theory': An Introduction to Organizational Behavior in Human Service Organizations." *Journal of Applied Behavioral Science* 15:449–469.

Merton, R. K. 1957. *Social Theory and Social Structure.* Glencoe, Ill.: Free Press.

Redman, B. K. 1976. *The Process of Patient Teaching in Nursing.* St. Louis: Mosby.

Richards, R. F., and Kalmer, H., guest eds. 1974. "Patient Education." *Health Education Monographs* 2(1).

Organizing Patient Education

Kolleen M. Biel, B.S.

This case study will describe my first position as a health educator. I'll tell you how I got the job, something about the setting in which I work, and what I do as a patient education coordinator.

HOW I GOT THE JOB

A friend from my hometown sent the classified advertisement of the opening for a patient education coordinator at Woodruff Hospital to me while I was away at school. The qualifications were a master's in health science or a bachelor's in nursing with two years of teaching experience. I had neither. However, I felt I had nothing to lose except one more résumé—of which I hoped I had more than I ever needed. The ad requested that the applicant come in person to complete an application. Because I was out of town, I called the Personnel Department and was told to send my résumé.

I did not hear anything for a few weeks, so I called and was told if they were interested they would have called. The following Sunday the ad appeared again; this time I went in person to complete an application. The director of education, who was doing the hiring, told me my résumé had been sent to another department because I did not have the qualifications, and it had since been misplaced. An interview was scheduled for the following morning.

During the interview, I explained my degree in community health education from Kent State University. The director of education stated she was unaware of anything like that at the undergraduate level. I described the courses I took, such as needs assessment, health behavior, and program planning. I also talked about the projects I had worked on during my internship at a local hospital. I had developed and implemented a safety program for hospital employees on preventing low back pain and a preoperative program for both inpatients and outpatients.

During the interview I asked about the hospital and found Woodruff Hospital was a private, non-profit, community-oriented psychiatric hospital with 98 beds. It is a special-treatment facility licensed by the Ohio Department of Health's Division of Mental Health and accredited by the Accreditation Council for Psychiatric Facilities (a wing of the Joint Commission on Accreditation of Hospitals) for the treatment of persons with psychiatric/alcoholism disorders. The hospital's mission is to provide (1) high-quality service to persons with psychiatric/alcoholism problems, and (2) education and consultation service to the community to promote early detection and treatment of psychiatric/alcoholism problems.

Located in Cleveland, the hospital serves the northeast Ohio area, with the highest concentration of patients from Cuyahoga County. Most patients are in their twenties and thirties, although those 13 years of age and over are admitted. Patients, admitted by an attending physician who is a member of the medical staff, are voluntary or involuntary. Involuntary admissions may be emergency referrals or probate referrals.

The full-time medical director handles clinical/administrative problems and is responsible for the clinical administration within the hospital. Department heads report clinically to the medical director and administratively to the executive director.

Kolleen M. Biel is a Patient Education Coordinator at Woodruff Hospital in Cleveland. She is working toward a master's degree in health education.

The hospital is governed by a board of trustees whose members are active in the community.

The services offered by the hospital include the following:

Nursing

Activities therapy: art, music, occupational, recreation, horticulture

Alcoholism services

Social services

Education: school, patient

Medical services

Nutrition services

Psychological testing

Ancillary services: plant operations

The philosophy of the Education Department includes these concepts: (1) Learning is a dynamic and lifelong process involving the whole person; (2) appropriate learning activities are necessary to positively affect growth and development of all persons; and (3) adult learners share responsibility for their learning.

THE BEGINNING

I accepted the position as patient education coordinator at Woodruff Hospital.

The patient education program is one component of the Education Department, supervised by the director of education. The job description for the coordinator was appropriate. It stated that the coordinator would be responsible for developing and consolidating patient education. This task included needs identification, program planning, training of patient educators, overseeing of the actual program, and evaluation. Although I have carried out these functions, my time is best used as a planner. Teaching patients would leave little time to plan new programs and to standardize and expand programs. Therefore I teach only very occasionally.

In school, I had been told to take things slowly. That was very good advice. Time was needed to get used to the new environment, the staff, and the way things were done; and the staff needed time to adjust to me.

I started by meeting with department heads and asking them what they thought patients needed to know. This process gave me an idea of the problem areas and gave people a chance to express their concerns. I did a lot of listening and let the staff talk, that is, get involved. This approach gave me the information I needed and contributed to gaining respect from the staff.

My next step was to review the patient education policy. After reading the existing manual on policy and procedures, I knew revisions were needed. But I waited to see how the system was working. The procedure for implementation was confusing and required excessive paperwork. Obviously, this was a deterrent; my files were filled only with blank forms. There would be no resistance to changing the policy. No one was following the current one!

The policy was that patient education would be coordinated through one department, but no reasons were given. I wrote down the following reasons:

1. Coordination guarantees that content is standardized. Patient A can be on 3 South and Patient B on 2 North, but the information they receive about a topic will be the same.
2. Continuity of patient education among disciplines can be assured. All health care personnel who come in contact with the patient have responsibility for patient education. Patient education is not solely the function of a nurse or physician. The patient learns about the low-salt diet from the dietitian, the range of motion exercises from the physical theerapist, and the community resources from the social worker. Each discipline plays a significant role in providing quality information.
3. Coordinated patient education provides a central resource for patient education. If a dietitian needs a program on nutrition for the alcoholic, she or he will check the central source. The dietitian will not have to think about who might have this information or where it might be found.
4. Duplication is avoided. A patient on one floor often has the same needs as a patient on another floor. The coordinator's office knows this. A staff member on a given floor will not necessarily know this; so it is easy to see how duplicate programs could be developed.

I also explained alternatives for initiating and implementing patient education programs. The Patient Education Planning Committee (PEPC) would play a major role, but that did not mean other staff could not be involved. So there would be two procedures for implementing patient education: one for the PEPC and one for staff who wanted to suggest or develop a program.

The policy and procedure manual is the bible of the hospital. Whenever a question arises, staff refer to the manual for the answer. For this reason, it was crucial to have a clear policy for patient education. When the policy was ready, I sent it to the executive director.

CHOOSING THE PATIENT EDUCATION PLANNING COMMITTEE

Selecting the PEPC members was crucial. An informal sociogram method was used to identify potential members. I started by asking people whose judgment I trusted for names of persons they thought would be appropriate for planning education, I also inquired about who was presently doing some patient education. To the names suggested to me, I added a few possibilities. One person from each discipline and one alternative was chosen. I took two names to each department head and stated that either person A or person B would be appropriate for the planning committee. The department heads were able to choose between the selected alternatives. By having the final selection made by the department heads, I hoped to help them feel involved in the formation of the committee.

I met with all the prospective representatives individually to confirm their interest, explain their responsibilities, and explore the days and times they would be available. Each person was enthusiastic and interested in planning patient education. The committee comprised a registered nurse, a mental health worker, a dietitian, a social worker, an activities therapist, and the patient education coordinator.

RESPONSIBILITIES OF THE PEPC

It was important for members of the committee to feel comfortable with one another so they could work well together. Therefore, at the first meeting of the committee, I used get-acquainted exercises: a brief autobiography, drawings of personnel definitions of health, and ranking of items such as wealth, beauty, fame, health, success, and intelligence. Committee members were queried about their personal health habits, such as smoking, eating, sleeping, exercising, and seat belt use. As the members discussed these, they recognized it was very difficult to do the healthiest things all the time. We concluded that patients would have the same difficulty.

After these activities, we used brainstorming to identify or assess the education problems of patients. Those identified included inability to express anger or feelings; poor nutritional status, specifically with alcoholic patients; lack of understanding regarding their medication; misunderstanding of child development; low self-esteem; ignorance about community services; poor physical fitness; and families' lack of knowledge about what to do or expect.

The needs/problems were then ranked. We considered the number of people affected and how serious the problem was. As the vast majority of patients were on medication and many returned to the hospital because they did not comply with medication instructions, we decided to start specifically with antipsychotic medications.

OBJECTIVES

During the next week, I formulated some possible objectives for the ranked needs and brought them to the next meeting. Everyone on the committee had additions or suggestions to make. The nurse said the patient should know both the name of the medication and the dose. We wanted the patient to know what the medication usually did. In our wording we were careful not to say why the medication was given, since we didn't know.

Everyone agreed the patient should know about possible side effects and be given helpful hints to alleviate them. The social worker suggested that the patient should be able to read the prescription label. She stated that, in the past, patients who were not informed about how much medication to take and when to do so could have found this information on the prescription label.

The objectives were patient-oriented and behavioral. They included more than the cognitive domain, for patients need to express their fears and concerns about taking medication. They also covered the involvement of patients with their own care (that is, seeing that patients completed personal medication charts) and the facilitating of communications between doctor and patient. After writing the objectives, the committee began developing the content. Throughout the weeks that followed, I researched all the points we wanted to cover. As the patient education coordinator, my job included the collection of information between meetings and the preparation of agenda and working materials, plus any leg work necessary to expedite the committee's work. I brought a draft to each meeting, and the content specifics were worked out after considerable discussion.

As chairperson of the committee, I used a democratic and informal approach. When I had a suggestion for the program I explained why it seemed worth considering and then let the committee express its opinions. Some ideas would be discarded and others immediately adopted.

The committee members worked together very well. They always listened to everyone's suggestions. When they did not agree with a suggestion, they would ask for an explanation as to why the proposed item should be incorporated in the program. They were very generous in sharing their experiences. Openness is essential in this type of committee planning.

METHODOLOGY FOR PROGRAM ON MEDICATION USE

My training in education was most useful in planning the methodology for the program. I followed the principle that a variety of methods and aids should be used. Transparencies and handouts were developed; discussion questions for the objectives were formulated; visual aids were reviewed and selected. The content of all materials was basic; words were short (i.e., syllables were limited).

At this point, I made a most useful discovery: There was a lot of talent around willing to help with the development of materials. For example, when I wanted illustrations on the transparencies, I discovered my secretary was a skilled artist.

We applied the "primacy and recency" principle. Information and options encountered at the beginning and the end of an education experience are more powerful than those encountered in the middle. We translated that principle into this message at the end of the program: Patients should continue taking their medication even if they feel better, because they feel better owing to the medication.

The principle of reinforcement was used as well. As part of follow-up, instructors would check the medication charts and offer positive feedback.

We also provided for relieving anxiety that might be produced in an educational activity. For example, when we described possible side effects, we emphasized they were possible but not definite. We also prepared a list of helpful hints for coping with the side effects.

For the first program we decided on a group setting, a class, so that patients could offer support and appropriate suggestions to one another. This informal environment gave patients a chance to ask questions and explore their points of interest. We summarized each group meeting. The summary pulled together and reinforced the important points.

TRAINING THE INSTRUCTORS

I presented an in-service session on policy and procedures for patient education to the patient care staff. Patients were referred to patient education by physicians, head nurses, treatment planning teams, or class instructors. During the in-service session, I identified staff interested in teaching specific patient education programs for all the problems described at the PEPC's first meeting. Three people in the nursing department were interested in teaching medication education.

The instructors were all registered nurses, so they were familiar with the content. We gave them several journal articles on major tranquilizers for reference. Those who were not familiar with operating an overhead projector were instructed and then provided hands-on experience. Handouts on strategies for changing behavior were also available.

In a brief training session, I reviewed the responsibilities of the instructors for this program: that is, secure necessary equipment, meet with patients before class to explain the program, and document attendance and responses on the patient's chart.

IMPLEMENTATION

To select the best time for classes, I met with the director of nursing. We decided to meet with the head nurses because they could determine the best times.

They suggested we wait until September to start so as to avoid being interrupted by summer vacations. They said morning was the best time and suggested that classes be limited to six patients at one time and be held in the classroom on the second floor.

I met with the three volunteer instructors who offered suggestions for time schedules for the floors. As patient education coordinator, I made the arrangements, that is, reserved the classroom and scheduled the classes.

The instructors asked for the names of patients who had been referred to the major tranquilizer program. These patients were notified about the program and given the day and time of the program.

The first program was held on October 7, 1981. Seating was arranged in a semicircle to aid discussion. Patients were given a personalized medication chart, along with handouts that listed the name, dose, and schedule of their medication; other information about the medication was summarized on the handout.

The lesson plan included such information as the name of the medication, the way it works, precautions, side effects, and helpful hints. The instructor explored how patients felt about taking the medication and their concerns in following instructions. The medication chart and prescription label were reviewed. Patients were encouraged to ask their physician questions in the future.

The patients asked questions throughout the program. They wanted further information on what the medication did and clarification of why the dosage varied from one patient to another. When they didn't understand what was said, the instructor gave examples they could grasp. They interacted with one another. When one was reluctant to take medications, another would talk about how much better he or she felt because of a medication.

EVALUATION

We decided to use a simple, individualized fill-in-the-blanks test. The committee felt that the patients should know the names of their medications, the dosages, and when they were to take them. The rest of the information was included on the handouts. As long as the patients knew where to get the information they wanted, the committee was satisfied.

The patients' reaction to the major tranquilizer program was positive. They thought it was a good idea and felt they learned a lot of useful information.

In addition to getting feedback from the patients, the instructors evaluated the program. They told me the concerns patients mentioned in class. The frequently asked questions were used to revise the program. For example, a few patients thought they were "sicker" than most other patients because they were taking a much higher dose of medication. A quick explanation settled that misunderstanding: 2mg of medication A equals 100 mg of medication B; people have different metabolisms; and just as food requirements may vary from one person to the next, so do medications. The committee responded to this and is presently working on a family education program that will include information on medications.

FULL CIRCLE: STARTING AGAIN

The PEPC developed programs for other medications: minor tranquilizers, antidepressants, and lithium. The committee then ranked the remaining needs/problems and the same process was started again. Among our other activities are the publication of a "Community Resource Guide," which gives names and descriptions of various agencies that could be helpful to patients, and an extensive physical fitness program. A family education series is being planned. Other programs will include assertiveness training, problem solving, parenting skills, growth and development, drug abuse, and hypertension.

Analysis

This case focuses on the health educator as the coordinator of patient education in a 98-bed psychiatric hospital. Her major responsibility in this position was planning educational programs.

Some of Bruner's (1971:43) concepts relative to a theory of instruction provide a frame of reference for this case. He states:

> Since learning and problem solving depend upon the exploration of alternatives, instructions must facilitate and regulate the exploration of alternatives on the part of the learner.
>
> There are three aspects to the exploration of alternatives. . . . They can be described in shorthand terms as activation, maintenance, and direction. To put it another way, exploration of alternatives requires something to get it started, something to keep it going, and something to keep it from being random.

The Patient Education Planning Committee provided the "activation." It got things started. The way in which the committee was appointed and organized generated interest among a number of staff members in the patient education program. The selection of a topic, the development of objectives for the program, the selection of a variety of materials and methods, the provision of patient and staff feedback, all helped maintain interest and enthusiasm. The direction for the program came from the health educator's and the PEPC's ongoing planning process.

The health educator functioned much like a classroom teacher preparing lessons for the first few sessions with a class she did not know. She applied principles of planning. But it was in trying out the planned program that the health educator learned whether she was on target for the class. Trying out the lesson is an on-the-spot needs assessment.

Planning *with* the target population and not *for* the target population is considered basic to the practice of health education. This health educator did not apply that principle, and she doesn't tell us why she didn't. We assume that to do so was not policy at Woodruff Hospital. The way in which she did proceed allowed her to get some sense of the patients' perceptions of need through exposure to patients who attended the medication sessions. Direct involvement of patients in identifying needs and in planning programs is the desirable route. Alternatives often have to be used until a program is well enough established to be able to challenge policy.

In carrying out the planning function, the health educator tells us several times about the things she did between committee meetings: refining the objectives drawn up at a meeting, following through on committee suggestions, getting the minutes of meetings together, hunting down resources, and so on. Competent staff work can make a difference in the planning and implementation of programs. This case illustrates that point well. Other cases in this book do, too (e.g., Ogasawara, p. 262; and Semura, p. 301).

Biel describes the program as though it was planned and implemented with ease. She does not report that there were any obstacles in her path. This is in contrast to all other cases in this book that describe health educators functioning in medical care settings. At least three reasons for this unobstructed path come to mind:

1. The health educator followed sound professional operating procedures. She became acquainted, involved relevant actors, developed credibility, and chose as a first project a noncontroversial clinical subject of interest to all.
2. Psychotherapy is a learning process. People learn to get better with the guid-

ance of the psychiatrist; therefore one would expect a greater understanding of education in a psychiatric setting than in other medical care settings.
3. The hospital's administration appeared to have a commitment to education. The hospital had a department of education; it hired and provided support staff for a health educator. These actions suggest support for the concept.

However, all these factors existed in the Davis, Bartlett, and Skiff cases (pp. 103, 134, and 143). Why did they encounter obstacles not encountered in this case? Possibly because in this case no demands were made on physicians, nor was established policy challenged. Davis, Bartlett, and Skiff were trying to change established ways of doing things. In the final analysis, if educational principles are to be integrated into the fabric of patient care, established practices and policies must be challenged. Davis, Bartlett, and Skiff waited until they had sufficient personal and professional credibility before venturing into the arena of policy change. Because one has credibility does not mean one will be successful in altering or adjusting established practices. It does mean one can try to do so and probably won't lose a job as a result of trying.

This case describes how one health educator began the process of developing a patient education program in a small psychiatric hospital. It illustrates that appropriate use of professional skills, administrative support, and the judicious selection of projects provide a basis for establishing a patient education program.

References/Select Resources

Bruner, J. 1971. *Toward a Theory of Instruction,* Cambridge: Harvard University Press, Belknap Press.

This volume includes eight essays that the author describes as "efforts of a student of the cognitive process trying to come to grips with the problems of education." Although Bruner writes about the education of children, his thoughts are applicable to adults as well. All the essays provide the health educator with useful and thought-provoking ideas about teaching and learning. The essay of particular interest for this case is "Notes on a Theory of Instruction." According to Bruner, a theory of instruction has four major features: (1) "the experiences which most effectively implant in the individual a predisposition toward learning"; (2) "the ways in which a body of knowledge should be structured"; (3) "the most effective sequences in which to present the materials to be learned"; and (4) "the nature and pacing of rewards and punishments in the process of learning and teaching." Bruner's essays are clear and concise and offer a sophisticated treatment of the issues. Students will be rewarded for stretching their minds to understand—and make their own—Bruner's gems of useful ideas.

Cosper, B. 1977. "How Well Do Patients Understand Hospital Jargon?" *American Journal of Nursing* 12:1932–1934.

This report on a study in one hospital reveals considerable frustration felt by patients because they could not understand hospital jargon. Simple terms assumed to be understood by everyone, such as "pre-op," were found to be confusing to the patients. The study reported on could easily be replicated in any medical care setting.

Hillman, S. 1976. "The Health Educator—A Resource for Nurses." *Supervision Nurse* (September): 7:18–22.

The author provides a good description of the role of the health educator in contrast to that of other health professionals, for whom the educational component is not paramount. She illustrates this with three vignettes drawn from both community and hospital nursing. The article refers only to health educators prepared in schools of public health, although just a small percentage of the total number of health educators working in community and hospital settings received their training in such schools.

Mager, R. 1975. *Preparing Instructional Objectives.* Belmont, Calif.: Fearon.

This volume enables the reader to learn what instructional and behavioral objectives are, how to develop them, and how to use them. It is useful because it provides numerous examples and work sheets in every chapter.

Mathews, B. P. 1982. "Administrative Climate: Its Implications for Health Educators." In *SOPHE Heritage Collection of Health Education Monographs,* vol. 1: *The Philosophical, Behavioral, and Professional Bases for Health Education,* edited by S. Simonds. Oakland, Calif.: Third Party Publishing.

This article is directed primarily at the health educator whose work in an organization may include either education of or assistance to other members of the organization. Fundamental to this role is an adequate diagnosis of the administrative situation or climate. Variables necessitating analyses include influence, communication, decision making, leadership, and personal relations. Although Biel did not formally carry out an administrative diagnosis, we see elements of it taking place as early as her initial interview for the position and through her meetings with staff and department heads.

Discussion Questions

1. Assume you were appointed to the position of patient education coordinator at Woodruff Hospital. Describe a way in which you could fulfill your responsibilities that differs from the method described.

2. Prepare in detail the training sessions for the nurses in this case who were to teach the patient classes; include objectives, methodology, and evaluation.

3. As a patient education coordinator, write a letter to the administration describing the need for a change in patient education policy.

4. Assume you are being interviewed by a hospital administrator for the position of patient education coordinator. What would you say to convince the administrator that you had the knowledge and skill to fill this position effectively? Write out your statement.

5. Assume the following scenario at a Patient Education Planning Committee. Two members of the committee don't like each other; their animosity is well known in the hospital. For the first few meetings of the committee, their personal feelings did not intrude. But now they have clashed on the issue of interviewing patients about their interests for future programs. One threatens to go to the chairman of the board (a neighbor) and tell him the committee is disrupting hospital procedure. The two do a bit of shouting at each other about this issue. How would you, the health educator, handle this, immediately and in the long range?

Interdisciplinary Team-Building for Hypertension Patient Education in an HMO

Paul A. Davis, M.P.H.

Patients with hypertension are expected by medical practitioners to make complex and varied behavior changes in their lives to comply with medical regimens. Lack of compliance with these changes has been well documented (England, Alderman, and Powell 1979). The medical care system, particularly the ambulatory care centers where a majority of hypertensive patients are seen, is slowly realizing that specialized educational interventions are required to aid and support the patient confronting these difficult changes.

Interdisciplinary efforts, involving all health professionals concerned with hypertensive patient care, have been recommended (Bernheimer and Clever 1977). Ambulatory care clinics and health maintenance organizations (HMOs) are particularly suitable for building interdisciplinary educational teams for hypertension and other chronic illnesses.

This case study will highlight the practical steps in initiating, recruiting, building, and sustaining such an educational team effort; the central role of the health educator in this team-building process; and the organizational factors that either facilitated or inhibited team-building.

THE SETTING

A 14,000-member HMO in a rural, academic community offered subscribers two models of primary care: the family practice model and the internist/pediatrician model. The former was the larger of the two since the HMO was started by a family practice group. The medical care staff in the family practice group included eight physicians, six nurse practitioners, three R.N.'s, one full-time and three part-time pharmacists, one half-time nutritionist, and several clinic aides. Three pediatricians, one pediatric nurse practitioner, two internists, and two R.N.'s made up the remaining medical care staff. This case study concerns only the family practice segment of the HMO, although the final product reported in the case was adopted by all staff.

From its inception in 1976, this HMO had had a health education component with two master's-level health educators. I came on the scene in mid-1977 and began work on the case reported here in mid-1979. Until that time, health education activities centered on preventive programs like smoking cessation and weight control. These health promotion programs were planned and implemented by the health educators with little direct involvement by medical staff. There were no formalized educational programs for patients with an identified chronic disease. Patient education consisted of traditional patient counseling by the medical provider.

A goal of the health education department, therefore, was to involve medical staff in patient education—from initial planning to evaluation. However, the medical staff had shown little interest in patient education projects.

GETTING STARTED

The health education staff devised simple needs assessment questionnaires that asked for the clinicians' perceptions of their patients' educational needs in regard to preselected topics such as dia-

---

Paul A. Davis is a Health Education Coordinator for University Health Services at the University of Massachusetts and for the Valley Health Plan in Amherst, Massachusetts.

betes, arthritis, and high blood pressure. It was designed to raise the clinicians' awareness of patients' needs and to serve as a first step in physician involvement. Not surprisingly, hypertension emerged as a foremost topic of need and interest.

The summarized data from this needs assessment were presented first to the medical director, a pediatrician. Although he was not particularly interested in high blood pressure, he gave the go-ahead to pursue it as a topic for formalized patient education programs at the clinic. He also presented the data to the medical staff and supported the idea for a hypertension project with them.

TEAM-BUILDING: A PARTICIPATORY PLANNING PROCESS

Until this effort in high blood pressure education was started, clinical involvement in health education activities was minimal. The first step was to enlist a "volunteer" team for planning. The team was to include a family practice physician, nurse practitioner, pharmacist, nutritionist, and health educator. The greatest barrier to organizing the team was the clinicians' perception that there was no time in their schedules for planning a patient education program. This was painfully apparent as I was repeatedly turned down when I asked clinicians to help. Comments like "It's a wonderful idea; we need a high blood pressure program, but I'm just too busy right now" were typical. The problem was an organizational one.

Although all clinicians' job descriptions mentioned responsibility for patient education, no time was scheduled to accomplish anything but the traditional one-to-one patient counseling. The clinic administration was unexcited about allotting clinical time, and the clinicians were reluctant to add to already busy schedules by "volunteering" on their lunch hour.

The initial effort at recruitment of a team for high blood pressure education floundered until "volunteers" were persuaded to participate during lunch hours, cancellations, and other "extra" times. The doctor and the nurse practitioner who joined the planning group had three reasons for doing so:

1. A personal commitment to patient education
2. A particular interest in high blood pressure as a disease
3. Familiarity with the health educator as a person and a professional from previous encounters

The pharmacist and the nutritionist who made up the remainder of the team had more flexible schedules, so participation was easier for them.

A WORK PLAN

Given the great time constraints and difficulties in scheduling meetings with such a group, I drew up a tentative step-by-step plan (Table 1) to do the following:

1. Educate the planning group about the extent of the job and the steps required in the planning process.
2. Reduce anxiety about unknown tasks and work loads. In general, clinicians do not deal with ambiguity very well; therefore a flexible, concrete plan to which they can react avoids a sense of floundering.
3. Make the most of the limited time available.
4. Clarify the role of each team member, especially the health educator, whose role was the least well understood by other members. As one team member said, "This plan is great; now I'm beginning to see what a health educator does besides order pamphlets."
5. Use the plan as an aid for planning discussions. I made it very clear from the beginning that the plan was not written in stone; it was meant to be only a guide for action.

REINFORCING THE COMMITMENT

Once the planning group was determined and the general plan of action agreed on, I needed to ensure that the members would continue to "buy in to" the planning work. Initially, it was obvious that some members were dubious about the need for what seemed to them a long-drawn-out and unnecessary planning process. Some regarded a "quick and dirty" approach as adequate. Again, the lack of commitment of time and effort was a barrier. Scheduled one-hour lunchtime meetings

Table 1
Pilot Project for Hypertension Patient Education

Step/Task	Things to Consider	Who's Primarily Responsible?
1. Identify target group (hypertensives) and assess its needs	Referrals? Newly diagnosed? Already diagnosed? Spouses (care partners) to be involved? What are lower limits of blood pressure?	Planning group
2. Set goals and objectives	Examples: (a) X% of participants will be able to identify their drugs; (b) X% will reduce sodium intake	Planning group
3. Determine budget	Cost of materials (audio visuals, etc.) and mailings.	Health educator
4. Decide on format of educational intervention and logistics	Possibilities: (a) group education, (b) one-to-one educational consultation, (c) use of A-V and learning tools, (d) combination of above	Planning group
5. Determine evaluation strategy/details	What needs to be measured? What can be measured? How?	Health educator
6. Develop curriculum	What needs to be shared, taught, reinforced?	Planning group
7. Provide/arrange staff training	Ongoing orientation and information about program. Training in two areas: (a) hypertension and its treatment (indicated on recent staff survey) (b) educational, counseling, and referral techniques	Planning group
8. Prepare and/or purchase written and audiovisual materials		Health educator
9. Conduct pilot program		Designated staff
10. Evaluate		Health educator

often became half-hour work sessions as people apologetically came in late and had to leave early because of patient demands. However, during these brief meetings a group consciousness developed. I encouraged brainstorming as a way of establishing trust and defining roles. The lunch meetings became jocular and stress-free. In contrast, I had observed that medical staff meetings were often tense and frustrating because intergroup competition and lack of good group facilitation prevailed.

I was not concerned, initially, with accomplishing the task, but rather with developing group trust and cohesiveness. The first meetings were crucial. Continued participation by the members who were not yet a team had to be ensured. It was important that what seemed to be a burden became viewed as enjoyable, creative, and stress-reducing. Therefore I provided leadership for the group, initially set agendas, and monitored group process. Later, after the group began to function as a team, I facilitated the shifting of responsibility for those functions to the team itself.

TEAM DEVELOPMENT

It took about four meetings for a fully functioning team to develop. In the beginning, in addition to developing trust, discussions tended to center on treatment modes for hypertension. These discussions, though time-consuming, were important in establishing consensus about "what we are telling the patient." The team members tended to agree on major treatment issues. At the same time, the individual member's areas of expertise became apparent. These were appreciated by the other team members, and they began to *listen to* and *learn from* one another. This kind of sharing and exchange had never happened in the clinic before.

HEALTH EDUCATOR'S ROLE

My primary role in the process of the development of this team was facilitative. One example of how this role was staged was the task of setting program goals and objectives. All health educators will agree that setting sound goals and objectives is essential to any program planning process. However, other health professionals may not know how to set program goals and objectives. As a result, they may feel incompetent and unprepared, and therefore reticent, to join a team effort to do so. This was true of the hypertension planning group.

Consequently, I attempted to demystify the task of setting objectives. Prior to a meeting scheduled to work on goals and objectives, each team member was given a "homework" sheet to complete. The sheet asked three questions designed to elicit responses relevant to cognitive, attitudinal, and behavioral objectives:

1. As a result of the program, what new information do you expect the patient *to know*? (cognitive-knowledge)
2. As a result of the program, what do you expect the patient *to believe*? (attitudinal)
3. As a result of the program, what do you expect the patient *to do* differently? (behavioral)

I explained that the answers to these questions would become the basis of program objectives and emphasized the importance of answering as specifically as possible. Examples of responses were given for each question: for instance, the patient will believe that his/her hypertension medication lowers blood pressure.

At the next meeting, the team members shared and discussed their responses, which I wrote on newsprint. Because the questions were worded to elicit patient *outcomes* rather than educational *activities*, the group learned about the nature of program objectives. As the nurse practitioner commented, "I thought an objective was something *I* was supposed to do with the patient, not what *he* was to do!"

During the discussion, I made sure that the objectives were relevant, realistic, measurable, and time-specific by posing questions like "do you think this is possible to accomplish?" "How will we know the patient has done this?"

Once the list of objectives was organized and ranked by the group, I polished some of the language before the next meeting, being careful not to change the intent of the team's work.

This process ensured that the group was invested in the program, because it had created and therefore "owned" the objectives. An important task was accomplished, and the team coalesced around that task.

I could have sat alone at my desk and written more sophisticated goals and objectives. If this had been done, team members would not have learned about objectives, and the development of the team, which progressed around the task of setting the objectives, would have halted.

A FUNCTIONING TEAM

Once established as a functioning group, the team was able to carry out the necessary planning and implementation tasks. Among the characteristics of this viable fully working team were the following:

1. Punctual attendance at meetings
2. Shared responsibility for discussions about issues and participation in meetings
3. Completion of delegated tasks between meetings
4. A willingness to commit additional time to the project

Once functioning with these characteristics, the team was able to establish an effective hypertension education program that has continued for over two years.

As the team worked together for those two years,

the members identified the benefits of an interdisciplinary approach to education of patients with a chronic illness. Among these benefits were the following:

1. The roles of various health professionals, especially the role of the health educator, are better understood and appreciated in an organization.
2. By the diffusion effect, the rest of the clinic staff is kept aware of the team's efforts by their peers (e.g., the physician member reported on progress to the medical staff).
3. Distrust of the program is reduced.
4. Referrals to the program are increased as a result of item 3.
5. The clinic organization as a whole takes responsibility for patient education problems.
6. The interdisciplinary nature of chronic disease management is emphasized.
7. Organizational changes affecting patient care are more likely to take place (e.g., reminder cards for appointment keeping).
8. Because support for the program is broad-based, its continuation and longevity are enhanced.

CONCLUSION

The health educator's role is central to the team-building process. The health educator serves as the initiator for demonstrating the need for a team, for recruiting the team, and for "coaching" it. In many respects the efforts of the health educator need to be greater during the formative stages of team-building than later, when the team has learned how to function as a team. The health educator functions as a change agent by facilitating the process of learning how to integrate one's knowledge and skills with those of other disciplines so as to present a unified approach—a team approach to patient education.

REFERENCES

Bernheimer, R. E., and Clever, L. H. 1977. *The Team Approach to Patient Education: One Hospital's Experience in Diabetes.* Atlanta: Center for Disease Control, Division of Health Education.

England, A. L.; Alderman, M. H.; and Powell, H. B. 1979. "Blood Pressure Control in Private Practice: A Case Report." *American Journal of Public Health* 69:25–29.

Analysis

This case focuses on the health educator as a teacher, a facilitator of the learning process. His primary tasks were to help medical care personnel learn how to function as members of a team and value the team approach in the education of hypertension patients. He encountered two major barriers in carrying out this task: The medical care personnel, his students, felt they didn't have time for the task; and they did not think that detailed planning of a hypertension education program was necessary. Persistence and intimate understanding of the culture of the target population were essential in overcoming these barriers.

Davis's strategy was based on Lewin's force-field analysis (Jenkins 1961). Since he could not affect the "restraining forces," his decision was to strengthen the "driving forces." These were the personal commitment of the members of the team to patient education, their interest in hypertension, and their view of the health educator (they liked him; he had credibility).

Force-field analysis is a useful tool in a situation with identifiable barriers and facilitating factors. The analysis of how to proceed in a given project is often clarified

```
Driving Forces                              Restraining Forces

Interest ─────────▶   ┌──────────┐  ◀───────── Time
                      │ Patient  │
Commitment ───────▶   │education │  ◀───────── Perception of no
                      │          │              need to plan
Credibility of health ▶│         │
    educator          └──────────┘
```

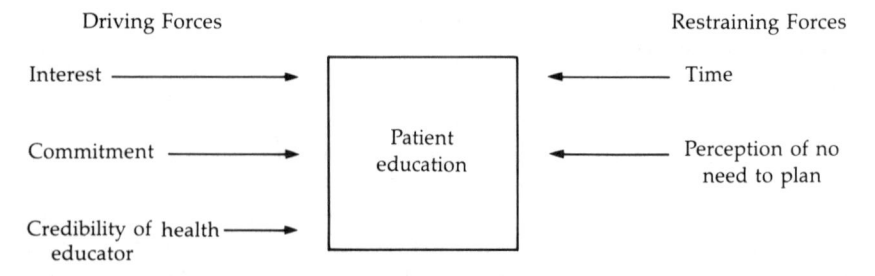

Figure 1 *Force-Field Analysis Applied to Team Building*

and focused by "drawing" the field. Figure 1 illustrates the "field" for this case.

The drawing does not take into account the strength of the forces. We have to assume the health educator thought that, because of his interaction with and observation of potential team members, the positive valences were strong enough if reinforced to withstand the pressure of the negative valences. It was clear to him he could not affect the time issue. He could, however, influence the team's perception of education if he could interact with the members long enough for them to experience the meaning and value of a team. The health educator therefore concentrated on maximizing their interest and commitment by developing "group trust and cohesiveness." This process, rather than the task, had priority in his plan.

In this respect his task was similar to that of the schoolteacher. Both have "students" (although the schoolteacher's students are less likely to walk out or come late because they have other things to do); both have to plan their first few lessons so as to gain the interest of their students as quickly as possible (Bruner 1971).

To capitalize on the driving forces, the health educator provided leadership for the team: He set the agenda, kept the discussion focused, involved everyone in the discussion, provided positive feedback, did not let anyone dominate, told a few jokes. In other words, he applied group process skills to develop a "creative, enjoyable, stress-reducing" environment. People will return to a situation that makes them feel good.

Note his first action. He presented the team with a chart (Table 1) that explained what had to be done and who should do it. The use of this chart was directly related to his understanding that any addition to their workload was a major concern of potential team members and that physicians have difficulty with ambiguity. The chart was a concrete, practical way to deal with these issues.

Creating an environment conducive to learning and involving the learners in the process through both team meetings and homework *allowed* individuals to learn how to function as part of a team. As team members began to catch on, responsibilities were gradually transferred to them. They needed the guidance but no longer the strong leadership of the health educator.

Note that team members were usually late or left early during the first few meetings of the team. However, once the team was organized and the members assumed ownership, they managed to be on time for the meetings. People will spend their time in ways they think are important.

The health educator obtained administrative support for high blood pressure "as a topic for formalized patient education programs." Administrative support is considered essential for all health education programs.

What does administrative support mean? We'd like to think it means administration will be a strong advocate for health education programs. It may, but not necessarily. There are degrees of support ranging from toleration (Donnelly case, p. 352) to advocacy (Biel case, p. 95). The degree of advocacy for a health education project that accompanies administrative approval for the project depends in part on the style of the individual administrator, in part on the administrative style acceptable to a given organization, and in part on the priorities of the organization at a given time. The administrative style acceptable to the organization has the greatest influence on the type of support that can be expected in a medical care organization.

In this case, the medical director of the HMO gave his go-ahead for the program, presented the data to the medical staff, and supported the idea. That does not mean the medical director will intervene for a program with a physician who is not cooperative. That kind of action is generally not acceptable in the physician culture. Only under rare circumstances does one medical doctor ever tell another one what to do. The most you can hope for in a medical care setting is permission to do a program and periodic verbal and/or written support. You are then on your own to sink or swim.

The issue of "no time" for patient education is one we hear constantly from physicians and nurses. It is important to realize that time is a real issue in an HMO. An HMO's income is fixed, that is, the number of enrollees times their insurance premiums. Therefore every minute of the clinician's time is scheduled so as to ensure staying within the fixed income. Since most health insurance plans do not pay for providers to spend time on patient education, it is understandable why an HMO administration may not allow clinic time for this activity.

But where does this leave the health educator hired to develop patient education programs? A successful program requires, as we have seen, commitment, persistence, and innovative and creative approaches. Innovation and creativity are desirable under all circumstances. However, to be forced to work around a barrier as formidable as "no time for patient education" makes the work of the health educator much more difficult than need be. Unfortunately, until the payment system changes, it is unlikely that the time providers can devote to patient education will change.

This case study describes a methodology for capturing the interest and commitment of a group of providers of medical care for a patient education project. The group's interest was captured despite the members' conviction that they didn't have time and that they were being used by having to meet on their lunch hour. One by one, the potential members became committed because they were interested, saw that others were as well, and realized that, by joining forces, they could maximize their contribution and accomplish more than if they worked alone.

References/Select Resources

Benne, K. D., and Sheats, P. 1945. "Functional Roles of Group Members." *Journal of Social Issues* 4(2):41–49.

Roles related both to the group's task and to group-building are identified and defined here. The article also deals with the issue of individual agendas brought to all groups and how these relate to both the group's task and to group-building.

Bernheimer, R. E., and Clever, L. H. 1977. *The Team Approach to Patient Education: One Hospital's Experience in Diabetes.* Atlanta: Center for Disease Control, Division of Health Education.

This monograph offers a description of the development of an interdisciplinary team for teaching inpatients who have diabetes. The authors provide a detailed picture of the process of team-building. It was slow and frustrating but rewarding. The material is clear, explicit, and rich in the quality and quantity of detail. For example, descriptions of the organization and the implementation of team meetings are offered.

Bruner, J. 1971. *Toward a Theory of Instruction:* Cambridge: Harvard University Press, Belknap Press.

Bruner describes the essays in this volume as "efforts of a student of the cognitive process trying to come to grips with the problems of education." Although he writes about the education of children, his thoughts are applicable to adults as well. All the essays provide both the student and the health educator with useful and thought-provoking ideas about teaching and learning. They are written clearly and concisely and offer a sophisticated treatment of the issues. The essay of particular interest for this case is "Notes on a Theory of Instruction." According to Bruner, learning depends on "the exploration of alternatives." This exploration "requires something to get it started" (in this case the chart), "something to keep it going" (in this case the homework), and "something to keep it from being random" (in this case the focus on the objectives.) Bruner says curiosity is a major condition for the exploration of alternatives. One reason Davis had to work so hard to get the learning process started was that this condition was not present.

Cathcart, R. S., and Samovar, L. A. 1979 *Small Group Communication: A Reader.* Dubuque: Wm. C. Brown.

This volume offers a comprehensive treatment of small groups. It provides basic definitions and deals with the structure, function, and evaluative process for both task and growth groups. The section on task groups offers a useful framework for problem solving, that is, problem identification, analysis, and specification of options. The authors illustrate the use of this framework with different situations in which the problem solvers make different kinds of mistakes.

Jenkins, D. H. 1961. "Force Field Analysis Applied to a School Situation." In *The Planning of Change,* edited by W. G. Bennis, K. D. Benne, and R. Chin. New York: Holt, Rinehart & Winston.

This article provides the student with a clear picture of the Lewinian concept of force-field analysis. The application of the concept to a practical problem aids the student's understanding. Lewin contributed a number of concepts useful to the practicing health educator. Sometimes the original articles are difficult to understand because most of them were written as notes. His untimely death prevented Lewin from fully developing some of his ideas.

Rubin, I. M.; Plovnick, M. S.; and Fry, R. F. 1975. *Improving the Coordination of Care: A Program for Health Team Development.* Cambridge, Mass: Ballinger.

This is a training manual for interdisciplinary team-building. It leads the reader from the initial step, identifying the need for a team, through the detailed process of team-building. The material is easy to understand. Worksheets and diagrams are provided for every step in the process. The reader can learn, cognitively, how a team develops from this manual. However, the affective component of team development can be learned only experientially.

Wolle, J. M. 1974. "Multidisciplinary Team Develops Programming for Patient Education." *Health Service Reports* 39(1):8–12.

This article describes the organization and implementation of a workshop designed to "assist interdisciplinary teams from hospitals and other health organizations to develop patient education programs." Of interest here are the requirements for attendance at the workshop.

Those attending had to have administrative support to develop and use interdisciplinary teams; they had to be members of an interdisciplinary team; and the team had to be willing to devote three days to the workshop.

Discussion Questions

1. Can you suggest other ways of getting the providers together to plan the hypertension education program than the one employed in this case?
2. Once the team was organized, how would you as the health educator work with the team to develop the hypertension education program for patients? Identify the first five steps you would take in helping the group plan. That is, what would your role be versus the provider's role in planning?
3. Note the type of administrative support usually available in a medical care setting. Why is support provided in this way in this setting?
4. How would you try to convince the administration in an HMO that clinician time should be spent on patient education? What arguments would you use and how would you support them?
5. Develop an outline of a training program for providers in working with groups of patients.
6. What would you call the program outlined in item 5? What would be the content? What methodology would you use?

Liaisons: Using Health Education Resources Effectively

Judith R. Miller, M.P.H.

BACKGROUND

How do you maximize limited health education services to 290,000 enrollees, 350 physicians, 12 outpatient centers, 3 specialty centers, 2 hospitals, and 5,000 employees? The Health Education Department (HED) at a large, consumer-governed northwestern HMO struggled to find a system. The one chosen is called the liaison assignment.

The HED is a centralized department responsible to the vice-president for health promotion and evaluation. In the early days of the HMO, there was often only one person responsible for the educational services of members (enrollees). In 1976 the board of trustees examined the organization's educational needs that had resulted from a period of rapid growth. The board prepared a charge for the department to work in the areas of consumer, employee, and patient education (Green et al. 1976). Ten full- or part-time health education specialists at the master's degree level now provide those services. Underlying all the department's activities are three assumptions:

1. Education is an integral part of good medical and health care.
2. Learning occurs through experience and participation in decision making, problem solving, and planning.
3. As an extension of items 1 and 2, it is essential that the HED cooperate with many and diverse individuals, departments, and committees (Mullen, Kukowski, and Mazelis 1979:57).

Because most medical services are provided in the outpatient primary care facilities, the department was committed to providing the majority of the health education services there.

EVOLUTION OF THE LIAISON ROLE

The liaison role has had four phases:

1. Assignment
2. Community organization
3. Education plans
4. Contract for specific phases

In 1976 the HED provided several group programs: prenatal education, smoking cessation, weight control, and diabetes education. Each program had a coordinator, and classes were held at most of the outpatient clinics. Clinic managers needed someone to call about security in the clinic on the nights that the groups met; physicians often did not know whom to call to discuss education for teens with scoliosis. Since all the education specialists were new to the organization, they had to quickly learn about the needs and interests of enrollees and providers in order to set appropriate program priorities.

To meet all the needs, one health education specialist was designated as a liaison to each outpatient clinic, and the clinic manager and clinic personnel were told the name and phone number of their "contact person" from the HED. The clinic personnel made very few requests, and the HED still did not have its planning information.

Judith R. Miller is a Health Education Specialist for the Group Health Cooperative of Puget Sound in Seattle, Washington.

The author gratefully acknowledges the assistance and advice of her colleagues who have experimented with being liaisons.

In analyzing the lack of response to our availability, we saw that the explanation was clear and that the logical next step was to take a community organization approach—to have the liaisons go to their assigned clinics on a regular basis, gather data about who was in the clinic or specialty center, and determine how they perceived the educational needs there. Whenever possible, formally in meetings or informally in conversations, the liaison provided information about the HED or about other HMO services. The health educators found opportunities to say, "I'd like to work with you on that," or "I know someone who has dealt with a similar problem."

In a few months, the liaisons began to be expected at their locations on their regular day. Comments such as "It must be Wednesday, our health educator is here" or "We missed you last week" gave notice that health education specialists were becoming a regular part of the facility's personnel.

Although the community organization approach led to people knowing the name of their liaison and when the liaison was expected at the facility, it was not always clear *why* the liaison was expected. Some locations had staff who were convinced that education could solve organizational problems, such as how to handle large volumes of telephone calls. Many locations looked to their liaisons as information experts and asked for pamphlets or slide/tapes on given health problems. Others knew their liaison had a particular area of expertise and asked for help in developing programs to solve a particular problem—consumer orientation, cancer education, employee health promotion.

These specific requests came from a variety of individuals and groups. Liaisons had to decide priorities, the ways different projects would be related, and what needs the requests would fulfill. To bring some order into the request process, we asked the managers to work with the liaison to prepare an educational plan. The plan would be based on the objectives of the medical center and would include budgets, completion dates, and the names of those who would be responsible.

The idea was a useful one, but too time-consuming for providers of direct care. Liaisons noted a general impatience with the details of planning and a lack of staff time to resolve the questions of resources, numbers of patients with given problems, desired behaviors following the educational service, and so on.

The lack of plans led to another assessment of the liaison role. Several details were clear:

- Liaisons' names and skills were known.
- Liaisons knew what the specific educational needs were.
- Many needs were common throughout the HMO.

It was also very clear that among the providers there was a wide range of interest in accepting educational services. At one end of the spectrum was a regional manager who wanted a full-time health educator to be involved with all the activities of that region (one of the three that comprised the HMO's organizational structure). At the other extreme were locations where, in spite of the liaison's clearly identifying educational needs and recommending solutions, no one cared whether the needs were met. In between were places where staff had concern but could not arrange the time to plan or make the commitment to try a new approach. The community's economy and the HMO's budget would not permit an ever-increasing supply of health education personnel to meet the demands of the very interested while continuing to change the attitudes of the disinterested. One solution was to reallocate the HED's most important resource, people. The liaison role reached its fourth stage of evolution—the contract for specific negotiated products. Because the HED receives the most requests for service from all levels of the organization, the contract becomes a useful way to distribute scarce resources.

To develop a contract, a manager makes a request. The liaison and manager negotiate outcome dates and products *and* the resources each party will commit to reaching the outcome. The advantage of this approach is that the expectations are clear and the service of the liaison and clinic personnel can be measured according to the terms of the contract. If either party cannot fulfill its agreement, a reassessment can take place and corrections can be made.

Liaisons are more satisfied that their skills are used; managers are more understanding of the resources needed to provide education as an integral part of good health care. Contracts allow liaisons to make use of colleagues in meeting needs.

USEFULNESS OF THE LIAISON

The liaison function is and will remain key to meeting the educational needs of this large and diverse HMO. The role serves as an example of good health education: assessing needs, determining resources, starting where people are, and defining meaningful objectives. Evaluation has changed from number of hours spent to number of contracted services completed or even expanded from a single location to part of overall HMO services.

Through taking a developmental approach to the liaison role, the HED has identified a useful approach for defining and responding to educational needs. Liaisons have taught managers, consumers, and health care providers what educators do. Liaisons have identified issues that affect the organization and the HED and have provided the educators with an understanding of the HMO's needs and services that few other professionals have. The three-year experience has shown the effectiveness of a centralized department from which well-trained and experienced professionals can be deployed to solve problems. Using liaisons to facilities who contract to provide specific services is a reasonable way to serve a large, widely dispersed constituency.

REFERENCES

Green, L. W.; Mathews, B.; Mazalis, S.; and Mullen, P. D. 1976. *A Study of the Needs and Opportunities for Health Education and Related Educational Functions in a Group Health Cooperative.* Seattle: Group Health Cooperative.

Mullen, P.; Kukowski, K.; and Mazelis, S. 1979. "Health Education in Health Mainitenance Organizations." In *The Handbook of Health Education*, edited by P. Lazes. Germantown, Md.: Aspen Systems Corp.

Analysis

This case describes the allocation of health education resources in a large HMO. It illustrates the process of selling or advocating health education. The central task of the Health Education Department was educating the consumers of health education services, the providers of medical care, and the managers of inpatient and ambulatory facilities about the usefulness of health education services to their goals.

The adoption-diffusion process (Rogers 1983) provides a good theoretical fit for the planned approach to the central task. The presence of the health educators in the clinic created an awareness of their availability; the data they collected and their offers to assist set the stage for developing interest and provided an experience that the "consumers" could evaluate and try out if they wished. Some "adopted" health education services and some did not.

The HED had limited staff and so did not try to force the issue with those who were not interested. They worked with those who were and allowed the diffusion process to work with the others.

The health educators on the liaison assignment took the time—6 to twelve months—to get acquainted with the clinic personnel and let clinic personnel get acquainted with them. This step is part of the process of developing credibility. The other part of this process is a recognition of professional competence. The opportunity to demonstrate the latter is much more likely if one takes the *time* to deal with the former. As we will see in other cases (e.g., Thomas, Israel, and Steuart, p. 225), health educators working under the limitations of a short-term grant are restricted in the time they can devote to getting acquainted.

The health educators on the liaison assignments did not wait to be invited to participate in clinic projects. They asked to be included. They had decided that they had not been invited because the clinic staff didn't know they could contribute; so they let the staff know how much they had to offer. The practice of health education demands that the health educator be assertive.

Note the creative use of the contract mechanism in this case. It was a tool that forced the HED members and those with whom they contracted to be *accountable*. Lack of accountability has been a serious drawback to the acceptance of health education services.

Note also the placement of the HED in the HMO structure. It was in a centralized position that allowed it to cut across all other departments in the organization. This is a sine qua non because health education services cut across all departments. The health educator must not only be able to move freely among departments, but also know the issues of importance to departments and to the organization, because these influence what the health educator can do (Mathews 1982).

The HED "sold" health education to those who were providing services that could benefit from education. It did so by persuasively communicating the fact that the health educators knew services could be improved with education, and the providers of medical care did not. Advocacy is essential under these circumstances. The methodology used to "sell" was based on a concept of the learning/social change process: "People will adopt those practices they can try out to see if they work."

References/Select Resources

Deeds, S. G., and Mullen, P. D., eds. 1981. "Managing Health Education in Health Maintenance Organizations: Part 1." *Health Education Quarterly* 8:(4)279–375.

Deeds, S. G., and Mullen, P. D., eds. 1982. "Managing Health Education in Health Maintenance Organizations: Part 2." *Health Education Quarterly* 9:(1):3–95.

This two-part study might be titled "All You Want to Know about Health Education in HMOs." There are six articles in each part. Part 1 deals with health education in regard to the state of the art, acceptability, advocacy, opportunities, and innovative ideas for programming. Part 2 offers descriptions of specific health education activities. One article deals with professional issues for the health educator. What is it like to be a health educator in an HMO. What kind of training does one need? Although the articles in both parts are written from the perspective of HMOs, much of what is said is applicable to the practice of health education in any medical care setting.

Mathews, B. "Administrative Climate: Its Implications for Health Educators." In *SOPHE Heritage Collection of Health Education Monographs*, vol. 1: *The Philosophical, Behavioral, and Professional Bases for Health Education*, edited by S. K. Simonds. Oakland, Calif.: Third Party Publishing.

The author discusses the difference between a technological and social administration and the implications of each for the practicing health educator. She provides the reader with a frame of reference with which to analyze the administrative climate. The variables included are influence, communication, decision making, leadership, and personal relations, all of which can be identified in Miller's case study. Finally, she discusses the relationship between the climate and the learning process.

Mullen, P. D., and Zapka, J. G. 1982. *Guidelines for Health Promotion and Education Services in HMOs.* Washington, D.C.: U.S. Department of Health and Human Services, Public Health Service.

This is a must book for anyone responsible for managing health education programs in HMOs. The appended material is particularly valuable because it provides protocols and management tools in use at a number of HMOs around the country.

Rogers, E. M. 1983. *Diffusion of Innovations.* 3d ed. New York: Free Press.

In this third edition of Roger's work on the diffusion of an innovation, he notes the tremendous increase in diffusion research since his first publication in 1962, when he reported on 405 studies on diffusion. For this edition, he reviewed 3,085 studies. The major difference between this edition and the second one is the extension of diffusion theory to include factors that antecede and follow the adoption process. For example: Where did the diffusion come from? Which comes first, the need or the innovation? What kinds of problems are encountered, and how are they solved as the innovation is implemented? Rogers makes a distinction between an organization's and an individual's adoption of an innovation (chapter 10). Although the innovation, in the Miller case, was promoted in an organization, its use in the organization required that it be adopted by individuals.

Discussion Questions

1. Assume you have been assigned to one of the clinics for one day a week and have collected the data the Health Education Department required for that clinic. Specify your steps in advocating health education in that clinic.

2. Suppose a physician in the clinic to which you are assigned told you, "You can do the education, but I'll do the doctoring." How would you respond?

3. Can you identify disadvantages to the contract mechanism described?

4. Note the indicators that the HED used to measure its acceptance by clinic staff. How can you distinguish between levels of acceptance by the type of conversation/interaction you have with staff?

5. Assume you are on a liaison assignment and the providers in your clinic perceive health educators as providers of materials, pamphlets, films, and so on. Write out the issues you would raise with them to try to change their perception. Specify exactly what you would say and do.

A Self-Care Unit for Management of the Common Cold in a Prepaid Setting

Barbara B. Estabrook, M.S.

THE PROBLEM

Heavy utilization of medical services for care of the common cold has been documented in college health services and other prepaid settings. The University Health Services at the University of Massachusetts–Amherst sought an efficient and effective means to care for minor, uncomplicated upper respiratory tract infections.

THE SETTING

The University Health Services at the University of Massachusetts in Amherst offers a comprehensive prepaid health plan to over 30,000 students, their dependents, and university staff and their families. Services include primary care, mental health care, dental health care, and specialty services. Inpatient facilities, laboratory and X ray, physical therapy, health education services, and a pharmacy are also provided. In the late 1970s there were approximately 100,000 outpatient visits annually, with a primary care staff of 30. This health service has a strong orientation to individual responsibility in health, reflected in programs for contraception, wart care, dental health, and other areas.

Barbara Estabrook is Manager of Member Services for the Multi-Group Health Plan, Wellesley, Massachusetts. She was formerly Patient Education Coordinator for the University Health Services at the University of Massachusetts at Amherst.

THE SITUATION

Numerous approaches to the problem of overuse of health services for common colds were tried at the University Health Services and elsewhere. Education, direct service, and self-care methods were employed. At the University Health Services, the first attempt to address the problem was made in the early 1970s. Persons wanting cold medications reported to the pharmacy, where over-the-counter preparations were available. Some of these items were prepaid; for others there was a charge unless a clinician "prescribed" them. Thus there was a financial incentive to use professional time for cold care. A folder on cold care and information sheets on the use of the drugs were available. This program was modified by making cold pills and aspirin available on tables in the clinic area and in some dormitories on campus. Under this arrangement, consumption of these items was so great that it can be assumed there was much waste and/or misuse. There was also the question of whether the University Health Services was legally responsible for the proper use of drugs dispensed under such free distribution.

It became evident that a revised system of cold care was needed. The matter was considered over several years, and finally the solution was precipitated by difficulty in achieving a full staff of physicians for the 1975–1976 academic year. Several modifications in clinical procedures to address the short staffing included increased nurse practitioner hours in the clinic, institution of a 50 cent copayment for all pharmacy items, and establishment of a self-care unit for colds. This strategy was developed by the University Health Services' executive director, medical director, and director of health education and approved by the interdisciplinary Executive Committee.

THE DEVELOPMENT PROCESS

Members of the health education staff, working with an administrative intern, designed the self-care unit. It was very generally modeled after a successful system at the University of Southern California, although with considerable modification (Klotz 1974). The following objectives were established for the unit: (1) to offer expanded education about the care of colds, (2) to ensure medical attention for more serious health problems, and (3) to ensure user acceptance of the system.

After drafting a philosophy, a format, and rudimentary materials, the developers held a series of three meetings attended by directors of medical, nursing, pharmacy, and administrative staffs. The basic approach and materials were examined, and specific content suggestions for the symptoms check sheet and recommendations for self-treatment were solicited. In such a multidisciplinary team context, the health educator served as a coordinator, an organizer, an evaluator, a liaison with other resources, and a source of educational expertise. Input and support of clinicians and pharmacy staff were seen as critical. There was considerable approval of using the general concept already in place for building support for this particular implementation. It was expected that because they had provided and reviewed the unit's mechanisms for patient screening and its health information, professionals would be more comfortable in referring patients to the unit. In addition to the meetings with the development team, the health education staff held a meeting with the nurse practitioners to engender input and support. Time in the meeting schedule of physicians was not available, so communication with them was by memo.

Finally, other aspects of the system for obtaining care and drugs were examined to anticipate built-in factors that might affect use of the unit. These aspects included policies and procedures for pharmacy operation, appointment making, and the walk-in clinic. As already described, pharmacy policy had created a financial incentive to use professional services. The policy was changed to eliminate this incentive. Consumers with colds who made appointments or appeared at the walk-in clinic were to be encouraged by support staff and professional staff to use the self-care unit whenever possible.

Thus the Cold Self-Care Center was instituted with the University Health Services staff using principles of organizational development through attempting to both incorporate the expertise and meet the needs of all the staff. The user evaluation and cost effectiveness evaluation that concluded the development process will be described later.

THE COLD SELF-CARE CENTER

The Cold Self-Care Center consists of a series of large posters mounted over a specially designed counter with handouts and other materials. The unit helps the user answer two basic questions: (1) Is what I have really just a common cold or do I need professional care? (2) If I don't need professional care, what can I do to help myself feel better? In answering these questions, the center emphasizes the self-limited nature of the illness, and the limitations of the available medications, deemphasizing their use and favoring the use of "home remedies," such as saltwater gargle and extra rest and fluids. Users of the center are provided with the opportunity to choose and obtain appropriate medications if they so desire.

The process for use of the unit, which takes about five minutes, is summarized in Figure 1. The user enters the system from any one of several sources and receives general information on colds. Symptoms are assessed on the basis of a checklist. If serious symptoms exist, the user is directed to see a clinician (in a walk-in clinic for urgent problems). If no serious symptoms are present, the user proceeds to information about specific home remedies and medications that might, on the basis of symptoms, be chosen. Finally, a self-prescription blank is completed and presented to the pharmacy if cold drugs or supplies are desired. Printed handouts are available that enlarge upon and reinforce the information presented. The user makes the diagnosis and prescription, maintaining the option to receive professional care at any point in the process.

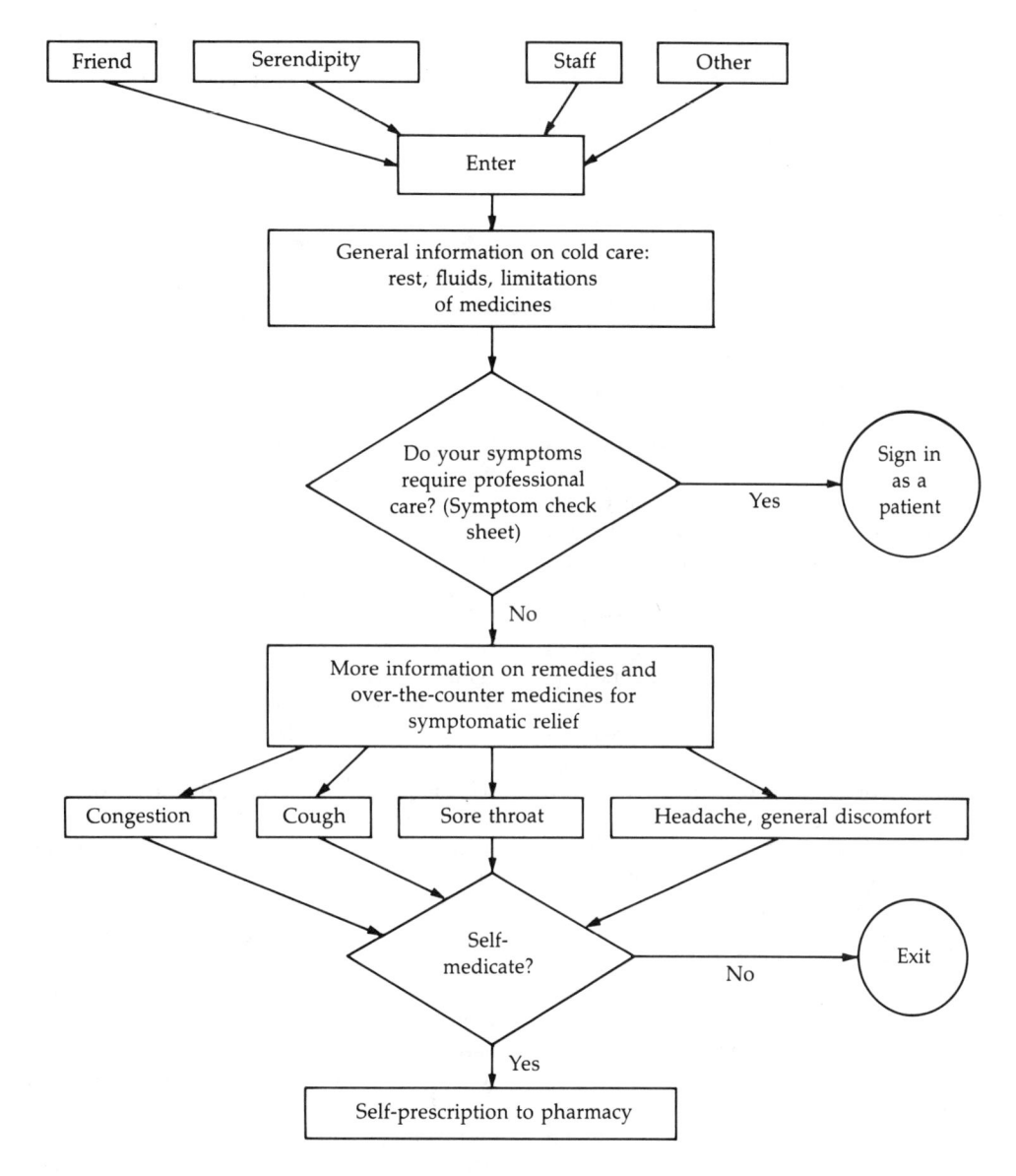

Figure 1
Patient Flow of Cold Self-Care Center

THEORETICAL AND RESEARCH CONTEXT

In addition to situational factors, relevant data and theory influenced the development and design of the Cold Self-Care Center. Self-care programs and materials have become increasingly common. Self-care is defined as the consumer's self-initiated and self-controlled performance of those activities traditionally carried out by providers. It is a means of contributing to the efficacy of care, thereby improving the outcome of health services, particularly ambulatory care, in which consumer behavior is a key to successful outcome. Self-care approaches have been effective in some health problem areas resistant to change by other methods, such as obesity, smoking, and alcohol abuse. Self-care training programs are also a means for introducing information and skills into a community's informal network of advice. In addition to these benefits, positive effects can be realized by the individual's taking responsibility for his or her own health and decreasing dependency needs. Thus there was a documentation to support a system in which consumers rather than professionals perform assessment and drug choice.

The posters and handouts that compose the system are essentially programmed instruction (although there is no feedback mechanism). This system has been viewed as a technique with some potential for health education, offering the opportunity to receive information at an individual speed and in small steps (Skiff 1974). One possible barrier to the unit's effectiveness, the limited amount of information that can be absorbed by someone who is ill, was anticipated (Mullen 1973). The information presented is reduced to an absolute minimum and is organized according to each symptom (e.g., what to do for a cough, what to do for a sore throat). This was seen as an appropriate scheme, because symptoms are the way in which people tend to view and interpret colds. Moreover, at present the only treatment available for colds is relief of symptoms. The unit's brevity also addresses another potential problem: patient dissatisfaction with long waits at a clinic or doctor's office (Comstock and Slome 1973). In fact, the unit's use becomes a benefit to the user in this respect because any wait at all is highly unlikely.

The facility maximizes the user's decision-making role. The attempt was to follow the human resources model of management, in which everyone in a system or organization is assumed to be capable of responsible, self-directed, self-controlled behavior (Miles 1965). The task of providers thus becomes the creation of a situation in which individuals can use their full capacities to the achievement of goals. The expectation of this model is that the overall quality of decision making will improve and satisfaction of individuals will increase.

As we have seen, the user of the Cold Self-Care Center is given several opportunities and tools for decision making. The user gains access also to the important power of diagnosis. This is done by using the symptoms checklist, a modified version of an algorithm, which has been hailed as a means to reduce pressure on the ambulatory care system, enabling consumers to perform routine tasks and make decisions (Green Werlin, and Schauffler 1977).

EVALUATION

Members of the health education staff conducted two evaluations. A sample of the self-selected user population was compared with a random sample of university students. This evaluation examined consumer satisfaction and impact on behavior, knowledge, and attitudes (Estabrook, 1977, 1979).

Users of the Cold Self-Care Center differed in several ways from nonusers. They had higher levels of knowledge about cold care, indicated more dependency on professional resources, and differed in health-related attitudes and cold-care behavior. They did not differ from nonusers in their self-medication behavior. Knowledge of criteria for seeking professional care was greater among users than among nonusers, and anticipated future use of professional care for colds was extremely low among users. General satisfaction with the program was quite high. Speed and ease of use were most often cited as reasons for satisfaction.

The second evaluation was a cost analysis of the Cold Self-Care Center. Development and maintenance costs were calculated, and the cost per user was compared with the cost of an outpatient clinic visit. The ratio of outpatient care costs to self-care costs was 14.7 to 1. Analysis of records of outpatient visits for colds and sore throats for three years prior and two years following the center's implementation indicated a reduction in visits of over 2,500 per year. Dollar savings to the institution are estimated at over $46,000 for the first two years of the center's operation (Zapka and Averill 1979). The evaluation of this program illustrates the great potential of health education to control costs of medical care and yet not compromise consumer satisfaction.

REFERENCES

Comstock, L., and Slome, C. 1973. "A Health Survey of Students: Prevalence of Perceived Problems." *Journal of the American College Health Association* 22:150–155.

Estabrook, B. 1977. "Evaluation of a Patient Education Program for Self-Care of Colds." Master's thesis, University of Massachusetts–Amherst.

Estabrook, B. 1979. "Consumer Impact of a Cold Self-Care Center in a Prepaid Ambulatory Care Setting." *Medical Care* 17:1139–1145.

Green, L. W.; Werlin, S. H.; and Schauffler, H. H. 1977. "Research and Demonstration Issues in Self-Care: Measuring the Decline of Medico-centrism." *Health Education Monographs* 5:161–189.

Klotz, A. 1974. "The Establishment of a Self-Help Clinic as Part of a College Student Health Service." University of Southern California. Typescript.

Miles, R. 1965. "Human Relations or Human Resources?" *Harvard Business Review,* July–August:148–152.

Mullen, P. D. 1973. "Health Education for Heart Patients in Crisis." *Health Services Reports* 88:669–675.

Skiff, A. 1974. "Experiences with Methods for Patient Teaching from a Public Health Service Hospital." *Health Education Monographs* 2(1):48–53.

Zapka, J., and Averill, B. W. 1979. "Self-Care for Colds: A Cost-Effective Alternative to Upper Respiratory Infection Management." *American Journal of Public Health* 69:814–815.

Analysis

This case describes a cold self-care program at a university health center. The program, however, could be applied in any medical care setting.

The task of the health educator in this case was that of planner, coordinator, and liaison with other health team personnel. In addition to familiarity with educational planning models and knowledge about medical self-help and appropriate treatment of upper respiratory infections, the health educator needed to know what the skills of other medical care professionals were and what they could contribute to the project.

This case can be considered a model for dealing with a medical care problem through educational intervention. Any of several models of planning would fit the steps described in the case (Ross and Mico 1980:204–213).

The planning phase of this case is worthy of close scrutiny. Note that the policies and procedures of the University Health Services were examined to identify and try to remove built-in barriers to use of the Cold Self-Care Center. For example, the original pharmacy policy had created a financial incentive to use the University Health Service's clinicians. Care received through this health center's professionals, including prescriptions, was free, while there was a 50 cent copayment for self-prescribed medications. The only benefit of going through the pharmacy was time saved; but if the students felt they had more time than money, they would visit the clinicians, even if they had to wait to be seen.

The cold self-care program was adapted from similar programs at other university health centers. Adaptation not only helped provide a model but also lent credibility to the idea because it had been successful with a similar population elsewhere. Thus a critical principle of practice was applied: Don't reinvent the wheel.

Input from all relevant staff was sought and incorporated into the program. Since the staff's attitudes could influence the use of the Cold Self-Care Center, it was important to involve them in the planning. Staff attitudes and behavior would be identified under the reinforcing factors in the PRECEDE model if that model were used for planning.

In this case as in others (Semura, p. 301; Ogasawara, p. 262), we have an example of competent staff work. The health educator kept the project moving, organized meetings as needed, kept those who could not attend informed of decisions, contacted staff individually as necessary, collected background information, identified issues, and so on. As has been noted in other cases, these activities alone will not result in a successful project, but their lack can seriously impair a project.

Some of the limitations that arise in clinical practice are also illustrated. For instance, the health educator was not able to meet with the medical staff and had to rely on written communication. Another example is the design of the evaluation. A comparison group of cold sufferers who received professional care for their colds was desired but could not be obtained because of clinic procedures.

The concept of self-care is central to this case. Informed self-care is new; prior to the self-help movement, the message from the medical profession was to rely on health professionals to diagnose and prescribe, rather than to self-medicate. Nonetheless, people did use home remedies and were heavily influenced by advertising for over-the-counter medications. Patient self-care, education, and responsibility for prevention are now much more widely accepted. They have an increasing effect on the cost of medical care and on philosophies and beliefs about the medical care system.

The concern for costs in a prepaid health center is obvious. This type of facility has an incentive to decrease inappropriate use of services. But this might not be the case in a fee-for-service setting. The educational goals described in this case would not be consistent with the financial goals of that system. As Ross and Mico (1980:222) say, "The goals must accord with the client system's existing policy."

Beyond the issue of cost for the health center is the larger question of cost analysis and health education. Green (1974) was one of the first to suggest that cost analysis was a component of health education. Cost studies in conjunction with impact evaluation can provide strong justification for health education. Impact evaluation alone tells us only the results of the program. Cost analysis obviously yields information on the cost of the program—overall costs as well as unit costs. This knowledge permits determination of whether resources were effectively and efficiently expended. Decisions about continuation or expansion of a program thus can be made in a more informed context.

Cost analysis includes a number of methods. Prominent among these are cost-benefit (CB) analysis and cost-effectiveness (CE) analysis. In CB analysis, both the input and output of a program are valuated, and a ratio of input costs to dollars saved or some other benefit is developed. In health education it is often difficult to valuate program outputs. In CE analysis, outputs are not valuated; rather, the costs of two or more methods that achieve the same outcome are compared. In the Estabrook case, a ratio of outpatient costs to self-care costs was developed, which provided the evidence to determine that self-care for colds was a cost-effective method.

By increasing emphasis on cost analysis, health education will be able to compete successfully for its share of scarce resources. The Estabrook case provides an excellent example of how cost analysis can be implemented without sophisticated cost accounting, grants, or additional staff. Administration made the decision to allocate staff time to do this study.

This case takes a perennial problem—the pursuit of professional care when self-care would suffice—and offers a tidy solution that is applicable to many medical settings. For example, physicians in private practice could educate their patients in appropriate self-care measures.

The value of education as an intervention strategy was demonstrated in this case on many levels: appropriate use of services, user satisfaction, knowledge of appropriate care, and cost benefit.

References/Select Resources

Avery, C. H.; Green, L. W.; and Kreider, S. 1976. "Reducing Emergency Visits of Asthmatics: An Experiment in Patient Education." Testimony presented before the President's Committee on Health Education, Regional Hearings, Pittsburgh, Pa.

This article offers another example of how health education can be cost-effective. Fifty-eight patients with asthma were randomly assigned to an experimental and a control group. Group discussion was the educational method. Use of the emergency room for problems related to asthma was monitored for four months. During this time the control group used the emergency room twice as often as the experimental group.

Green, L. W., 1974. "Toward Cost-benefit Evaluations of Health Education: Some Concepts, Methods, and Examples." *Health Education Monographs* 2 (suppl. 1):34–64.

This article is a landmark in the field of health education evaluation. Green challenges health educators to develop a rigor in program planning that will allow for cost-benefit analysis and offers measures for this purpose. What is known today as the PRECEDE model for program analysis was first published in this paper.

Levin, L. S.; Katz, A. H.; and Holst, E. 1976. *Self-Care: Lay Initiatives in Health*. New York: Prodist.

In the late 1960s and early 1970s, a vigorous self-care movement began in this country. To a great extent it was fueled by grass-root efforts such as the women's health movement. The goal at that time was to diminish the mystique of medicine to enable people to gain more control over their bodies. As the control of health care costs became increasingly important, decision and policy makers in health care viewed self-care as a way to control costs. Levin was one of the first academics to actively chart the course of the self-care movement and document its impact.

This book reports the discussion of an international symposium on the role of the individual in self-care. The conferees addressed three topics related to the main theme: (1) economics, social planning, and administrative practice; (2) health and educational practice; and (3) social and behavioral sciences. In addition to discussing these issues, the authors identify research issues in self-care.

Ross, H. S., and Mico, P. R. 1980. *Theory and Practice in Health Education*. Palo Alto, Calif.: Mayfield.

Chapter 11 of this book describes many of the planning models currently used in health education practice. These include the PRECEDE framework developed by Green and his associates, Sullivan's comprehensive program development model, and Mico's six-phase health education planning model.

Sieten, A. M., and Levin, L. S. 1979. "Self-Care Education." In *Handbook of Health Education*, edited by P. M. Lazes. Germantown, Md.: Aspen Systems Corp.

This article offers a comprehensive review of self-care issues. It covers definitions; the development of self care; different types of self care activities; and sponsorship, funding, resources, methods, and evaluation of self-care programs. It is a good starting point for anyone unfamiliar with but interested in self-care.

Zapka, J., and Estabrook, B. B. 1976. "Medical Self-Care Programs." *Health Care Management Review* 1(4):75–86.

This article describes the potential of self-care programs to control costs in prepaid medical care settings. It is based on the cold self-care study reported in this case. Cost impact was determined through cost-effectiveness analysis. In this analysis the costs for two programs that lead to the same outcome are compared. Cost consists of personnel, medications, supplies, and indirect items necessary for the maintenance of any program.

Discussion Questions

1. What other self-care programs might a health center institute?
2. What is the difference between cost-effective analysis and cost-benefit analysis? Which method was used to evaluate this case?
3. Why might some medical practitioners resist the introduction of a self-care program?
4. Describe some methods that could be used to influence consumers to use a self-care unit.
5. How would you introduce a self-care program in the community? How would the planning differ from that described in this case?

Patient Education in a Rural Ambulatory-Care Setting: The Patient Education Reimbursement Project

Randy H. Schwartz, M.S., and Paula Sanofsky Morris, Ph.D.

This paper is based on a study of patient education in 22 ambulatory care centers in rural Maine. The problems faced by these health centers closely reflected problems of the rural communities in which they operated—limited resources, isolation, lack of transportation, a sparse population base, and depressed conditions of the local and national economy. Rural America has traditionally suffered a scarcity of health care resources and has had difficulty recruiting and retaining health manpower (Roemer 1976).

Two federal programs were instituted to improve health care provision in rural areas: the Rural Health Initiative Program and the Health Underserved Rural Areas Program. Through these programs, the government sought to (1) coordinate existing resources, (2) encourage innovative programs, and (3) support research/demonstrations (Henderson, Bates, and Sliepcevich 1978). Among the ten health priorities cited in the National Health Planning and Resources Development Act, P.L. 93–641, was this one: "The provision of primary care services for medically underserved populations, especially those which are located in rural or economically depressed areas." The Rural Health Initiative Act (1976) listed as a goal: "To emphasize programs of prevention and health education to gain full utility from the medical resources available to a rural area" (U. S. DHEW 1976).

Maine, New England's largest state, has many "rural areas" as defined by these programs. When the project began, 31 of Maine's 35 ambulatory care centers were situated in medically underserved rural areas.

PROJECT DESCRIPTION

With a grant from the Health Underserved Rural Areas Program, the Maine Department of Human Services proposed to develop and implement the Patient Education Reimbursement Project (PERP) (Mullane et al. 1980). Operation of the project was subcontracted to the Health Education Resource Center (HERC) of the University of Maine at Farmington in December 1977. The agreement between the HERC and the Department of Human Services listed the following goals:

1. Demonstrate that focused health education services delivered to patients having selected chronic disorders or other problems which result in consistently high rates of care utilization can, under controlled circumstances, reduce the total per capita expenditure for health care for these patients and/or improve health outcomes.

Randy H. Schwartz is Project Manager for the Maine Diabetes Control Project, in the Maine Department of Human Services. He was formerly Project Evaluator of the Patient Education Reimbursement Project at the University of Maine, Farmington. Paula Sanofsky Morris is Assistant to the President at the University of Maine, Farmington. She was Evaluation Consultant to the Patient Education Reimbursement Project and later Coordinator of Research and Evaluation at the university.

The authors wish to thank Mr. Edward Miller, Director of Health Education, Maine Department of Human Services, for his assistance during the course of the evaluation and for his review of the manuscript.

2. Develop guidelines for specification of health education services which would be routinely reimbursed by Medicaid, including consideration of:
   - provider qualifications
   - diagnosis or characteristics of eligible patients
   - reimbursement procedures
   - rate setting
   - quality assurance
   - service models

Patient education programs funded by the PERP were initially restricted to two disease entities: diabetes and hypertension. These were chosen because they have a high incidence and prevalence among the general population and are amenable to change or control through patient education in conjunction with clinical care. Educational material about diabetes and hypertension was already available to serve as references for newly emerging programs.

In the project's first year, 13 of the 33 eligible health centers were funded, and 10 implemented programs. In the second year, 9 new programs were initiated. Six were based on the CORE Communications in Health Package, a marketed cassette/slide program. One other health center contracted with a local hospital for the provision of patient education services. During the third year, 14 more programs began, making a total of 33 programs in 22 health centers. Over the course of the project, programs were allowed to address a wider array of topics. By year three, programs had been developed for hypertension, diabetes, chronic obstructive pulmonary disease, cardiac care, prenatal care and childbirth, weight reduction, and smoking cessation. Over 1,200 patients had been served.

PROJECT EVALUATION

In February 1980, two years after the project began, the Health Education Resource Center undertook an evaluation of the PERP. A health educator was hired to conduct the evaluation, and an evaluation specialist served as consultant to the project. Together they planned and implemented the evaluation. This work included developing the design, using instrumentation, interviewing, doing data analysis, and generating reports. Almost no project data had been collected before that time. This situation posed serious problems. As is often the case, project administrators overlooked evaluation until they needed answers to specific questions. By then, important information had been lost. Given the lack of data from the first two years of the project, many significant questions could not be answered. This flaw, in itself, taught an important lesson: planning and evaluation go hand in hand. Both must be given ample attention at the outset of a project. Under the circumstances, a study was planned that would (1) review project strengths and weaknesses, (2) document accomplishments, and (3) capture subjectively what had been learned about providing formalized patient education in rural settings.

Six sets of variables were used to examine how the PERP and the health center programs evolved and operated:

1. *Organizational variables*—administrative arrangements, political forces (internal and external), agency characteristics, and service populations
2. *Program model variables*—health education program characteristics, referral patterns, and monitoring and evaluation procedures
3. *Personnel variables*—staff size, mix, training, attitudes toward health education, and turnover
4. *Planning and implementation variables*—reasons for participating, proposal development, staff involvement and determination of needs
5. *Patient variables*—characteristics of health center users and program participants
6. *Project grant variables*—administrative structure, advisement, staffing, political pressures, and planning and evaluation procedures

Data were collected by review of project documents and face-to-face interviews. Representatives of the 22 participating health centers, particularly persons responsible for the health education programs, composed most of the sample. When a health center operated under the aegis of a larger parent or umbrella agency, relevant personnel at the administering agency were interviewed. Interviews were also conducted with administrators, advisory board members, and staff of the PERP.

A structured interview guide was used to help focus the interviews. Questions addressed the appropriateness of patient education programs, their adequacy, effectiveness, efficiency, and side effects. Information was also gathered on program characteristics, the program planning process, and recommendations for the future. Each interview included an analysis of factors that helped or hindered program development.

FINDINGS ON PATIENT EDUCATION PROGRAMS

The programs funded by the PERP used a wide variety of educational methods and materials. Both one-to-one and group sessions were conducted. Centers that chose one-to-one programs (programs matching one health care provider with one patient) did so for the following reasons. First, they felt that in small, rural communities, where everyone knows everyone else, patients are not comfortable discussing personal matters in a group. Second, providers preferred doing education at the time of the patient visit. Third, few patients had the same need for the same kind of education at any given time. Fourth, providers felt more comfortable working with individuals. Group sessions were preferred in other health centers for two reasons: They were more cost-efficient, and they provided an important source of support to participants.

Patient educators in the programs funded by PERP included nurses (R.N.'s and L.P.N.'s), physician assistants, physicians, and dietitians. In most cases they were responsible for providing clinical care and considered organized patient education an added responsibility. Most felt their time was too limited and would have preferred hiring separate personnel for patient education. Only a few centers could afford this arrangement.

One of the major mistakes of the project was assuming that health centers already provided formal patient educaton. Many health center staff saw patient education as a new responsibility—one for which they were not prepared. In some cases they had not wanted to participate in the project, but their administrators sought PERP funding and insisted. Direct care staff were often delegated the job of planning and implementing educational programs. Lack of involvement in decision making about patient education, insufficient time, and inadequate training were commonly cited as problems. Many providers felt they were not effective educators, particularly when their programs first began.

One health center solved the manpower problem by contracting with a local hospital for the services of a trained health educator. The health center staff felt their own time was severely limited and preferred this arrangement. Most respondents said that planning and providing health education programs was demanding work. Many resented taking time away from individual patient care to do educational programs. Several respondents felt that negative consequences would result if the patient's regular health care provider did not act as educator as well. They noted that the trust established between patient and care giver is a critical factor that enhances the educational encounter.

APPROPRIATENESS OF THE PROGRAMS

The clear and consistent sentiment was that organized patient education is a highly appropriate activity for rural health centers. By their very nature, community-based, ambulatory health centers were seen as particularly well suited to the provision of formal patient education. Respondents regarded patient education as an activity that is directly related to the health center mandate. Most felt that educational activities should be expanded beyond patient education to include community health education.

ADEQUACY OF THE PROGRAMS

Questions about the adequacy of programs were met with confusion and uncertainty. None of the health centers had reliable data on the need for specific programs. Most were operating on untested assumptions. Some respondents reported that once the most highly motivated patients passed through a program, they were unable to fill enrollment. Others reported that they could not meet the demand and were seeing only the tip of the iceberg in regard to need. Factors that would influence the adequacy of programs included the size and composition of the service population, other available sources of care and education, and the disease entity or medical condition being addressed. Without community-based needs assessment data, the adequacy of the programs funded by the PERP remains uncertain.

EFFECTIVENESS OF THE PROGRAMS

None of the health centers had empirical data on the effectiveness of their programs. Although there were early attempts to collect data on patient knowledge and satisfaction, these data contributed little to evaluating program effectiveness because the relationship of these variables to behavior change is so tenuous. No data on health status or utilization were systematically collected.

On the basis of subjective impressions, most respondents thought that their programs were effective. They could not, however, explain the criteria they used to define effectiveness. Many respondents reacted to questions about effectiveness with disdain or bewilderment. While some recognized the importance of the issue to funding and program planning, others thought that even broaching the topic was inappropriate—that patient education was always of value and should not be subject to scrutiny.

Overall, the findings suggest that program effectiveness (what it means, why it is important, and how it can be measured) is poorly understood and generally neglected. It is an area in which education, training, and technical assistance is sorely needed.

EFFICIENCY OF THE PROGRAMS

None of the health centers collected data on the efficiency of their programs. Factors perceived as affecting cost included the time required for planning and start-up, staff time invested in providing the program, space, audiovisual aids, and printed materials. There were few ideas on how to measure program "benefits." Respondents seemed unaccustomed to thinking in terms of efficiency; many said they did not know how to begin addressing the question. Most surprising was the lack of cost or efficiency data from people at administrative levels.

Programs were funded by the PERP on an administrative cost basis in relation to the projected number of patients. Per patient costs varied tremendously. For example, a diabetes education program cost $110.54 per patient in one center and $30.00 in another. A major cost factor was the type of personnel who provided the program.

There was considerable disagreement among respondents about the importance of program efficiency. Some felt that programs should be altered or abandoned if inefficient; others regarded patient education a valid endeavor regardless of program efficiency. Program efficiency must be attended to, however, particularly given the concerns of third-party payers. It is one of the areas of the project that should have received the greatest attention but in fact received the least. One of the major shortcomings of the PERP was that it failed to provide participating health centers with the information, education, training, and technical assistance they needed to measure the efficiency and effectiveness of their programs.

SIDE EFFECTS OF THE PROGRAMS

A number of positive side effects reportedly resulted from institution of the programs:

1. *Attitudes*—an increase in awareness, understanding, and support of patient education on the part of health center staff and administrators
2. *Communication*—more and better communication between patients and providers; also improved communication among providers as they worked together planning and implementing programs
3. *Public relations*—improved image of the health center as an agency concerned about the community's well-being
4. *Utilization*—improved utilization as patients learned to use services more appropriately; also increased enrollments as a result of favorable publicity
5. *Quality of care*—an improved medical encounter due to better communication between patient and provider and increased attention to whole-person care; also more attention to issues such as nutrition and the coordination of care

DISCUSSION

Although the PERP was successful in supporting the development of patient education programs, the project failed to accomplish what was originally intended. There were four major reasons for this failure. First, given the state of patient education in rural Maine, the goals were overly ambitious, that is, the goals of (1) demonstrating that patient education can reduce per capita health care expenditures and/or improve health outcomes, and (2) developing guidelines for third-party reimbursement. Second, three major assumptions upon which the project rested proved incorrect:

1. That rural health centers already had organized patient education programs, so that PERP funding would be a simple financial transition
2. That physicians and other primary care personnel had experience in organized patient education and felt comfortable in a teaching role, so that no training would be necessary
3. That health center staff had both the time and the interest needed to develop and implement patient education programs, so that funding would be a sufficient incentive

These false assumptions set the project awry. No resources were directed to helping the health centers learn how to develop and implement programs. The need for training and technical assistance was not satisfied, and the time required for start-up was substantially underestimated. Problems associated with offering programs in spite of skeleton staffs, high staff turnover, limited service hours, and poor transportation were overlooked.

It took the first three years of the project to recognize and address these errors. By the spring of 1980, patient education was geared up to where it was thought to have been at the project's outset. Health centers were operating patient education programs, and the interest and enthusiasm of health care providers had increased tremendously.

Third, a host of historical and political factors contributed to the project's false start. The major political issue was whether any health center or only a select few could participate in the PERP. Health center advocates who sought additional resources for all health centers pushed for open participation. They won out over those who argued that the project would be more manageable and effective if alternative model programs of a few health centers were compared.

Another political issue was whether program criteria should be carefully defined or left broad and general. Those who saw the project primarily as a means of obtaining federal dollars for the health centers did not want to impose rules and regulations. The project advisory board, which consisted of experienced health educators, disagreed. But the board was overruled and few program criteria were set.

These decisions had major implications. They minimized the provision of technical assistance, eliminated quality control, and emphasized the provision of service at the expense of demonstration and evaluation.

Fourth, on an operational level, the project suffered from lack of an adequate project design. Well-defined objectives, measurable, time-limited objectives, sound project management and evaluation were virtually impossible. There was no clear description of the activities that had to be accomplished, no assessment of the resources needed, and no clear allocation of responsibility. Without this basic framework, the project advanced willy-nilly, falling farther and farther behind schedule.

Lack of a clear implementation strategy also left the project director unable to defend the need for additional staff. Without adequate manpower, some of the most important project activities could not be implemented. This was another reason that needs assessments, training, technical assistance, data collection, monitoring, and evaluation were partly or totally ignored.

The PERP tried to wed service provision and demonstration in the context of political pressures and the realities of rural life. It had mixed success. Despite the many problems encounterd, the project made a significant contribution to patient education in Maine's rural communities. It increased awareness of the importance of patient education and mustered new support for organized programs. It made possible the provision and expansion of patient education programs in rural health centers, many of which otherwise would not have had start-up capabilities.

Many lessons were learned over the course of the project. For example:

- A politically influential board may be an asset or a liability. Political clout lends strength to a project, but political pressure can misdirect project efforts.
- Voluntary participation by health centers and health center staff is essential. When providers are impelled to participate, additional fears and resentment have to be overcome.
- Programs need to be clearly defined. Otherwise it is impossible to measure the impact of alternative models.
- Standards of third-party payers need to be specified and integrated into program designs if reimbursement is desired.
- Greater expertise is needed in program planning and evaluation if the impact of patient education is to be documented.

The PERP eliminated funding as a barrier to developing patient education programs. The project's experience showed, however, that providing funds does not eliminate other problems or make the provision of patient education a simple process.

CONCLUSIONS

As the PERP demonstrated, the mere infusion of dollars does not make patient education possible or necessarily effective. Not all medical personnel are comfortable with or qualified for the role of patient educator. Adequate training and technical support are necessary before providers in isolated rural areas can meet the challenge.

The availability of resources, the staffing patterns, and the population base also affect the ability of health centers to develop and implement programs. Old and new alternatives for program arrangements should be considered at the regional and state level. These might include the following:

- Contracting with local hospitals for education services
- Hiring state level consultants to provide technical assistance to the health center staff
- Developing regional teams of health educators to travel among the health centers
- Sharing health education staff among several centers

Furthermore, assistance is essential regarding such issues as teaching methodology, program planning and evaluation, and disease-specific content areas. Expertise in these areas could be obtained from state, regional, and local agencies such as health departments, hospitals and medical centers, public and private institutions of higher education, consulting firms, and groups such as the Cooperative Extension Service.

Other social, political, and economic factors that are beyond the health centers' ability to control also influence the provision of patient education. These include manpower training programs, federal grants, state budgets, licensing, health care legislation, national heatlh insurance, unemployment, gasoline prices, and third-party reimbursement policies. All have effects that trickle down to the health center level and affect the need for and feasibility of offering various forms of patient education.

So many factors affect the success or failure of a new program that many facets of a health center's situation must be taken into account. This necessitates a solid planning process in which evaluation is an integral part. There is no universal prescription for implementing organized patient education, but a prospective plan for evaluation will anticipate key questions, and a sound project design will address them. The experience of Maine's rural health centers and the PERP would have been strengthened significantly had such planning and evaluation occurred.

REFERENCES

Henderson, A.; Bates, I.; and Sliepcevich, E. 1978. *Developing Health Education Programs in Rural Health Projects*. Carbondale: Southern Illinois University at Carbondale. Department of Health Education.

Mullane, M.; Duby, L.; Reynolds, R.; and Gold, R. 1980. "Patient Education Reimbursement: An Experiment in Maine." *International Quarterly of Community Health Education* 1(1):87–102.

Roemer, M. I. *Rural Health Care*. 1976. St. Louis: Mosby.

U.S. Department of Health, Education, and Welfare. Human Services Administration. Bureau of Community Health Services. 1976. *Rural Health Initiative: Program Guidance Material for RHI/HURA Grants*. Rockville, Md.

Analysis

This case describes the evaluation of an innovative patient education reimbursement project in which a health educator functioned as the project evaluator in consultation with a professionally trained evaluator. The focus of this case was evaluation. We do not know quite enough about the internal functioning of the programs at each site to determine their theoretical bases. We can assume, however, that sound theory was probably not a concern or an interest in developing and implementing the program and that the training needs were unsatisfied.

In contrast, the evaluation appeared to have a well-defined theoretical foundation in qualitative research. This research paradigm was chosen mostly out of necessity rather than out of allegiance to any paradigm. As the authors state, the evaluation did not begin until two years into the project, which eliminated the possibility of collecting many valuable data. In this evaluation, as in many qualitative evaluations, structured interviews were widely used. As Patton (1980:205) notes, "The fundamental principle of qualitative interviewing is to provide a framework within which respondents can express their own understandings in their own terms." The structured interview, also known as the standardized open-ended interview, has the following strengths, according to Patton: "Respondents answer the same questions, thus increasing comparability of responses: data are complete for each person on the topics addressed in the interview." Interviewer effects and bias are reduced when several interviewers are used. Decision makers are able to see and review the instrumentation used in the evaluation. Finally, the structured interview facilitates the organization and analysis of the data (Patton 1980).

Document review was the other prime method of data collection for the evaluation. Superficially, this seems like a straightforward process. However, there are a number of concerns that must be addressed if document review is to serve a useful purpose. There must be access to needed documents, which is predicated on knowing what is needed. Access to the complete document record is particularly crucial when dealing with multiple sites, as in this case. Negotiation for access to documents should take place before the evaluation and ideally before the program even begins. The documents, however, may be inaccurate, incomplete, and selective of only positive aspects of the program. They are likely to be of uneven quality, especially when many people are responsible for documentation, as is true with multiple sites. Information received from documents should therefore be triangulated with information from other sources to ensure reliability.

Although data collection is obviously an important issue in evaluation, this case highlights a number of other issues. For instance, there is the issue of reimbursement for patient education. Since the mid-1970s, several groups and individuals have been promoting third-party payment for patient education services. The hope is that patient education, for at least some diseases, will have a demonstrable effect on medical outcome, with accompanying cost savings. Therefore, if third-party payers covered patient education, this would stimulate further patient education programming, which would lead to further cost savings. So the task has been to determine whether patient education could affect outcome and cost; hence the program documented in this case.

However, implicit here is the question: When do you throw out the baby with the bath water? That is, if the intended medical outcomes and cost savings don't occur, does that mean that patient education has less potential than assumed? Not necessarily. It may mean that the methods utilized to carry out the program were inappropriate. Another question is whether the research or evaluation design is adequate for detecting the intended changes. In addition, questions must be directed to selection of subject, staff qualifications, resource allocations, administrative support, and the way the educational program fits in with total institutional goals.

A final issue is that of the health educator as evaluator (see the Windsor case p. 273), as well as the health educator's relationship to a professional evaluator. A professional evaluator is someone whose graduate training has specifically prepared her or him for upper-level evaluation positions. The truth is, however, that many evaluators of programs have no experience or training in health education. Very often they have research or evaluation backgrounds in sociology, psychology, or education. The evaluation team in the present case consisted of a graduate-level trained health educator and a professional evaluator. Such a combination is one way to ensure an adequate evaluation for a health education program. Another way is to train health educators in evaluation. Health educators who have had both evaluation training and direct program experience probably make the best evaluators of health education programs. Although some training of health educators in this regard is beginning to take place, the master's-level student is often exposed only to a research course that masquerades as an evaluation course, emphasizing experimental and quasi-experimental design without exploring levels of evaluation, or discussing how to manage and triangulate data and how to function in a practice setting.

References/Select Resources

Patton, M. Q. 1980. *Qualitative Evaluation Methods*. Beverly Hills: Sage Publications.

This book is widely recognized as the best introduction to qualitative evaluation. It is an excellent source on methods that are readily adaptable by the practitioner. It also provides the practitioner with the necessary background to convince others of the need for and the appropriateness of qualitative methods.

Windsor, R. A.; Baranowski, T.; Clark, N.; and Cutter, G. R. 1984. *Evaluation of Health Promotion and Education Programs*. Palo Alto, Calif.: Mayfield.

This is the first book-length treatment of evaluation methodology for health education. It provides the practitioner as well as the academician with the necessary tools and skills to evaluate programs ranging from the simple to the complex.

Zapka, J.; Schwartz, R.; and Giloth, B. 1982. *Locating Resources for Evaluation*. Chicago: American Hospital Association/Centers for Disease Control Health Education Project.

This annotated bibliography of evaluation resources is designed primarily for those responsible for evaluating patient education. However, it is very useful in any setting for anyone charged with evaluating health education.

Discussion Questions

1. What baseline data would you have collected in this case if you had had the opportunity to do so?
2. You have a meeting with the president of your state's Blue Cross Association to lobby for third-party reimbursement of patient education. What will you say?
3. Document review was one method of data collection used in this case. What are some other unobtrusive or nonreactive methods of data collection?
4. Besides diabetes and hypertension, what other diseases might be amenable to third-party reimbursement?
5. What problems could occur if an evaluation team consisted of a health educator and an evaluation specialist from another discipline?

Health Hazard Appraisal in a Family Practice Residency

Edward E. Bartlett, Dr.P.H.

In the 1940s the pendulum of American medicine began to swing away from the generalists and toward the specialists. The legacy of the esteemed "G.P." became fainter, and general practice came to be viewed as an anachronism by many. But this trend began to reverse itself in the 1950s and 1960s, aided by general practitioners' fear of their imminent demise, and later by the public's dismay at impersonal, fragmented specialist care and by governmental impatience about physician maldistribution. Ultimately, the American Board of Family Practice was established in 1969, which allowed physicians to pursue three years of residency training in order to sit for their "boards" in family medicine, and thus be viewed as specialists by their peers and the public.

Considerable effort was expended to identify the attributes that distinguished family medicine both from general practice and from the parallel specialty of internal medicine. The tenets of the primary care movement dictated that family medicine provide first-contact, whole-person, and longitudinal care. But family medicine philosophers went beyond those three essentials: not only should family practice take a family-centered approach, it also should place emphasis on the behavioral sciences, preventive medicine, and health education (Stephens 1976).

On July 1, 1980, I accepted a position as director of health education on the faculty of the Department of Family Practice at the University of Alabama in Birmingham. At that time, the faculty included seven other persons: five physicians (one part-time), a social worker, and a physician assistant with an M.P.H. who was working as an administrator in the department. There were 12 residents, 6 in their first year, 4 in their second year, and 2 in their third year.

The department had never employed a health educator before (or a nonphysician with a doctoral degree on the faculty). The principal health education activities were pamphlet racks in the waiting room and by the examination room; a collection of photocopied handouts on a variety of topics, stored in a file cabinet in the laboratory; and a motley collection of cardboard boxes filled with pamphlets, stored in an unused exam room. The task of the health educator was to develop "a comprehensive health education program," including preventive medicine activities. This case study details the evolution of one facet of this comprehensive program: health hazard appraisal (HHA).

Health Hazard Appraisal, also known as health risk analysis, is a means of identifying disease risk factors before a person becomes ill (Hall and Zwemer 1979). For example, a patient who smokes and eats a high-cholesterol diet would be at high risk for heart disease. The identification of these risk factors then serves as a basis for health education counseling and selected therapeutic interventions (e.g., control high blood pressure). Because of its importance for primary prevention and its applicability to clinical practice, I decided to attempt to implement HHA in the practice.

CHRONOLOGY OF EVENTS

The following chronology traces the evolution of the efforts to implement HHA in the Family Practice Center:

Edward E. Bartlett is an Assistant Professor in the Division of Health Education–Health Behavior, School of Public Health, and in the Department of Family Practice, School of Medicine, at the University of Alabama at Birmingham.

October 24, 1980 Noon lecture on "Integrating Prevention into Medical Practice: Health Hazard Appraisal or Periodic Health Screening?" for residency and faculty. Lecture compared HHA and periodic health screening and recommended the former for adult medical practice.

November 1 Special Saturday morning meeting called by chairman for all interested faculty, residents, and staff to select various forms for the medical record, including HHA. Agreed to use one of the computerized HHA forms developed by Medical Datamation, located in Bellevue, Ohio (exact version of HHA form not decided upon).

November (whole month) Met individually with M.D. faculty and residents to ascertain preference for length of HHA (possible lengths ranged from two to eight pages, costing $6–10 each). Most persons preferred the four-page version.

December 2 Chairman met with health educator and decided to order 100 copies of the two-page version of HHA. The two-page form was selected because of its lower cost.

December 16 Health educator knew that the chances of success with HHA would be greater if more people actively supported it. Therefore health educator proposed a research project to evaluate the effectiveness of HHA, in which interested faculty members and residents could participate. Chairman approved this idea.

January 2, 1981 First meeting of HHA Research Group. Two M.D. faculty members, two residents, nurse practitioner, and health educator attended. Basic research methodology was discussed and agreed upon.

January 7 Health educator met with nursing staff and receptionists for one hour to explain the use of HHA form.

January 15 Presentation at noon meeting to faculty and residents to formally present the form and answer questions.

February 4 One receptionist refused to make more telephone calls to arrange patient follow-up visits to discuss results of the HHA, stating that patients didn't want to have to come in just to discuss the HHA, especially if they would be charged extra for the visit. (This appointment-making responsibility subsequently was taken over by the secretary for the health educator).

Mid-February Generalized problems become apparent when patients fail to keep follow-up appointments and complain about being charged for the HHA.

March 4 Problems in implementation of HHA were discussed at meeting of HHA Research Committee; decided to try to charge patients for HHA at initial, not follow-up, visit, and to keep a list of patients who were given the form to improve follow-up. A hand-scored version of HHA ("Healthstyle," developed by the federal Office of Health Information and Health Promotion) was presented to the committee, which gave it a favorable response.

March–April HHA used less consistently than before in the clinic.

April 17 At its weekly meeting, faculty approved use of the hand-scored Healthstyle instead of the computer-scored HHA.

May 18 Computerized HHAs were removed from the clinic (125 had been distributed to patients during the previous four months) and data collection for research project was concluded. Healthstyle was placed in all clinic examination rooms with the sign: "To Our Patients: If you want to learn about ways to promote your health, fill out this paper and discuss it with your doctor today."

June–July Five to ten HHA forms used each week in the clinic (about 50 new patients were seen each week during this time).

July 31 Learned of "Request for Proposals" for the Robert Wood Johnson Foundation for innovative medical care projects; began to consider various projects to propose.

August 14 Preliminary results of HHA research project were presented to faculty and residents; consensus of discussion that followed indicated that HHA should be a part of medical practice, but the physician often might refer this task to others (e.g., the nurse practitioner).

August 21 Chairman decided that the RWJ Foundation proposal should focus on research of the effectiveness of HHA.

September 22 RWJ proposal mailed.

October 5 Nurse practitioner proposed to the medical director to implement a "Health Promotion Flow Sheet" (HPFS) to be used in conjunction with the HHA, which listed such screening procedures as blood pressure, weight, Pap smear, rectal exam, hemoglobin, and cholesterol.

October 19 After several discussions, medical director agreed to use HPFS and to have receptionists give HHA to all new patients in the waiting room and to place HPFS in their medical records for their physician to implement.

October 22 Upon trying to arrange meeting with receptionists to carry this out, health educator was informed by a departmental administrative assistant that "we are not ready to implement the forms." (This statement probably was the result of the perception of the administrative assistant's supervisor that the medical director did not have the authority to approve the inclusion of HPFS in patients' charts.)

October 30 Implementation of HHA and HPFS approved by chairman and faculty at weekly meeting, as agreed on October 19.

Early November Nurse practitioner met with each resident to ascertain his or her preference for use of either HHA or HPFS and whether the resident wanted to do it or refer this to the nurse practitioner. Virtually all residents stated they did want this to be used in their practice and that they preferred to do it themselves.

November 11 Meeting with receptionists held to discuss faculty decision of October 30 and to solicit their input about specific details of implementation.

November 12 Implementation of HHA and HPFS by receptionists began.

December 9 Letter received from RWJ Foundation that proposal had not been approved.

January 29, 1982 Completed review of medical records of selected new patients seen since January 1. Of the 20 charts with a completed HHA form in them, *none* of them indicated that any HHA counseling had been done by the physician, as suggested by the absence of any notation in the Progress Notes, in the Problem List, and in the HPFS. Only one HPFS was found on which the physician had made an entry of any sort.

DISCUSSION

The principal advocates of HHA were the health educator and the nurse practitioner. The medical director also was interested in HHA partly because of its potential for marketing the services of the Family Practice Center to prospective patients.

During the second year of continuous effort to implement HHA, one acquired a feeling of déjà vu: a repetitive cycle of discussions and negotiations with faculty; meetings with receptionists to explain revised procedures; no overt resistance by residents during discussions but glaring indications of benign neglect when they saw patients; more data collection; discussions with faculty; revised procedures; and so on.

Consideration of the reasons for the difficulties in implementing the HHA leads to an examination of the issue from several perspectives. A review of comments by faculty and residents and reflection on my experiences in this position provided several insights. An analysis of the health educator/resident relationship from the perspective of power casts further light on the issue. Finally, an analysis of the adoption of an innovation by the individual residents and the diffusion of an innovation in an organization (the Family Practice Department) offers additional answers.

COMMENTS BY FACULTY AND RESIDENTS

Comments made by various faculty and residents help to explain why difficulties were being encountered:

1. "It might be because of the source."—M.D. faculty member, referring to fact that the health educator is not a physician.
2. "The results of the HHAs are very similar—the patient is overweight, smokes, doesn't

use seat belts, and doesn't exercise. Once you've told the patient to quit smoking, etc., what else is there to do?"—M.D. faculty member.

3. "All this stuff about prevention is full of crap."—Resident.
4. "I wouldn't know what to say to the patient if a patient had a high score in one of the risk areas."—Resident who was an active member of the HHA Research Committee.
5. "Nobody is going to tell me how to practice medicine."—Resident.
6. "The doctors don't want another burden."—M.D. faculty member.
7. "Doctors don't want to do clinical activities for which they will end up in the poorhouse."—M.D. faculty member, referring to the fact that preventive medicine and counseling are sometimes not reimbursed by third-party payers.
8. "Maybe the physicians don't have enough time to do HHA."—Statement of several people.
9. "Patients don't want to pay just to get the results of their HHA—they prefer to pay for procedures and prescriptions, not advice."—Resident.
10. "The patients don't understand the meaning of figures and statistics. How can the numbers be true, because the patient could be killed in a car wreck tomorrow?"—Resident.
11. "I didn't understand the meaning of all the numbers on the computerized results form."—Resident.

Not all physicians in the department would agree with all these comments, but they do provide insight into the attitudes and perceptions of some.

In reviewing these comments and reflecting upon other experiences, I concluded that the following factors contributed to HHA being viewed as peripheral rather than central to medical practice by the residents:

1. Physicians are paid for treating sick people, not for keeping them healthy. Thus HHA was not perceived to be financially rewarding in real-world medical practice.
2. Residents see their residency training as primarily a means of gaining experience in diagnosing and treating illness. They believe that knowledge about topics such as health education and prevention can be "picked up" once they get into practice. Because preventive activities will inherently reduce patient utilization, HHA was perceived as basically inimical to the residents' educational goals for their residency experience.
3. Physicians are less comfortable with *educational* approaches to patient care than with procedure-oriented *medical* approaches. Giving an immunization to prevent polio is a precise task; counseling and educating about life-style is hazy, unpredictable, and perhaps superfluous. The intricacies and challenges inherent in life-style modification are not perceived as such by most physicians.
4. Patients who believe strongly in health promotion see physicians infrequently, their reasons being both attitudinal (they don't like to go to doctors) and biological (they are healthier anyway). Physicians therefore see a biased sample of the population who are less interested in prevention and are less willing to pay for such services.

It is questionable that lack of time is a valid reason for not using HHA. The average American physician now works 49.6 hours a week (Goldfarb 1981:146). This figure will probably decrease as the physician surplus increases. In the Family Practice Center, high-level administrators believed that most residents had time to see twice as many patients as they did. Even if a physician did not have the extra few minutes to discuss HHA with the patient, this responsibility could be referred to a mid-level practitioner or the health educator.

Although there are other reasons why using HHA poses problems to the average medical practice (e.g., difficulties in explaining the meaning of statistics to patients, imprecision of statistics), the four reasons just listed are believed to be the most important.

BEHAVIORAL SCIENCE PERSPECTIVES

POWER

Power is defined as the ability of agent O to influence the state of agent P; "agent" refers to a person, organization, political party, or nation, and "state" includes the agent's behavior, beliefs, attitudes, or politics. Power has been studied from the perspectives of community politics (Rossi 1966) and interpersonal relationships (French and Raven 1968). This discussion rests on the second approach.

In their classic paper on the bases of social power, French and Raven cite five sources of interpersonal power:

1. *Reward Power*—ability of O to influence P with desired material incentives (e.g., salary, gifts)
2. *Coercive power*—ability of O to punish P (e.g., impose a fine, revoke privileges)
3. *Legitimate power*—based on the internalized values of P that O has a legitimate right to influence P
4. *Reference power*—based on the psychological identification of P with O
5. *Expert power*—based on P's perception of O's expertness in a given area of knowledge

These five bases of power are applied to the association of the health educator (O) with the family practice residents (P) in Table 1.

The questions of legitimate, referent, and expert power of the health educator in medical education were found to revolve around the issue of whether a person has completed four years of medical school, not issues of clinical acumen, relative contribution to a person's health, research abilities, community service, administrative contributions, or service orientation to patients.

The paramount importance granted to the possession of an M.D. degree highlights the difficulties of the non-M.D. in influencing an M.D. This recurrent problem brings out the latent issue of medical chauvinism, which implies that other bodies of health-related knowledge are believed to be either a subset of medical knowledge (e.g., nursing, pharmacy) or a genus substantially irrelevant to clinical practice (e.g., behavioral science, epidemiology). There are several corollaries to this belief:

1. Medical care is the most important contributor to a person's health and is virtually identical with health care.
2. Physicians are preeminent in all matters pertaining to health, and all health professionals should work under a physician's direction.

Table 1

Health Educator's Influence on Family Practice Residents by Type of Power

Type of Power	Degree of Power		
	High	Medium	Low
Reward			X
Coercive			X
Legitimate			X
Referent			X
Expert		X	

3. Only physicians can make important contributions to training medical students and residents.
4. Physicians should not be held accountable to other health professionals or to patients.
5. Physicians should be paid a higher salary than other health professionals.

These beliefs are basic to the feelings and actions of most physicians in their interface with other health professionals. The effect is to lessen the credibility and power of the nonphysician in a medical setting.

ADOPTION OF AN INNOVATION BY INDIVIDUALS (RESIDENTS)

Among the important factors that determine whether an innovation will be accepted are the characteristics of the innovation itself (Rogers 1971):

1. *Relative advantage*—medium to high relative advantage of HHA to improve a person's health, but low relative advantage to help treat the patient for the patient's medical problem. It is not clear whether physicians' main interest is to improve persons' overall health or to treat their immediate medical complaint.
2. *Compatibility*—low to medium compatibility with values and needs of physicians, for the reasons cited earlier (see pp. 136–137).
3. *Complexity*—very high complexity because of the nature of the educational-behavioral ap-

proaches required for life-style modification.
4. *Trialability*—high trialability by residents to see how HHA can fit into their practice habits.
5. *Observability of benefits*—low to medium because health education's attempt to influence life-style is not always successful, and because the health benefits of behavior change may not become apparent for years.

This analysis suggests that to the extent that physicians are interested in treating patients for their immediate problem, and to the extent that they prefer medical over educational approaches to patient care, HHA will have a poor chance of being adopted. But some physicians have a greater commitment to preventive medicine and therefore will be more likely to use HHA.

DIFFUSION OF INNOVATIONS IN AN ORGANIZATION (FAMILY PRACTICE DEPARTMENT)

Zaltman, Duncan, and Holbek (1973:185) suggest that the following steps occur in the adoption of an innovation by an organization:

1. Change in structure and/or function of the external environment
2. Performance gap
3. Felt need to change structure and/or functioning of organization
4. Use of persuasion to get others to see that change is needed
5. Search for solution: use (modify) existing solution or develop new solution
6. Identification of most appropriate alternative
7. Decision making to adopt most appropriate solution
8. Sustained implementation of solution
9. Change in organization

Steps 1–7 are considered the *initiation* phase, and steps 8–9 constitute the *implementation* phase.

Zaltman and colleagues identified five variables that are crucial to the successful diffusion of innovations in organizations:

1. *Complexity*—number of occupational specialties, degree of task differentiation
2. *Formalization*—degree of emphasis on following specific rules and procedures in the organization
3. *Centralization*—extent to which authority and decision making are delegated to others lower in the organizational hierarchy
4. *Interpersonal relations*—ability of persons to maintain good personal relationships with others
5. *Dealing with conflict*—ability to address and resolve differences of opinion

Examining these five variables in terms of the initiation and implementation phases of the adoption process, we see that the last two variables—good interpersonal relations and ability to deal with conflict—are important during *both* phases. However, the three other variables operate in opposite directions during the two phases (Zaltman, Duncan, and Holbek 1973:159). The following are conditions most favorable to the adoption of an innovation by an organization:

Initiation Stage	Implementation Stage
Higher complexity	Lower complexity
Lower formalization	Higher formalization
Lower centralization	Higher centralization

For example, during the initiation stage a greater range of innovative ideas can be generated when persons from a variety of professional backgrounds are involved, when greater flexibility of rules and procedures is permitted, and when decision making is less centralized. However, the opposite occurs during the implementation stage.

Applying the five variables to the department of family practice, the following analysis emerges:

1. *Complexity*—medium to high
2. *Formalization*—low
3. *Centralization*—low centralization in generation of new ideas, high in having them approved, and low in implementation stage
4. *Interpersonal skills*—medium
5. *Conflict resolution*—low to medium, depending on the personalities and issues involved

This analysis indicates that innovation is facilitated better in the initiation stage than in the implementation stage in this organization; the low centralization apparent in the implementation phase makes it extraordinarily difficult to accomplish permanent organizational change. This situation accounts for the repeated problems encountered in implementation of the HHA in the clinic, including the residents' tepid response and the receptionist's lack of cooperation.

SUMMARY

This case study has reviewed the process of implementation during a 16-month period of HHA in a training program for family practice residents. What might appear on the surface to be a fairly simple innovation to implement (a one-page form to practice preventive medicine) proved to be much more difficult to integrate into the practice than one might expect. These difficulties then were analyzed from the perspectives of power and diffusion of innovations, which shed considerable light on the roots of the problem.

It is believed that as long as physicians have no financial incentive to practice preventive medicine, and as long as organizational patterns of authority and decision making remain the same, HHA certainly will be tolerated, but probably never enthusiastically embraced.

REFERENCES

French, J. R. P., and Raven, B. 1968. "The Bases of Social Power." In *Group Dynamics*, edited by D. Cartwright and A. Zander. New York: Harper & Row.

Goldfarb, D. L., ed. 1981. *Profile of Medical Practice, 1981*. Chicago: American Medical Association.

Hall, J. H., and Zwemer, J. D. 1979. *Prospective Medicine*. Indianapolis: Methodist Hospital of Indiana.

Rogers, E., and Shoemaker, F. 1971. *Communication of Innovations: A Cross-Cultural Approach*. 2d ed. New York: Free Press.

Rossi, P. H. 1966. "Power and Community Structure." In *Political Sociology*, edited by L. A. Coser. New York: Harper & Row.

Stephens, G. G. 1976. "Reform in the United States: Its Impact on Medicine and Education for Family Practice." *Journal of Family Practice* 3:507–512.

Zaltman, G.; Duncan, R.; and Holbek, J. 1973. *Innovations and Organizations*. New York: Wiley-Interscience.

Analysis

This case focuses on the health educator assessing a means to integrate health education principles into medical practice. Bartlett selected a strategy and devised a plan to meet the need. The case illustrates that although there may be verbal expression of interest in meeting a need, a target population may not be committed to pursuing that interest. It also illustrates the dichotomy between research and practice. The health educator was forced to modify the research aspects of the project to accommodate the practice aspects.

Bartlett analyzes the reasons for the failure of the Health Hazard Appraisal project from the perspectives of power, the adoption of an innovation by an individual, and the diffusion of an innovation in an organization.

Concepts in learning/social change theory also explain the nonacceptance of HHA by the residents. For example: the source of information was not considered credible; the residents did not perceive HHA to be useful or meaningful for them; the environment in which they worked, the medical care setting, did not support the use of HHA by paying for preventive activities; this new behavior was not acceptable to the residents' social group (note their comments about it); and because learning has an affective dimension, often more powerful than the cognitive dimension, some saw HHA as threatening to their livelihood (see p. 137).

The strategy employed by the health educator to introduce HHA to the residents was one with which the residents were familiar—soliciting their input and suggestions regarding desirable approaches and procedures and providing them with information. Medical education depends heavily on the lecture and other types of information-giving as a methodology.

Zaltman and Duncan (1977:198–200) list a number of basic qualifications for the change agent, such as technical qualifications, administrative ability, interpersonal relations, motivation and drive, commitment, character, personal security, poise, and backbone. In this instance the qualifications of the change agent were not the issue. It wouldn't have made a great deal of difference how qualified the change agent was. The target population was not interested in changing, and that is the central point this case makes.

The quoted comments of the residents and faculty regarding HHA certainly suggest that HHA was not a priority in their practice. Granted, the misunderstandings or lack of information about the use and interpretation of HHA would interfere with their using it. But anyone interested in HHA could easily learn how it should be interpreted and what to say to the patient.

It may seem incongruous that these physicians were not interested in a preventive tool such as the HHA. In fact, though, their disinterest was totally consonant with the goals and training of physicians. Physicians are trained to diagnose and treat disease. The system rewards diagnostic ability and effective treatment. It does not reward prevention of disease. Most medical students are not exposed to prevention in their training. If it is included in the curriculum, it is given minimal time. One cannot blame medical students for thinking it is not important. To their mind, if it were important, it would command more time in the medical school curriculum.

Individual physicians may be interested in prevention. But to expect the medical care system to be interested is probably unrealistic. The Rosenberg case (p. 216) illustrates ways of carrying out preventive activity within the system. However, in that case, very little involvement was required by the physician.

References/Select Resources

Katz, D., and Kahn, R. L. 1978. *The Social Psychology of Organizations.* New York: Wiley.

This book is an excellent resource on organizations and organizational theory. It is a comprehensive, meaty volume about organizations as members of social systems. It deals with the effect of organizations on individuals; the environmental forces that impinge on and are created by organizations; organizational changes; organization models; and the structure and development of organizations and research in these areas. It is probably most appropriately used at the graduate level.

May, J. T.; Durham, M. L.; and New, P. K. 1980. "Professional Control and Innovation: The Neighborhood Health Center Experience." In *Research in Sociology of Health Care*, vol. 1, edited by J. A. Roth. Greenwich, Conn.: JAI Press.

This paper reports on a study of policy formulation, both formal and informal, associated with "innovative" health care programs. It focuses on the role of physician control in this regard. Data were collected through focused interviews of Neighborhood Health Center leadership. Grounded theory was the analytical tool. The study's findings support the conclusions about the introduction of an innovation in a medical setting that were arrived at in the Bartlett case.

Robbins, L. C., and Hall, J. H. 1970. *How to Practice Prospective Medicine.* Indianapolis: Slaymaker Enterprises.

This document provides useful historical data on the development of the Health Hazard Appraisal. It offers a rationale for its inclusion in primary care, specifically family medicine. It also presents the statistical data on which the risk appraisal is based and describes the method of calculating risk.

Zaltman, G., and Duncan, R. 1977. *Strategies for Planned Change.* New York: Wiley.

This basic resource for the health educator as change agent defines and describes the steps in the process of change. Part 2, "Strategies for Change," is particularly relevant to this case. It offers a more detailed explanation of the issues that hindered change than is provided in the case study.

Discussion Questions

1. Do you think the true response of the family practice residents to the HHA could have been known before implementation of the project?
    a. If you do think so, how could their expected response have been determined?
    b. Justify the practicality of your approach or specify why you believe your approach would have identified the real feelings of the residents about the HHA.
2. What early clues did the health educator get that the project was not going to fly?
3. Develop an education program for a group of patients who have taken the HHA. Describe the theory and methodology you would use to help the patients understand the meaning of the HHA to them and take necessary action.
4. Identify the value and the limitations of an instrument such as the HHA.
5. Identify preventive procedures that you believe could be integrated into medical practice. Describe how you think this could be done.

A Health Education Service in an Acute Care Hospital

Anna W. Skiff, M.S.P.H.

This case discusses patient education activities of a health education service in an acute care hospital. It outlines the hospital system, the population served, and certain special features of the setting. The origin, organization, and responsibilities of the the health education service are sketched, as is the rationale for program emphasis on patient education. Events and forces that shaped educational opportunities are identified, and issues related to the health educator's role in an acute care setting are considered. Although the health educator also had responsibility for work in the community and for employee health education, these aspects will not be described here.

BACKGROUND

This 400-bed U.S. Public Health Service Hospital cared for the acutely ill on its medical, surgical, psychiatric, and pediatric services, maintained a dialysis unit for those with end-stage renal disease, and treated persons with Hansen's disease. There was no obstetrical service. There was a large active ambulatory service. The hospital conducted education and training programs for several categories of health personnel and carried on basic and clinical research. Medical and dental leadership was supplied by full-time staff.

Several special features of the hospital system need to be mentioned because they may have influenced how the health education program developed and functioned. First, as already stated, the medical and dental staff were full-time and salaried. Most were members of the Commissioned Corps of the Public Health Service, one of the five uniformed services of the United States. Therefore they were more easily available to staff than other physicians and dentists in most voluntary hospitals. Further, because patients were the clients of the system rather than of any individual practitioner, some of the tensions stemming from proprietary concerns were less likely to occur.

Second, financial considerations rarely impinged on health professional/patient relationships. Beneficiaries, either as ambulatory or as hospitalized patients, received needed treatments and medications without cost.

Third, continuity of care was ensured for most because both ambulatory care and hospitalization were provided. In many respects the system functioned like an HMO offering total care in a closed system. The full benefits and promise of continuity could not always be achieved because, although senior clinicians remained relatively constant, the intern and resident staff rotated periodically. However, opportunities for follow-through and follow-up were facilitated by having the persons discharged from the hospital scheduled for return to a clinic. The integrated medical record helped link all aspects of care.

Fourth, for a number of years the future of the Public Health Service system in providing direct medical care through its own hospitals and clinics was uncertain. Would the hospitals continue? If so, what should be their mission? Should they be closed? Seemingly settled in 1972, these questions resurfaced in 1977 and in 1980. The system was dissolved in 1981. The instability engendered by debate hampered optimal program planning and

---

Anna W. Skiff is the former Chief of the Health Education Branch of the Division of Hospitals and Clinics, Health Services Administration, U.S. Public Health Service. She is now retired.

implementation. There was too much tentativeness, too many "ifs," too much time spent putting out fires.

THE HEALTH EDUCATION SERVICE

Several factors converged to bring about the establishment of a health education program at the Public Health Service Hospital, Staten Island, in 1967. One was the increasing attention nationwide to the responsibility of health care institutions for education of patients. Another was an enlarged mandate for the Public Health Service hospitals, which encouraged and authorized them to become more active in providing service in the communities where they were located—an involvement that would require expanded outreach efforts. Last was the attitude of the hospital's director, who was personally convinced of the importance of health education and who had, in previous public health assignments, worked with health educators and knew what they could do to interpret health programs and goals.

The program was in place from 1967 until November 1981, when the federally conducted Public Health Service system of hospitals and clinics was terminated. The new program was launched with the formation of an Office of Health Education within the Office of the Director and the employment of an education specialist for health to head the effort. In 1977, in an administrative reorganization, the Office of Health Education became the Health Education Service, reporting to the associate director for hospital services. All hospital departments except medicine, dentistry, and administrative services were part of Hospital Services.

The program was fortunate in having strong administrative backing both initially in the Office of the Director and in later years from the associate director for hospital services. This support took the form of explicit reference to the importance of the program at professional staff meetings and recommendations to those planning educational projects to seek assistance from the health educator. The educator was also appointed to membership on a number of hospital committees.

When the health education unit was formed, the administrative placement was designed to permit the program to work across departmental lines, and the educator's position was classified at a sufficiently high level to make possible easy interaction with heads of other departments. In the course of the program's existence, it was headed by two persons. The first person who filled the post was an education specialist with several years of successful experience in a large city health department. He held the position for three years, during which time he not only established the program within the hospital but also became deeply involved in community health affairs. He was particularly effective in linking the hospital's resources and mission with pressing local community concerns of the 1960s before moving on to another position within the Public Health Service. In June 1971, after the post had been vacant for about a year, I came on the scene and remained until the hospital passed from federal management. My prior experience included a 10-year stint as a medical technologist and 20 years in community health education.

GOALS

The Health Education Service had the following responsibilities:

1. Provide consultation in the planning and execution of coordinated health education services for inpatients, outpatients, employees, and community agencies and organizations.
2. Stimulate hospital staff to give greater priority to the performance of educational tasks essential to the provision of personal health services.
3. Serve as a resource to staff by aiding the health team in developing and appraising the educational component of health services.
4. Identify resources that might be used in carrying out educational activities.
5. Assist the hospital staff in planning and executing health education aspects of pre- and in-service training programs.
6. Participate in education programs in cooperation with community organizations related to health protection and promotion.
7. Serve as a liaison between the community

and the hospital to interpret community services provided by the hospital.

In this listing of responsibilities, the emphasis on a "staff," as opposed to a "line," role is striking. The position description that was developed with consultation from an experienced community health educator reflected a sophisticated view of the task to be undertaken and invaded little turf of other health professionals already on the scene. From the formulation, it followed that the educator would work primarily through others in a supportive and consultative role.

In 1981 the direct outlay for the service, including the educator's salary, the pro-rated salary of the secretary (which was shared), employee benefits, and materials, was about $60,000.

The service was initially located in a small office on a well-traveled corridor close to the director's office and on the path to the medical library. This placement and my open door favored many informal communications with staff and eased the way for our explorations of what activities might be of mutual interest. Later, relocation to another building off the beaten track put an end to these casual but important exchanges. Getting visibility and earning credibility and acceptance are essential first steps and ongoing requirements in program development.

Although the stated responsibilities of the Health Education Service directed that attention be given to patient, employee, and community health education, I gave highest priority to improving communications with patients for several reasons:

1. The health care institution has a direct responsibility to assure that the patients who come to it can manage safely when they leave.
2. The proper management of many conditions requires patient participation and understanding for optimum results.
3. The hospital as a training institution is the setting where most staff learn what is expected of them as practicing professionals, and education of patients represents such an expectation.
4. Patients and their families learn from hospital experiences how to behave in other circumstances vis-à-vis the health system and its providers.

For these reasons and others, I realized how important it is to make teaching and learning a part of the hospital experience.

In addition, to concentrate on patient education, I knew that I had to resist my own background. It would have been far easier for me to divert my attention to community affairs, in which I was experienced and comfortable—to retreat to the familiar—than to tackle the job at hand. In addition, at that time in the evolution of health education in the hospital setting, it was important to try to show administrators what could be done with patient populations. Administrators across the country had to be persuaded (many still do) of even the relevance and practicality of education for patients and shunned the notion of health or community education as a proper function of a hospital. In 1971 only a handful of hospitals had an organized patient education service. Concrete achievement in patient education in the Public Health Service Hospital might be helpful in stimulating programs elsewhere.

Strong beliefs shaped my approach to patient education. First, there was my conviction that almost every patient has some learning needs. Second, I believed that the teaching/learning experience should occur in, and be the responsibility of, each department or service providing service to a patient. I agree with a statement made by Linda Aiken (1970:1918): "If we view patient teaching in terms of formal instruction, it is possible to delegate the responsibility to one or two persons. If we believe that patient teaching is an on-going process, then each [staff person] providing a treatment or service must assume this responsibility. Since in my opinion patient teaching *is* an on-going process, all staff need to be prepared to carry out this function." Third, it is in an atmosphere of caring that the sharing of ideas and information can be most effective. Unless this climate prevails—a climate of caring, respect, and trust in the ability of most persons to manage their own affairs—effective patient education cannot occur.

In a successful translation of these beliefs, the hospital as an entity would be engaged in patient education. Patient teaching would no longer be restricted to providing information about just a few disorders or be viewed as the domain of only one or two professional groups.

IMPLEMENTATION

What happened as program responsibilities were carried out and assumptions tested? A special health education committee was not established. Instead, work was undertaken on an ad hoc basis with departmental people and with existing and newly created hospital committees to resolve problems that their work identified.

A look at involvement with other staff and departments shows that at some time or other the Health Education Service had worked with almost every unit in some capacity. Some encounters were brief and quite superficial; others were more sustained and substantial. Often the opening wedge was a request to help prepare an exhibit or to provide a pamphlet or film. (The Health Education Office stocked a large supply of pamphlets on many topics.) Relationships built upon satisfying these requests often led to other joint efforts.

In my experience, most health workers are well aware of or sensitive about their deficiencies in helping patients understand their conditions. However, they are action-oriented, sometimes pressed for time, and sometimes lack the necessary content or skills to help patients learn. The resulting anxiety propels them to seek an all-purpose instructional method or tool or protocol that will do the job for them. The Health Education Service had available a variety of teaching tools—flip charts, outlines, leaflets, protocols, and a series of video tapes. Except for brief flurries of interest, they remained unused. Somehow they did not fit well into the practitioner's system of working. Seldom did they exactly match a particular patient's needs.

One of the tasks of the educator, and one I came to realize only after a long time, is to help staff members gain confidence that they have the information patients need; that most learning needs of patients are not complex; that most teaching is just explaining, not a lecture in Biology 301; that a number of disciplines share responsibility for helping patients learn; and that techniques such as effective interviewing and listening can be acquired to help do the job. With more experience, I saw indications that most hospital stays allow the transmittal of only minimal essential information and that it is in an ambulatory setting that more extensive educational interventions can be undertaken.

I was involved in all but a few of the hospital staff's educational ventures. The initiative usually came from a clinical service or department, but at some point (often, at first, to provide materials for the project) I had a chance to shape what happened. For example, not long after several different health professionals began meeting regularly to try to improve their service to patients with progressive cancer, I was invited to join them. This group gradually developed a multifaceted program that included a support group for patients and their families, a sporadically published newsletter, continuing staff- and self-development, and patient and family education. On a few occasions, I became more aggressive or assertive in working with them than was my custom. For example, when the group was planning a practical training session for families caring for the terminally ill, I insisted that they rehearse their presentations to help ensure conformance to time constraints and objectives. At a meeting during which the program was evaluated, I pointed out to the very satisfied presenters our deficiencies as well as accomplishments. But only rarely did I assume such an assertive stance with any group.

Some of the biggest boosts that health education received was through the good offices of the frequently maligned regulatory bodies. Demands for informed consent and quality assurance, which involved requirements of the Joint Commission on the Accreditation of Hospitals and Professional Standards Review Organization, highlighted the need to communicate more effectively with patients. I was called on to participate in the development of tools and approaches to meet these demands.

In respect to informed consent, as a member of the hospital's Research Committee, I came to be an advocate for clear explanations to potential subjects to ensure their informed participation. From time to time I assisted in revising the consent forms to simplify and clarify them. This role gave me access to researchers and physicians to discuss issues related to communication and understanding. A knowledge of ways to assess readability and comprehension levels was helpful here as well as in reviewing other written materials used in the hospital.

An audit had demonstrated how poorly many patients were informed about practices to be followed after discharge. Therefore, to help satisfy requirements of quality assurance, a multidisciplinary group prepared, and the hospital adopted, a form on which the physician's discharge instructions were to be recorded and given to each patient. A physician assumed responsibility for explaining to the medical staff the importance of the form and the requirements for its use. It was easier to get the form prepared and adopted than to assure its correct and routine use by the staff. Illegible, unintelligible documents were often given to patients. Ways needed to be devised to monitor use and identify and discipline those who failed to use it well. How to achieve proper completion of necessary documents is an ongoing problem, as most medical records departments will attest. Paperwork can be a burden. Nevertheless, for some physicians and for some patients in this instance, the process proved worthwhile.

Another problem was one uncovered by the Discharge Planning Subcommittee, a multidisciplinary group that proposed policies, objectives, and procedures for discharge—work in which the education of patients formed a large component. The subcommittee's work disclosed a great gap in physician-nurse communication that not only restricted effective communication of the nurse with patients and family members but also impeded scheduling of treatments, nursing home placement, and so on. And remember, this was a hospital where the medical staff was full-time! To help close the gap between the professionals, weekly physician-nurse conferences were scheduled. Members of the subcommittee monitored these sessions for some months to encourage their occurrence. The nursing service coached its head nurses to assist them in making the best use of this conference time with physicians. And again, some services responded well and maintained their weekly conference, while others encountered all kinds of difficulties and meetings petered out with no adverse repercussions on the professionals.

Next, at the request of staff nurses, the Discharge Planning Subcommittee developed precisely defined instructional objectives for three commonly occurring conditions: hypertension, chronic obstructive pulmonary disease (COPD), and diabetes. An educator provided leadership here by introducing nominal group process as a method for identifying the topics to be covered and for setting priorities among them.

The different perspectives and understandings of the disciplines represented on the subcommittee resulted in a brief yet surprisingly comprehensive set of practical instructional goals. Responsibility for meeting them was to be shared among disciplines, with "lead" responsibility assigned for a particular topic and performance verified through sign-off. Each discipline made systematic efforts to prepare staff to use these forms. Compliance was spotty. Staff shortages, staff turnover, and other unit upheavals reportedly contributed to the poor response. Still another factor in the failure to use these outlines may have been the unwieldiness of using separate forms for each situation requiring intensive instruction or assessment of the need for instruction.

As I think back, one of the outstanding characteristics of the ten-year experience was the number of multidisciplinary activities that took place. The Discharge Planning Subcommittee, the weekly pediatric conference, the weekly rehabilitation unit meeting, and the cancer support group come immediately to mind. They were invaluable in helping ensure the delivery of consistent messages to patients and families, with attention to the many dimensions of need.

In delivery of information to patients and families, one-to-one conversations were the most frequently employed mode. This approach is the most adaptable to the time slots available and permits the greatest response to individual need. Its weaknesses are well known; unless it is expertly used, omissions and misunderstandings abound.

Group sessions were conducted for only a few conditions. Classes for hospitalized diabetics were held regularly throughout the ten-year period and had antedated the establishment of the Health Education Service. From time to time educational group sessions were initiated for persons with other conditions, notably heart ailments and weight control problems, but these sessions tended to lapse as staff enthusiasm waned, assignments changed, and other demands interposed. There are a number of very real obstacles in carrying out classes for hospitalized patients: short lengths of stay, variations in severity and seriousness of the same disorder, recency of onset, discomfort and/or weakness of the "student," lack of suitable location, transportation problems, and scheduling conflicts, as well as wide variations in the health professionals' skills and aptitudes for instruction.

The group of health professionals who presented a group program for patients with COPD gave the most educationally sound program, in my opinion, thanks to the leadership and ability of the physician. It was a *series* of sessions involving the *same* group of invited patients—most being followed on an ambulatory basis. Each session included practice of a skill, the provision of information about some aspect of care (e.g., medications, nature of illness, nutrition, or early detection of problems), and opportunity for questions. The multidisciplinary group that developed the program met to evaluate its progress at the conclusion of each series and made changes based on its review. Some concrete positive outcomes were observed in some patients who took part. This group, like others working with patients, sometimes had the discouraging experience of poor responses to their invitation to attend sessions.

One of the most difficult tasks in working in the health care setting was to impress upon eager would-be teachers what is involved in planning and implementing an educational program—to help them see that "an idea is not a program." The physician's firm leadership and his understanding not only of what constituted a program but also of the need to plan and review as well as to present made the COPD instructional sessions unique. The Health Education Service was not involved in this program except to secure needed materials. Here was the instance in which a staff member (the physician) was eminently able to organize and carry out a program.

One of the stated functions of the Health Education Service was to stimulate staff to carry out their educational responsibilities. When I began to work at the hospital, I wrote down for myself my objectives. First among them was the intent to influence physicians in training to fulfill their educational responsibilities. In all honesty, I must confess almost total failure in that regard. The steps taken to achieve the objective were as follows:

1. Each year at professional staff meetings formal presentations called attention to the need for education of patients, the contribution of education to desired outcome and professional satisfaction, and the resources available to help.
2. Attempts were made on two occasions to interest the director of medical education (a part-time responsibility) in including, as a planned part of physicians' postgraduate training, discussions of the education role and the attainment of proficiency in its performance.

My recommendations fell on deaf ears. One reason for this might have been that the director of medical education saw his role as primarily an administrative one, that is, scheduling and routing trainees, with little responsibility for the trainees once they were dispatched to various chiefs of service. In fact, these chiefs might well have resisted any intervention in their training programs. It occurs to me now, that the stronger approach might have been to talk to the chiefs individually to make a case for developing educational skills.

An important factor in the unsuccessful ventures with the interns was their need to concentrate on developing and strengthening basic clinical skills. The nursing staff, harassed by turnover and short-staffed, was not in a much better situation, although its leadership expressed interest in improving patient teaching. The nurses as a group were responding to pressures in their profession to extend their role and were by and large accepting education of patients as part of that role. The leadership was capable and experienced, but it was constantly faced with the need to train in routine procedures because of the uneven preparation of its staff nurses.

Several times during the ten-year period, I was involved with formal efforts of the nursing service to improve the ability of nurses to instruct patients. Carefully planned programs designed by the in-service nursing staff with my participation were presented to create awareness of the importance of teaching, to provide information about the teaching/learning process and about the availability of resources, and to develop skills in setting instructional objectives. A variety of teaching techniques were used in these sessions.

How well the information and skills acquired in these sessions were applied is not clear to me. Hindsight suggests that much more follow-up by head nurses back on the units was required to encourage use of the approaches recommended and to overcome system obstacles to their use. A continuing problem for the nursing service was the turnover among head nurses and staff nurses, which made it extremely difficult to have people available who were prepared to provide education or any other component of care in a consistent fashion.

From time to time trainees in the pharmacy and diet departments also sought help from the Health Education Service in carrying out educational projects. The nutritionists who were deeply engaged in diet counseling were eager to increase their teaching skills. Pharmacists, recognizing that patients lacked sufficient instructions about medications, identified the need for system change as well as staff development to increase opportunities for instruction. Physical and occupational therapists called on the service periodically for materials and other assistance.

Still another area of responsibility was that of participation in aspects of pre-service training. For example, the training program for physicians' assistants, in response to requirements of its accrediting group, included in its very first weeks a session on the health education responsibilities of health workers. Throughout the year of their academic work, the trainees, with the help of the social work staff, examined the psychosocial impact of various conditions on the behavioral aspects of illness. This approach was developed in joint discussion with the director of the program, the social work department, and the Health Education Service.

Important as the early presentation of the education lecture was as a conditioning influence, the program might have offered periodic "booster" sessions as specific topics were discussed. Such sessions, building on the psychosocial base, could have helped trainees develop and practice techniques for helping patients to learn.

Efforts to develop and appraise the educational component of health services took the form of medical record review and/or audit, anecdotal reports (usually horror stories), and formal study. With assistance from a consultant in health services research, two small projects were carried out to determine patient learning needs so that patient teaching might be more appropriately focused. Findings from these studies dispelled some myths about areas of patient ignorance while revealing areas of real weakness. For example, one finding was the frequent occurrence of multiple disorders in a single patient. This finding illustrated the difficulty of automatically or mechanically using highly specific teaching protocols and pointed to the need for flexible, individualized information tailored to the situation. Though this problem was, I am sure, no surprise to practitioners, it had by and large escaped the attention of those developing packaged teaching tools. Almost without exception all staff were highly cooperative as these studies were carried out. The medical records staff, unit clerks, nurses, and physicians all assisted in the process. Study findings were shared with them.

The study instrument itself was later adapted for use in one ambulatory clinic by a physician and nurse as a way of quickly determining matters about which patients needed instruction. The use of the tool was another attempt to find ways of integrating an educational function into the practitioner's role. Documentation of the use of the tool was required, and I periodically prepared brief summaries of the results of its use and shared them with the staff. Difficulties experienced in its use were noted and discussed. For example, we considered whether it should be administered on each visit and when efforts at teaching should be terminated as fruitless. Interestingly, although the tool opened up dialogue between health professionals and patients, and sometimes revealed ignorance whose consequences could be serious, the health professionals grew bored with it, and only administrative leadership sustained its use. It's intriguing to speculate why health workers express little boredom with continuing assessments of vital signs but become dissatisfied with repetition of this sort of procedure.

CONCLUSIONS AND RECOMMENDATIONS

It is impossible to capture in this brief account all the elements that made up a decade's work. The range of activities described here give just a glimpse of what was involved. Omissions and distortions are perhaps inevitable. What should not be omitted is acknowledgment of the support and encouragement of a host of co-workers who shared the goal of improving service to patients.

What lessons do I draw from the experiences cited here?

First, some general observations:

- Patient education is here to stay, and attention will continue to be focused on improving com-

munications between patients and health workers.
- Much more work has to be done to find better ways for professionals to deliver needed information to patients.
- All health professionals are not villains and all patients are not angels. Both groups are made up of complex human beings with many similar needs. Both need to be respected and trusted.
- Frequent staff turnover and system instability are serious impediments to educational programming.
- If I had it to do over, I would still select work on patient education as a priority because it is ethically and strategically right.
- As previously identified by others, there are three levels of function for education—the institutional, the programmatic, and the direct-instruction levels. The health education specialist generally functions at the first two levels.

Now, some specific observations:

- The administrative placement of the health education service is important and advantageous.
- The director of such a service should be an experienced person prepared by training and experience to interact effectively with heads of other services. The directorship is not an entry-level position. The setting and job are tough ones.
- The "staff" role identified for the service is an appropriate one—but one that does present a dilemma in claiming a product or outcome and therefore can pose difficulties in assuring organizational survival.
- Although there are a number of allies in other disciplines, a one-person service in an adjunctive and somewhat alien field has an uphill job vis-à-vis a traditional service setting.
- An essential for improved patient education is staff development through education. Hospitals should consider integrating patient education and staff training in a single educational department to pool education and training resources and to improve the educational quality of staff training.
- A number of system changes are required for effective patient education and patient care. Administrators and health professionals have to face up to the need for increased staff communications with patients and schedule time accordingly. Educational performance needs to be assessed just as other qualities of a practitioner are.
- Reasonable expectations of what can be accomplished in teaching and learning during hospital stays need to be agreed on.
- The usefulness of one-to-one exchange will persist, but more attention must be paid to strengthening the interviewing and listening skills of health workers.
- Health educators in this setting should have or strengthen competency in applying educational methodologies. They should be able to cite with confidence research and studies that validate these methodologies. They should be equipped to recommend educational approaches useful for other workers and to instruct and monitor their application.
- Educators should be assertive in intervening in their area of competency—to assist and to correct. Educational programs should not be undertaken casually. The use of field trainees to organize groups or classes solely as field work exercises to be discontinued when that training ends should be terminated as educational malpractice (perhaps even medical malpractice). These programs *can* be planned steps in program trial and development and are appropriate as such.
- Teaching guides and protocols are needed, but they can do only a small part of the job.
- The ambulatory setting should be used for the extensive education that complex health problems may require. Appointments with health professionals could be scheduled for groups of patients with similar problems and characteristics. Health professionals need to be available for such meetings.

REFERENCE

Aiken, L. H. 1970. "Patient Problems Are Problems in Learning." in *American Journal of Nursing* 70:1916–1918.

Analysis

This case focuses on the health education specialist as the director of the Health Education Service in a 400-bed Public Health Service Hospital. The educator functioned primarily as a consultant. The goal of the Health Education Service, as Skiff defines it, was to integrate the educational function into the practitioner's role. She chose this goal rather than other possible goals such as community education because she believed that charity begins at home. One does not advise the neighbors how to educate their constituencies unless that advice is practiced at home.

Skiff indicates success in reaching her goal with the nursing profession. She attributes this both to the impetus from nursing leadership, which urged nurses to improve their patient education activities, and to an interest by most nurses in patient education. Unfortunately, because of a constant turnover in staff, developing a stable core of nurses who could carry on the nursing patient education function was difficult.

Skiff indicates somewhat less success in reaching her goal with physicians. She questions why this was so. In so doing, she raises an issue critical to the practice of health education in medical care settings. Much of this analysis will focus on that issue.

Diffusion of an innovation provides a theoretical fit for this case (Rogers 1983). Skiff's goal was to assist the providers of medical care to adopt the practice of communicating with patients about their health and medical care needs. Communicating with patients means learning how to interview and how to then translate both the patient's information and the professional's knowledge of the patient's health status into recommendations that the patient can understand and carry out.

In addition to diffusion theory, many principles of learning/social change are applied in this case. The principle most evident is: Begin where the learner is. That is what this health educator did, responding to every request whether or not it was relevant. As she notes, doing that opened doors for her and allowed her to ask appropriate questions. These questions helped raise the staff's awareness of and interest in patient education.

Also applicable here is Bruner's concept that readiness to learn is developed (Bruner 1971). The health educator's "curriculum" for developing readiness was making herself available and raising appropriate questions.

Involvement of the learner in the learning process was another learning principle applied. Through participation in ongoing hospital committees, the health educator involved the members of those committees in learning about patient education. She did this by raising questions, involving committee members in discussions, focusing on patient perception and need, and carrying out certain tasks with committee members. These activities contributed to the members' understanding of patient education. Much of this learning was informal. The committee members were probably unaware they had learned until they began to use the concepts and skills that the health educator had "taught" at committee meetings.

In addition to a theory on how a new practice was adopted or learned, we need to consider theories about the structure of the organization in which the case took place. The structure of the hospital clearly influenced what the health educator was able to do. The domain theory (Kouzes and Mico 1979), referred to in the introduction to Part 2, is useful in explaining the response of the physician population to health education services. Consider that the service domain is governed by "principles of autonomy and self-regulation" and that the health educator was hired by the management domain. She chose to work with the service domain. Therefore she was in the position which Squyres (1982) mentions as having responsibility but no authority. She did have some status by job classification, administrative placement, and previous reputation, but this was not always well exploited.

The major strategy employed to achieve the goal set forth for the Health Education Service was consultation. Lippitt and Lippitt (1978) describe the consultative process on a nondirective-directive continuum (Figure 1). Note that all the roles listed in the figure were played by the author and that on a given occasion she employed more than one. She cites one situation in which she was assertive but indicates that she rarely took this stance. Her preferred approach was nondirective. She did, however, advocate for education on numerous occasions with the Discharge Planning Subcommittee and with the Research Committee.

The consultation role as played out in this case differs from the role as described in the social science literature (Argyris 1973). Most consultants contract with an organization for a time-limited task. In this case, the consultant was an employee of the organization, an internal consultant. The members of the service domain with whom she chose to work did not ask for her services. Many were unaware that these services could benefit their patient care activities. And of those who were aware, some were conscious of their deficiencies in patient education and yet found it difficult to seek help.

In most consultant relationships, the client has some knowledge of the issue or problem that brings the consultant to the organization. In this case, not only did the clients, the service domain, not know they were clients, but their perception of the issue on which the consultant was to work created barriers to successful consultation.

The health educator's modus operandi did fit the consultative process as described in Figure 1. But the organizational structure to support that role was missing.

Lack of administrative support has been blamed for lack of progress in many health education programs. This health educator had strong support from the hospital's administration, and so doors were opened for her. She was put on appropriate committees, was given materials she needed, was placed in a position in the hospital's structure so she had access to all departments and services, and was identified by the administration as a valuable staff member whose services should be sought by other hospital staff. In addition, the medical staff were full-time and on salary. Time, availability, and money were not issues in this hospital.

Yet the availability of the medical staff, strong administrative support, and the professional competence of the health educator were not enough to ensure the attention, interest, and commitment of the majority of physicians in integrating the concepts and skills of patient education into patient care. Why? The structure of medical care organizations, referred to earlier, offers some answers, as do the norms and values of the physician culture, discussed in the introduction to Part Two.

This case raises two issues for the practice of health education. One is the role of the health educator in the acute/chronic care hospital, and the second is the difficulty health educators seem to have in reaching physicians. These issues too are discussed in the introduction to Part Two.

This case describes a sophisticated view of the health educator's role in a large

MULTIPLE ROLES OF THE CONSULTANT

Objective observer/ reflecter	Process counselor	Fact finder	Alternative identifier and linker	Joint problem solver	Trainer educator	Informational expert	Advocate

CLIENT ⟶ CONSULTANT

LEVEL OF CONSULTANT ACTIVITY IN PROBLEM SOLVING

Nondirective ⟵⟶ Directive

Raises questions for reflection	Observes problem-solving process and raises issues mirroring feedback	Gathers data and stimulates thinking interpretives	Identifies alternatives and resources for client and helps assess consequences	Offers alternatives and participates in decisions	Trains client	Regards, links, and provides policy or practice decisions	Proposes guidelines, persuades, or directs in the problem-solving process

Figure 1
Description of the Consultant's Role on a Directive and Nondirective Continuum

Source: Reprinted from Gordon Lippitt and Ronald Lippitt, *The Consulting Process in Action,* San Diego: University Associates, Inc. 1978. Used with permission.

acute/chronic care hospital. It chronicles the activities the health educator carried out in attempting to integrate educational principles into the fabric of medical care. The barriers inherent in the structure of the hospital and in the values of medicine allowed for limited success toward this goal.

References/Select Resources

Argyris, C. 1973. *Intervention Theory and Method: A Behavioral Science View.* Reading, Mass.: Addison-Wesley.
Argyris writes about direct involvement of the theorist/researcher in the process of organizational change. Ordinarily, the role of the researcher would be to provide consultation about how to change and how to test the results to demonstrate the relevance of the theory. The author suggests that the theory can be better tested if the researcher gets his or her hands dirty in the process. The volume is about consultation with organizations that wish to make changes in the structure or function of the organization. Although the book is written in organization development language, the principles are similar to the learning/social change principles with which the health educator deals. The book offers much of interest on the process of both social change and consultation. It is, however, a sophisticated treatment of the subject.

Bruner, J. 1971. *Toward a Theory of Instruction.* Cambridge: Harvard University Press, Belknap Press.

Bruner describes the eight essays in this volume as "efforts of a student of the cognitive process trying to come to grips with the problems of education." Although he writes about the education of children, his thoughts are applicable also to adults. All the essays provide the health educator with thought-provoking ideas about teaching and learning. Bruner offers a sophisticated treatment of the issues. His clear, concise essays are a gold mine of useful ideas, and students will be rewarded for stretching their minds to understand these ideas and make them their own. The essay of particular interest for the Skiff case is "Education as a Social Invention," in which Bruner discusses the need for each generation to redefine "the nature, direction and aims of education." He suggests that an increased understanding of the process of education is one reason for redefinition. Advanced knowledge of the concept of readiness to learn is one example he offers to support his thesis.

Kouzes, J. M., Mico, P. R. 1979. "Domain Theory: An Introduction to Organizational Behavior in Human Service Organizations." *Journal of Applied Behavioral Science* 15:449–469.

In the authors' view, the structure of human service organizations differs from the structure of organizations such as business and industry. They contend that the members of human service organizations fall into one of three groups: (1) the policy domain, the board members, (2) the management domain, the administrators and their staff, and (3) the service domain, the professional members of the organization. Each of the three domains has different norms and different decision-making modes, so there is constant conflict among them. The authors do not label the different modes of functioning as right or wrong, or good or bad. They are what is, reality, and must be dealt with. The Skiff case illustrates ways in which to deal with this conflict. Some of the strategies employed: forming interdisciplinary committees, developing relationships with members of all domains, and relating to the needs of each domain.

Lippitt, G., and Lippitt, R. 1978. *The Consulting Process in Action.* La Jolla, Calif.: University Associates.

The authors provide a concise, practical, and useful volume on the consultation process for the beginner. They offer a good deal of "how to" information, explaining the principles behind the suggested action. The book offers an excellent description of the skills and competencies needed by the consultant; a good discussion on the consultation process; and an introduction to ethical, research, and evaluation issues in consultation.

Rogers, E. M. 1983. *Diffusion of Innovations.* 3d ed. New York: Free Press.

Rogers reviewed 3,085 studies on diffusion for this edition, an indication of the great strides made in diffusion research since his first publication in 1962, when he reported on 405 studies. Because he now extends diffusion theory to include factors that antecede and follow the adoption process, he poses some new questions. For example, where did the diffusion come from? Which comes first, the need or the innovation? What kinds of problems are encountered, and how are they solved as the innovation is implemented?

Rogers identifies three ways in which decisions are made to adopt or reject an innovation: a decision by the individual independent of an organization; a collective decision made by consensus among members of a group; and an authoritarian decision made by a few members of a group for the group (chap. 1). In the Skiff case, decisions to adopt innovative health education practices were made by individuals.

Squyres, W. 1982. "The Professional Health Educator in HMOs: Implications for Training and Our Future in Medical Care." *Health Education Quarterly* 9(1):67–80.

In this article, Squyres offers a frank discussion of the issues of health education practice in HMOs. One of these issues is the responsibility—without the authority to support it—given the health educator by the medical care institution. The Skiff case illustrates this issue clearly.

Discussion Questions

1. Describe another way in which this health educator in this case might have interpreted her role, and identify the kinds of tasks that role would require.

2. Could this health educator have exploited the strong administrative support she received so as to give her greater leverage with the service domain? If so, how?

3. You are assigned to work with a discharge planning committee. Describe how you would assess needs.

4. The chief of pulmonary medicine has asked for a course for patients with chronic obstructive pulmonary disease (COPD). Describe how you would develop this course.

5. You are working in the ambulatory clinic of this hospital and you find that many nurses and doctors are not using the educational assessment form that has been developed. How would you proceed in trying to get greater utilization?

Management Functions of the Health Education Director: Examples of Data Management Activities

Jane G. Zapka, Sc.D.

Management has been defined as "the process of creating the internal environment for organized effort to accomplish group goals" (Koontz and O'Donnell 1955:26). It is an enormously complex endeavor involving a variety of processes, activities, and techniques.

Health educators do not often ascribe the role of "manager" to themselves. Yet the very activities of a manager, particularly planning and organizing, are essential processes and functions of health education practice. A health educator within an organization must usually coordinate activities across departments and across disciplines, as does a manager or administrator. In addition, recruiting staff, giving feedback, and conducting program evaluations are management activities usually performed by health educators. If managers are to construct organizations that "maximize efficiency and effectiveness" to various external constituencies and simultaneously minimize stress, dissatisfaction, and unhappiness to internal constituencies" (Goldsmith 1981:67), this challenge certainly applies to the health educator's role.

This case assumes that understanding basic managerial principles is critical from two major perspectives: (1) Understanding and applying these principles will improve effective and efficient performance of the education department of an agency; and (2) understanding the larger organization's managers and the "managed" environment will enhance the effectiveness of the educator's interactions with persons at all levels.

Management, similar to education, is an eclectic, applied field. It draws on the organized knowledge and theories of many disciplines, including psychology, sociology, mathematics, and operations research (Koontz 1968).

Obviously, one cannot do justice to the enormous literature on management and organizational theory and its applications, but it is hoped that this case study will stimulate further inquiry. Students are urged to explore further those theories and related skills that might not be part of their current repertoire and to consider which skills complement their management style and which ones might increase their effectiveness.

This study will focus first on the general functions and activities of management. Then an anecdote will focus on a broad management activity, the development of a departmental information system. The anecdote demonstrates the integration of several management functions by a director of a health education department within a larger service agency, in this case a university-based health maintenance organization.

FUNCTIONS AND ACTIVITIES OF MANAGEMENT

The functions and activities of a manager vary with the size of the enterprise of both the parent organization and the education department, as well

---

Jane G. Zapka is an Associate Professor of Health Administration in the Division of Public Health at the University of Massachusetts at Amherst.

The author wishes to acknowledge the helpful comments on earlier drafts by Diane Wolfe, M.P.H., Director of Health Education, University of Massachusetts Health Services; and Seth Goldsmith, Sc.D., Associate Professor and Chair, Health Administration Program, University of Massachusetts—Amherst, Division of Public Health.

as according to organizational needs and idiosyncracies, environmental pressures, and personality characteristics. Although managerial functions cannot be neatly isolated and the detailed categorization of managerial functions varies among authors, a general consensus has evolved.

Planning involves the processes and activities related to the selection of objectives, policies, and programs, as well as the procedures for achieving them—in other words, deciding what work must be done. Within a health organization, planning can be considered at three levels (Deeds, Hebert, and Wolle 1979):

- The organization-wide or systems level, which encompasses the department within the entire organization and within the context of the community
- The programmatic and activity level, which considers specific groups of clientele (target groups) or certain disease categories
- The face-to-face, individual level, which involves direct personal interaction with the client

This study discusses functions that are applied to all levels, but primarily the organizational and departmental levels. The development of an overall plan for an education department requires the systematic assessment of perceived needs from the consumer, staff, and organizational perspectives; determination of priorities among these needs; and the formulation of program activities based on finer diagnoses of specific problems. Planning is, of course, decision making and involves selecting among choices. What is the mission and role of the unit? What functions will the Education Department itself develop (e.g., staff training, coordination, direct service provision, consumer advocacy)? What activities should receive priority within those functions? What resource allocations are necessary? For the manager, planning generally results in the production of a written document that outlines objectives and activities according to short- and long-range time frames.

Organizing involves the determination of how to carry out those activities required to achieve the objectives of an enterprise. The essence lies in "dividing up the work" so as to accomplish the department's objectives (Rakich et al. 1977:20), that is, deciding who will do what with whom to achieve the desired end results. Organizing activities include task assignments to various individuals and groups, delegation of authority to carry them out, and arrangement of conditions for effective teamwork, horizontally and vertically, among organizational units. How can the health education director accomplish activities through the staff of other departments? How should tasks be assigned among several members of the health education staff to achieve maximum efficacy and effectiveness?

Staffing involves determination of the personal requirements to perform necessary work. It requires defining the manpower requirements for the activities to be done and includes inventorying existing personnel. It involves recruiting, selecting, and training new personnel and/or reorienting existing staff members. The monitoring techniques of this function are relatively standardized personnel approaches, such as defining job descriptions, job specifications, and budget limitations.

Staff development is also pivotal to meet changing personal and organizational needs. "Developing people suggests a high level of commitment to the maximal utilization of human resources, which becomes critical in a labor-intensive industry, such as health care" (Goldsmith 1981:72). Because the education director is usually in the position of accomplishing objectives through other people, over which he or she has no authority, the design of staff development programs aimed at improving education skills of clinicians is a familiar and difficult challenge.

Staffing, though sometimes considered a resource-consuming and discouraging activity, is perhaps one of the most critical functions of a good manager, because it is the staff that makes a labor-intensive unit like health education and promotion services successful.

Directing involves the leading and guiding of staff members, effecting the human activity to accomplish program goals. Although sometimes this managerial function is seen as a powerful force resulting from a supervisor/subordinate relationship, it is usually more related to a manager's ability to lead and motivate (Gibson, Ivancevich, and Donnelly 1982: chaps. 5 and 8). It reflects communications ability and the achievement of an effective flow of ideas and information in all directions.

Coordination is probably the essence of managerial success for the manager of an educational department. Even though health organizations are often highly bureaucratic, the education director almost always is in the position to guide, persuade, and coach rather than to supervise or "be boss" to the other health professionals whose cooperation is needed to make a program work, including physicians, nurses, and administrators. Achievement of group goals across departments often carries considerable responsibility, with little authority. To coordinate in such an arena, the education director must have extraordinary skills as a persuader. The manager's ability to receive, transmit, and act on information is critical to directing and coordinating functions. Skills in working with governing and advisory boards, volunteers, and committees are essential. However, the education director must have at least some apparent authority over the organizational placement of the department, plus a commitment to the program from upper-level administrators. (Mullen and Zapka 1982:chap. 7).

Controlling, or *monitoring,* relates to the comparison of performance against accepted and, ideally, predetermined standards. The director must monitor performance, correct deviations, and assure task completion in a timely manner according to professional standards of practice. As educational activities span departments and lines of authority are more diffused, an education director must anticipate needs, but create flexible plans to allow for inevitable readjustment of time lines. Control techniques, such as time/activity charts, program activity budgets, person-hour records or logs, and quarterly reports, are increasingly utilized. Management information systems must be designed to help monitor progress. On the programmatic level, evaluation of program-outcome objectives is also critical.

The *representing* function pertains to environmental relationships, broadly defined. The manager of an educational program certainly is the spokesperson for the department within the larger organization. This is a time-consuming function that requires political sensitivity not only to the needs of the department but also to those of the larger organization and of consumers. The skills of presentation, debate, analysis, negotiation, and articulation are critical. In addition, the educational function, particularly those activities that involve patient and community education, puts the educational staff in a visible, public position. In actuality, this staff represents the organization as a whole and has an indirect but overt public relations function. The health educator's traditonal role of mobilizing community support and managing planned social change is of utmost relevance to the organization's role as a sensitive, responsive service (Parlette, Glogow, and D'Onofrio 1981).

DEVELOPMENT OF A SYSTEM FOR MANAGING DATA

The director of the Health Education Department of a prepaid group practice within a large university is continually asked to justify the unit's five (full-time equivalent) staff members. Sometimes this is an explicit request from administration, but sometimes it is a derisive comment from other staff who wonder what she can possibly be doing with all that time, since her staff spend considerably less time on individual, direct client contact than the clinicians do. The director's usual response to such requests or comments has been to recite the activities and programs offered by the educational unit. Although she generally believes her staff to be dedicated and effective (and in several cases overextended), she realizes that to plan and allocate resources more effeevely she must develop an organized way to document and subsequently evaluate the directions in which staff energy is expended. She decides to implement a new and improved reporting system for the Health Education Department.

One inference from this brief anecdote is that clinicians do not understand the role, function, and activities of a health education department and/or that they do not support them. Hence the need to plan a strategy for unit "marketing" (a representing function). Another inference of the anecdote is that the time of six people (five staff plus the director) may or may not be justified in view of the activity output (perceived or otherwise) of the unit, or that energy could be better spent on other activities. The following discussion relates mainly to the latter inference and describes the development of an information system for monitoring staff activity as part of the manager's planning and control functions. If the department is perceived as an efficient, accountable group, such a system will also benefit the representing function in the long run.

BACKGROUND AND ANALYSIS

Good management requires understanding of data. Within many health education units, data are often subjective, assumed, unorganized, incomplete, and/or inaccurate. However, as health education becomes a defined organizational function, health educators are developing monitoring and reporting systems that will provide data needed for accountability, resource development and control, program planning, and program evaluation (Thompson and Handelman 1978). Use of such data can ultimately improve the efficiency and effectiveness of departments of health education and promotion.

A management information system is a systematic way to collect, process, store, retrieve, and transmit selective information on staff activities, clients, and fiscal transactions (Broskowski 1979). Such systems are operational in human services organizations in one form or another and are becoming increasingly sophisticated in prepaid practice. Although a system set up for an education unit should be consonant with that of the larger organization, special problems inevitably arise because of an education department's unique activities and functions.

Following are the three components of a basic management information system (Broskowski 1979):

- The *resource component* comprises data on the specific services the health education staff provides to clients—either to patients/members or to other staff—and the deployment of staff resources among specific program activities. Coordinating, planning, and evaluating time should be accounted. This component may also include data on utilization of other nonstaff resources, such as self-care manuals and other materials.
- The *client component* is composed of data on the clients serviced. It might include personal and demographic data, membership data to determine eligibility, and limited historical data, such as previous participation in special group programs.
- The *fiscal component* contains information on the sources, amounts of income, and amount and nature of expenses. It is recommended that standard cost-allocation methods be used with major program activities delineated as cost centers. (Berman and Weeks 1982:chap. 5).

There is an important distinction between the terms *data* and *information*. "Data are any record of events; information is data which have been manipulated and transformed into a meaningful guide for specific purposes (Thompson and Handelman 1978:136). Information has relevance and utility for specific purposes. Analysis of data is what makes them relevant and useful.

For data to become useful information, specific decisions must be made about what information is necessary. In making such decisions, the health education director was faced with the following problems:

- What are the specific department and intervention goals and objectives, and what data are needed to help evaluate whether they are achieved?
- What client information is necessary (e.g., demographic characteristics, enrollment information, history of previous service)?
- What service utilization data are necessary (e.g., number of clients participating in each activity, attrition rates, volume of direct and indirect services)?
- What data on staff activity are needed (e.g., staff hours devoted to direct and to indirect services, by type of activity; volume of services provided by individual staff members)?
- What fiscal information would be helpful (e.g., total direct service costs for each intervention, cost per unit of service for each intervention, cost per encounter)?

Once the health education director had outlined what data would actually be useful for management functions, she could assess the status of the existing system for collecting those data and develop a plan based on the gaps between the current system and the desired system.

The health education director carefully reviewed existing processes and reports, discussed needs with her staff and the administrator, and then identified the following issues:

- Although the total revenues and costs of the department were well accounted, the costs of various activities and programs were not objectively computed.
- The relationship of direct costs to activity benefits was not explicitly monitored. There was some indication that certain resource-consuming activities were reaching very few members.
- The level of activity by each staff member was largely anecdotal, and there appeared to be some disparity. Concrete data were needed for professional staff review and for program planning.
- The level of services to various client groups in the HMOs was unclear (e.g., in a university-based HMO, client groups, each with a separate fee structure, could include students, student dependents, faculty, and staff).
- There seemed to be little reinforcement of educational activities by clinicians. The education staff saw no notation of prevention/education programs in the members' health records.
- The contribution to health education activities by staff from other HMO cost centers (e.g., physicians, nurse practitioners, psychologists) was not formally recognized.
- Data collected from members participating in certain ongoing programs were not standardized and were not used efficiently for activity evaluation, by comparison to historical or normative standards (Green et al. 1980).

Considering the three broad components of data—resource, client, fiscal—the health education director decided to proceed as follows:

- Design a reporting system for the health education staff to document time allocation and track activity output (e.g., programs provided) of the Health Education Department.
- Better organize data collected from clients during ongoing program activities so as to facilitate documentation and evaluation.
- Use these data and the departmental budget to improve cost analysis of the department's activities.
- Incorporate in the medical record notes concerning a member's participation in organized educational activity.

DEVELOPING A REPORTING SYSTEM FOR STAFF'S TIME AND PROGRAM

Data for the resource components are usually collected by staff-reported activity logs; for example, each staff member submits a monthly or weekly log of his/her activities. Initially, a three-page standardized reporting form was designed. It captured the efforts in the obvious areas of service provision, such as community education (ongoing programs and one-shot efforts), individual client consultation, group patient education programs, and training activities. Data were kept according to population or target group (e.g., students, HMO members) so as to better assess the level of staff energies expended for each and to subsequently monitor the equitable distribution of resources on the basis of respective contributions to the department's budget. A documentation key was designed and orientation sessions were held with the staff. Keeping the form handy, staff members would note some encounters directly on the form at the time of occurrence and add others at the end of the month, reconstructing their activities from their appointment books.

Over the next several months of use, the form was debugged and refined to make reporting less tedious and to accommodate the task variations among staff members. As staff configurations, the program profile, and the level of management sophistication shifted over the years, the form was further refined (Figure 1).

A major issue continued to be the documentation of "planning and communication" time. Recording time in meetings, "desk time," and so on was tedious. As the department's activities became solidified over the years, the usefulness of such data decreased. The use of a constant as a multiplier for planning time was introduced and is currently being tested (Wolfe 1982). In this approach, direct activity is reported (e.g., eight sessions of a smoking cessation series for two hours each, with

Month _____   Staff _____

INDIVIDUAL MEMBER CONSULTATION	Career/Academic Advising	Personal Problem/ Patient Education		Academic Project	Member Relations	
		Student	VHP		Student	VHP
			AMA | UHS			AMA | UHS
Est. hours						

COMMUNITY PROGRAMS (include class guest lectures)	Topic	Group/ Location	Date	# Hours	Attendance	CH
	1. 2. 3. 4. 5. 6. 7. 8.					

GROUP EDUCATION (multisession, ongoing)	1. 2. 3. 4. 5. 6.					

OTHER COURSES AND COLLOQS	Topic	# Sessions	# Hours	Attendance	CH

OTHER TRAINING (UHS staff, RAs, HRs, etc.)	Topic	Group	# Sessions	# Hours	Attendance	CH

Figure 1 *continued*
Monthly Staff Activity Log (Computerized)
Source: University of Massachusetts Health Services—Amherst.

	Group(s)	# Hours	Attendance	CH
MEMBER RELATIONS Orientations	1. 2. 3. 4.			
Tours	1. 2.			
SHAB, MAC, and subgroups	1. 2. 3. 4. 5.			

	# People	Project/Topic(s)	Time
SUPERVISORY ACTIVITIES Academic (UWW, BDIC, individual study)			
Field trainees			
Other			

	Activity	With Whom?	Hours
COLLABORATION AND CONSULTATION In-house	1. 2. 3. 4. 5. 6. 7. 8. 9. 10. 11. 12.		
UMASS community	1. 2. 3. 4. 5. 6.		
Outside	1. 2. 3.		

Figure 1 *continued*

PEER PROGRAMS (PSE, health aides, student reps, contraception volunteers, alcohol peers, healthreach)						
STAFF TIME		# Sessions	# Hours	Date	# Students	SCH
Group classes	1. 2. 3. 4. 5. 6.					
		# Peers	# Hours			
Individual consultation and supervision						
PEER ACTIVITIES		# Programs	# Hours	Date	# Students	SCH
Group programs						
Individual consults						
PROFESSIONAL IMPROVEMENT	1. 2.					Hours
OTHER						

Figure 1 *continued*

15 clients). It is then adjusted, using a logical ratio, such as three hours of logistics/planning/communications/evaluation for each hour of direct provision of an established ongoing activity. The ratio is higher for innovative programs, for which planning and development time is greater.

During this phase of department and management maturity the use of a minicomputer for staff log summaries was also introduced. The staff log format was changed to ensure easy entry of data into the available terminal in the format necessary (Data Dex). Figure 2 on page 164 shows the revised

Code Sheet—Health LD Reporting System

1. Staff name
2. Co-facilitator: Use 2 or 3 initials.
3. Type of program: Use 2-letter code as follows.

Usually a group:

WO	workshop facilitation
PR	presentation (not a class)
CL	class lecture
TR	training (giving it)
OR	orientation/tours
OH	occupational health

Usually peer class–related:

PE	peer class
SP	supervision
IS	interviewing and screening
PD	poster distribution

Usually an individual:

AA	academic assistance
CC	career counseling
PC	personal counseling
MA	member advising
SS	social service

Staff/dept. activities/miscellaneous

CM	committee
CE	continuing ed
CS	consult with other agency or dept.
DP	displays

4. Date: MM/DD/YY, e.g., 01/15/82
5. # Hours: Use whole or decimal numbers, e.g., 1, 3, 1.5, 2.5, 8.
6. # Sessions: Use whole numbers, 1 or 2 digits.
7. Topic: Use title of topic up to 20 letters; try to standardize within your own area.
8. Location: Use a 3-letter code.

General

UHS	in UHS
AMA	at AMA
VHP	at VHP offices
HMP	Hampshire College
AMH	Amherst College
UMS	UMass on-campus (not dorm)

NES	Northeast/Sylvan
OHC	Orchard Hill/Central
SWT	Southwest
CCT	Campus Center
OFF	Off-campus

NHC	Northampton Center
NHS	Northampton Site
GRK	Greek Area
SPH	School of Public Health

9. Total attendance: Use 0–999 numbers; always complete this section. (Estimates are better than nothing!!)
10. UMass: 0–999
11. VHP: 0–999
12. Hamp: 0–999
13. Amh: 0–999
14. Other: 0–999
15. Male: 0–999
16. Female: 0–999
17. Dorm: A specific dorm or building. Make your own 3-letter code.
18. Misc: Up to 10 letter spaces. Use as desired. Tell Diane if you want a special report from this column.

Figure 2
Monthly Staff Activity Log (Computerized)
Source: University of Massachusetts Health Services—Amherst

NAME _____ MONTH, YEAR _____

Three Initials ____ ____ ____

Co-facilitator	Type of program	Date	# Hours	# Sessions	Topic			Location	

Total Attendance	UMass	VHP	Hamp. Coll.	Amh. Coll.	Other	Male	Female	

Co-facilitator	Type of program	Date	# Hours	# Sessions	Topic			Location	

Total Attendance	UMass	VHP	Hamp. Coll.	Amh. Coll.	Other	Male	Female	

Co-facilitator	Type of program	Date	# Hours	# Sessions	Topic			Location	

Total Attendance	UMass	VHP	Hamp. Coll.	Amh. Coll.	Other	Male	Female	

Co-facilitator	Type of program	Date	# Hours	# Sessions	Topic			Location	

Total Attendance	UMass	VHP	Hamp. Coll.	Amh. Coll.	Other	Male	Female	

Co-facilitator	Type of program	Date	# Hours	# Sessions	Topic			Location	

Total Attendance	UMass	VHP	Hamp. Coll.	Amh. Coll.	Other	Male	Female	

Figure 2 *continued*

reporting form, and Figure 3 is a sample annotated tabulation report.

In addition to the development of a staff-reported log, a departmental master calendar was posted to schedule service activity for all program delivery outside of individual consultation. With just a quick glance at it, one could tell which staff members were booked and for what date. This expedited scheduling of program requests by the secretary; it also facilitated emergency coverage, for it obviated individually tracking down a staff member who was not already scheduled.

The calendar also became a simple way to document contributions of staff from other organizational units. For instance, a pediatric nurse practitioner might be the speaker at an HMO-sponsored community lecture. The date, title, name, department, and direct time commitment were noted. Collated monthly were data on the number and nature of various programs, as well as data on contributions to health education programming from other organizational cost centers, which could be shared with other department managers.

IMPROVING ORGANIZED DATA COLLECTION FOR ONGOING INTERVENTIONS

Health education services develop within an HMO in three general stages: information, action, and stabilization (Vosen and Deeds 1981). The formative stage focuses on needs assessment, strategic planning, and capacity building. The action stage is operational, focusing on program content, implementation, and visibility building. During the stabilization phase, many interventions have been piloted and subsequently standardized, and teaching protocols established (Mullen and Zapka 1982:102–108; DeJoseph 1980). It is during this phase that standardized documentation and summative evaluation become priorities.

The anecdote under discussion occurred during this stage of development—the action phase. The protocols for several activities had been debugged and process evaluation was ongoing (Shortell and Richardson 1978). The data collection approach used for such activities as smoking cessation and weight management had been evolving. At this stage, the program staff was asked to clearly define the following:

- Specific program objectives (behavioral and learning objectives)
- Factors (attitude and cognitive skills) that theory and literature demonstrated were important to the behaviors in question (National Interagency Council on Smoking and Health 1974)
- Organizational variables of interest (e.g., membership category—student, faculty, family, community member)

Standardized reporting forms were then designed for specific activities. This would decrease staff time spent on reporting, standardize data for subsequent time series analysis (i.e., did process or outcome measures change from year to year?), and gather data that could be compared to normative data in the professional literature and/or compared to data from colleagues at other HMOs.

Examples of some of the forms are given in Figure 4 (on page 168). In addition to being clearly necessary for evaluation purposes, the summary charts derived for the forms proved very helpful in explaining and reporting the activity to administrators and other professional staff (Davis 1982). Figure 5 on page 169 is an example of a summary chart.

UNDERTAKING COST ANALYSIS OF SELECTED ACTIVITIES

Analysis of data is what makes them relevant and useful; analysis detects significant patterns. Cost analysis is one method. Once data on resource expenditures, service activity, and, in some cases, program outcome or effectiveness have been collected in an organized objective fashion, cost analysis becomes feasible. Although cost-effectiveness studies receive considerable attention in the literature, such studies are complex (Levin 1979; Shepard and Thompson 1979) and often not feasible for the practitioner. However, more basic cost analysis is both feasible and helpful for routine management decisions (U.S. DHEW 1979; Posavac and Carey 1980).

Cost finding requires the itemization of all relevant costs—direct and indirect—to be charged against a certain unit or program for an activity

```
                        HEALTH EDUCATION MONTHLY REPORTS
    ┌─1──┬─2──┬────┬─3─────┬─────┬──────────────┬─4────┬─────┬─────┬─────┬─────┬─────┬────┬────┬─────┐
    │STF │ CO │ TY │ DATE  │ HRS │ SE  TOPIC    │ LOC  │ TOT │ UMS │ VHP │ HMP │ AMH │OTH │M  F│MISC │
    │INT │FAC │ PE │       │     │ SS           │      │ ATT │     │     │     │     │ER  │    │     │
```

STF INT	CO FAC	TY PE	DATE	HRS	SESS	TOPIC	LOC	TOT ATT	UMS	VHP	HMP	AMH	OTHER	M	F	MISC
PAD		CC	100581	1	1	HEALTH ED	UHS	1	1						1	
		CM	100681	2.5		MBR ADVISORY OM	VHP	11		11				5	6	
		OR		2		PLAN ORIENTATION	UHS	26		26				12	14	
		AA	100781	1	1	SMOKING INFO	UHS	1	1					1		
		MA	101481	1		MBR ADVISING	UHS	1		1				1		
		CC	101581	1	1	HEALTH ED	UHS	1	1					1		
		CM		1.5		NAC - INFO/ED	VHP	5		5				2	3	
		AA	101681	1	1	EVALUATION	UHS	1	1						1	
		CN	102081	2.5		MBR ADVISORY CM	VHP	9		9				5	4	
				1		DIABETES TSK FRC	AMA	4		4				2	2	
		MA	102881	1		MBR ADVISING	UHS	1		1					1	
	DMW	WO		2		HOLIDAY STRESS	OFF	45		14			31		45	
		PC	108881	1	4	SMOKING - INDV	UHS	1						1		
		SP		1	4	STAFF SUPERVIS	UHS	1		1					1	
				1	8	SP INTERN	UHS	1	1						1	
	SJW	WO		2	4	SMOKING CESS	AMA	12	1	11				6	6	
		CM	110381	2.5		MBR ADVISORY CM	VHP	11		11				5	6	
		OR		2		PLAN ORIENTATION	AMA	34		34				10	24	
		TR	110581	2	1	DENTAL DIVISION	UHS	10	10					5	5	
		CM	111081	1.5		MAC - INFO/ED	VHP	5		5				2	3	
		AA	111681	1	1	EVALUATION	UHS	1	1						1	
		CM	111781	1		DIABETES TSK FRC	AMA	4		4				2	2	
				2.5		MBR ADVISORY CM	VHP	10		10				4	6	
			111981	1.5		NAC HEALTH PROMO	AMA	6		6				2	4	
	DLM	WO		1.5		FITNESS, SMOKING	UHS	14	14					6	8	
		PC	111881	1	3	SMOKING - INDV	UHS	1		1				1		
		SP		1	6	STAFF SUPERVIS	UHS	1		1					1	
				1	6	SP INTERN	UHS	1	1						1	
	PDS	WO		2	2	MAKING CHOICES	AMA	12	2	10				4	8	
	SJW			2	4	SMOKING CESS	AMA	12	1	11				6	6	
	PDS			2	2	BABY IS HOME	AMA	8		8				3	5	
			120481	2		STRESS	AMA	10		10				4	6	
		CM	120881	2		MBR ADVISORY CM	VHP	10		10				4	6	
		OR		2		PLAN ORIENTATION	AMA	28		28				15	13	
		WO	121081	2		FIT IN WINTER	AMA	18	8	10				10	8	
		MA	121581	1		MBR ADVISING	UHS	1		1					1	
		CM	121781	1.5		MAC - INFO/ED	VHP	3		3				1	2	
			122281	2.5		MBR ADVISORY CM	VHP	9		9				4	5	
		PC	128881	1	3	PATIENT ED - VAR	UHS	3	1	2				1	2	
		SP		1	3	STAFF SUPERVIS	UHS	1		1					1	
				1	4	SP INTERN	UHS	1	1						1	
	PDS	WO		2	2	SINGLE PARENTS	AMA	6		6				2	4	
PAD				**65.0**	61			**341**	46	264	0	0	**31**	**128**	**213**	

```
                    CONFIDENTIAL - INTERNAL USE ONLY
                         5                     6   7    8    9
```

1. Staff member's initials.
2. Reportable encounters/activities (see key in Figure 2).
3. Summary report covers three months or one quarter.
4. Location (this is a multisite HMO).
5. Total direct contact hours for all types of reportable encounters.
6. Total direct member contacts during reportable encounters.
7. During this quarter, this staff member provided services to more HMO members (Valley Health Plan) than students (UHS).
8. One community discussion on Holiday Stress attracted 31 nonplan members (69 percent of those attending).
9. A manager might wonder if the sex ratio of contacts remains disproportionate over time and/or between staff members.

Figure 3
Mock Computerized Staff Activity

Source: University of Massachusetts Health Services—Amherst

SMOKERS' LIBERATION

Participant Demographic Data

Program	Participants (#) Total	Male	Female	VHP AMA	UHS	Student	Student Dependent	Other Area Residents	Mean Age of Participants	Marital Status Married	Nonmarried
All enrolled											
Completed program											
Dropouts											

Participant Smoking Habit History

Program	Mean Age Start Smoking	Mean Length of Smoking Habit (Yr.)	Daily Amount Cigarettes Smoked (# Participants) 0–20	21–40	41–60	61+	Parental Smoking Habits Neither smoked #	Father only #	Mother only #	Both smoked #	Previous Cessation Attempts Never	1×	2×	3×
All enrolled														
Completed program														
Dropouts														

Mean Daily Consumption at Baseline and End of Treatment and Percent Reduction in Smoking at End of Treatment by Category

Baserate Daily Consumption	Mean Daily Consumption (# cigarettes) Baseline	End of treatment	Number of Subjects	End of Treatment: Percent Reduction 100% quit	75–99%	50–74%	15–49%	14% less or incr.	No information
Very light smoker 1–4									
Light smoker 5–14									
Moderate 15–24									
Heavy 25–34									
Very heavy smoker 35+									
TOTAL									

Figure 4
Sample Program-Monitoring Forms

Source: Adapted by Valley Health Plan from report of the National Interagency Council on Smoking and Health (1974).

STOP SMOKING PROGRAM
*Number of Cigarettes Smoked
Per Day by Participants
Spring 1978*

Participant	Pretest	Posttest	+ 1 Month	+ 4 Months	+ 12 Months
1	20	0	0		
2	30	1–2	2–3		
3	20–30	0	4–5		
4	30	3–4	5–10		
5	20	3	0		
6	20–25	0	0		
7	60	6	60		
8	70	0	0		
9	40	0	0		
10	11	3–4	2–3		
11	15–20	0	0		
12	20	10–12	10–12		
Mean	30.58	1.54	7.33		

FALL 1976

	Pretest	Posttest	+ 1 Month	+ 3 Months	+ 12 Months
	$N = 7$	$N = 6$	$N = 7$	$N = 5$	
Mean	32.9	16.8	15.7	25.0	No data

SPRING 1977

	Pretest	Posttest	+ 1 Month	+ 3 Months	+ 12 Months
	$N = 7$	$N = 7$	$N = 4$		$N = 6$
Mean	26.4	1.8	23.75	No data	28.6

Figure 5 *continued*
Sample Summary Tables and Graph
Source: Valley Health Plan, Amherst, Massachusetts.

STOP SMOKING PROGRAM

Group summary: Mean cigarettes smoked per day for participants who completed program

Mean number of cigarettes smoked per day

30.58 (N = 12)
1.54 (N = 12)
7.33 (N = 12)

Pretest　　Posttest　　+ 1 month　　+ 4 months　　+ 12 months

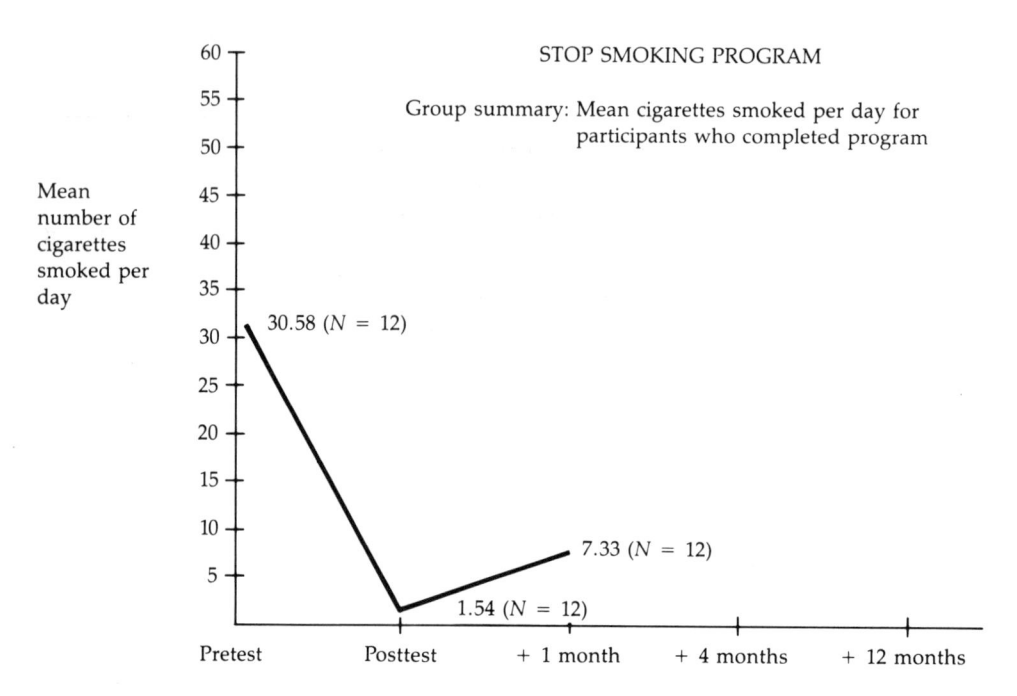

Figure 5 *continued*

(U.S. DHEW 1979). These costs are then considered with respect to select process and outcome indicators. The example in Table 1 illustrates how data collected from staff activity forms and specific programs are incorporated with budgetary figures.

The simple calculations allow the following:

1. Comparison with the same unit cost calculations in previous time periods
2. Comparison with similar cost calculations of other interventions
3. Comparison of fees (if applicable) to revenues
4. Calculation of the cost per encounter in a fashion similar to that made for clinical services
5. Documentation of the cost relative to selected criteria of output or effectiveness

Such an analysis provided information on which to base decisions not only about the activity itself (e.g., whether to try to decrease costs or increase revenues) but also about the activity in relation to other activities (e.g., whether the HMO should promote other activities and decrease availability of the smoking cessation program). Clearly, decisions about program priorities cannot be made solely on the basis of cost analyses of selected activities, but such analyses do provide an important dimension.

INCORPORATING HEALTH EDUCATION PROGRAM NOTES IN THE MEDICAL RECORD

Operational data can be distinguished from management data (American Association of Medical Clinics 1973). The former are data utilized in day-to-day operations; the latter are data that are subsequently used in planning and controlling the activity of an organization and department. The development of a process to incorporate notes in the medical records is primarily of an operational nature, distinguishing it from the other data management activities described here.

Notation in the medical record of a member's participation in an organized educational activity

Table 1
Cost Analysis—Smoking Cessation Program

Programs	Participants	Encounters	Costs Personnel	Materials	Cost per Participant	Revenues $25 per Participant	Net Cost per Participant	Net Cost per Encounter	Net Cost per Quitter*
3 (8 sessions each)	42	≈1008	144 hrs. @$15 12 hrs. @$ 8 2,256 hrs. Total $2,462	Folders $126 Postage 25 Xerox 10 Films 45 $206	$58.62	$1,050	$33.62	$1.40	$61.39

* Participant follow-up data indicated a 55 percent quit rate six months after the program.

was meant to complete the documentation of that person's receipt of, or participation in, preventive, diagnostic, and therapeutic services with the HMO. Documentation of participation in a group concerned with, say, weight management or lower back pain provides cues for the clinician's later reinforcement of positive health practices. From the perspective of management function, such notations also provide important visibility for the education unit's activities. Explicit health education connections to quality of care and quality assurance aid in the acceptance of health education programs. (Deeds 1981).

The health education director and her staff considered two types of approaches to making notations. In some instances a special form related to educational needs and interventions were inserted in the record (Figure 6). This insertion allowed a quick review of activity, dates, and pertinent process information. Other organizations have used a standardized rubber stamp to enter progress notes on participation in educational programs (Mullen and Zapka 1982:125).

SUMMARY

In closing, it is important to highlight two important issues in designing information systems: automation and the process of implementation.

There is a tendency to equate health data and information management with automation. Many data necessary for management of a health education department can be obtained by relatively simple documentation procedures, the dominant requirement being discipline to make brief, timely notations. Automation of any magnitude does represent a major investment of time, trouble, money, and management reputation (Thompson and Handelman 1978). Objectives, needs, and processes are rarely clearly defined at the beginning of any organized data-collection process. Considerable time for design and debugging is necessary.

In the organization under discussion here, the development of a computerized staff report evolved over several years. The result has been a usable system that not only provides data for accountability and planning but also is implemented with a minimum of staff resistance. The Southern California Permanente Medical Group has a well-developed form used by the health education staff at eight service delivery sites (Mullen and Zapka 1982:132). Mary Hospital in Illinois captures data entered by nurses and patient educators (Murphy and Finnegan 1980). The use of computers in health education departments will inevitably grow. Over the years, the computer capability (mainframe, micro, mini, and personal computers) of health care organizations will rapidly increase, and the feasibility of computerizing time and activity documentation for even small education departments will improve. It behooves health educators to become familiar with the potential of this technology (Taylor 1979). As such systems are designed and refined, the health education manager can seek consultation from those colleagues who have already struggled with data management system design and significantly decrease the time needed for development of their own system.

Focus on the technology and logic of a system can become engaging for some managers—so engaging, in fact, that attention to the administrative climate (Mathews 1972), to the process of involving staff in the design and implementation of data management activities, is underemphasized. As with any innovation, logical design and potential efficiency and usefulness do not make administrative excellence happen. The problems of restructuring reporting habits and reorienting people are the more difficult of the tasks involved in developing a management information system. Understanding the capacity of a staff to accept change is absolutely vital to the success of any information management project. The "whys" and potential advantages need to be shared. The perceived threat, the offensiveness at being monitored, the ascribed connotation of being "production-oriented" rather than "people-oriented"—all this resistance not only should be expected but should be planned for by incorporating efforts to address it.

In conclusion, attention to documentation and organized data collection clearly contributes to effective management of a health education department. Referring back to the main functions of management, relevant applications are obvious. In the case under discussion, the innovations in data systems helped the health education director to carry out the following tasks:

- Calculate the quantity of services being provided (useful in planning, controlling, and representing)

```
┌─────────────────────────────────────────────┐
│        Educational Encounter Summary        │
│                                             │
│                  To:                        │
│                From:                        │
│                                             │
│                Name:                        │
│      Referral Source:                       │
│     Nature of Inquiry:                      │
│       Date of Inquiry:                      │
│ Educational Intervention(s):                │
│           and Date(s):                      │
│             Outcome:                        │
│       Behavioral Plan:                      │
│                                             │
│             Comments:                       │
│                                             │
└─────────────────────────────────────────────┘
```

Figure 6
Medical Record Insert

Source: Valley Health Plan, Amherst, Massachusetts.

- Monitor the deployment of resources throughout the division (planning, staffing, controlling)
- Identify the participants or recipients of services and help identify accessibility or utilization issues (planning, controlling)
- Provide information to demonstrate accountability internally and externally (representing, controlling)
- Enhance communications internally with other departments within the organization (planning, organizing, representing)
- Provide a foundation for evaluation of the interventions (controlling)
- Assist cost accounting, rate setting, and budgeting (controlling, planning)
- Provide a foundation for staff performance reviews and staff development activities (staffing)

Attention to management functions by health educators will be an upcoming challenge to the field, if organized health education programs are to grow and flourish.

REFERENCES

American Association of Medical Clinics. 1973. *An Administrative Information System for a Group Practice Developing a Prepaid Health Plan.* Alexandria, Va.

Berman, H. J., and Weeks, L. E. 1982. *The Financial Management of Hospitals.* 5th ed. Ann Arbor, Mich.: Health Administration Press.

Broskowski, A. 1979. "Management Information Systems for Planning and Evaluation in Human Services." In *Program Evaluation in the Health Fields,* volume 2, edited by H. C. Schulberg and F. Baker. New York: Human Sciences Press.

Data Dex. 1981. Cupertino, Calif.: Apple Computer.

Davis, P. (Health Education Coordinator, Valley Health Plan, Amherst, Mass.). 1982. Personal communication.

Deeds, S. G. 1981. "Overview: The HMO Environment in the Eighties and Related Issues in Health Education." *Health Education Quarterly* 8(4):281–291.

Deeds, S. G.; Hebert, B. J.; and Wolle, J. M., eds. 1979. *A Model for Patient Education Programming.* Washington, D.C.: American Public Health Association.

DeJoseph, J. G. 1980. "Writing and Evaluating Education Protocols." In *Patient Education: An Inquiry into the State of the Art*, edited by W. D. Squyres. New York: Springer.

Gibson, J.; Ivancevich, J.; and Donnelly, J. 1982. *Organizations: Behavior, Structure, Processes*. 4th ed. Dallas: Business Publications.

Goldsmith, S. 1981. *Health Care Management: A Contemporary Perspective*. Rockville, Md.: Aspen Systems Corp.

Green, L. W.; Kreuter, M. W.; Deeds, S. G.; and Partridge, K. B. 1980. *Health Education Planning: A Diagnostic Approach*. Palo Alto, Calif.: Mayfield.

Koontz, H. 1968. "Making Sense of Management Theory." *Harvard Business Review* 40(4):24.

Koontz, H., and O'Donnell, C. 1955. *Principles of Management: An Analysis of Management Function*. New York: McGraw-Hill.

Levin, H. M. 1979. "Cost-effectiveness Analysis in Evaluation Research." In *Handbook of Evaluation Research*, vol. 2, edited by E. L. Struening and M. Guttentag. Beverly Hills: Sage Publications.

Mathews, B. P. 1972. "Administrative Climate: Its Implications for Health Educators." *Health Education Monographs* 12:19–31.

Mullen, P. D., and Zapka, J. 1982. *Guidelines for Health Promotion and Education Programs in HMOs*. Washington, D.C.: Department of Health and Human Services, Public Health Service.

Murphy, J., and Finnegan, M. 1980. "Hospital Harnesses Computers' Capabilities to Spot, Solve Problems in Patient Education Programs." *PROmoting HEALTH*, 1(6):1, 3.

National Interagency Council on Smoking and Health. 1974. *Guidelines for Research on the Effect of Smoking Cessation Programs: A Committee's Report*. New York.

Parlette, N.; Glogow, E.; and D'Onofrio, C. 1981. "Public Health Administration and Health Education Training Need More Integration." *Health Education Quarterly* 8(2):123–146.

Posavac, E. J., and Carey, R. G. 1980. *Program Evaluation: Methods and Case Studies*. Englewood Cliffs, N.J.: Prentice-Hall.

Rakich, J. S.; Longest, B. B.; and Donovan, T. R. 1977. *Managing Health Care Organizations*. Philadelphia: Saunders.

Shepard, D. S., and Thompson, M. S. 1979. "First Principles of Cost Effectiveness Analysis in Health." *Public Health Reports* 94:535–543.

Shortell, S. M., and Richardson, W. C. 1978. *Health Program Evaluation*. St. Louis: Mosby.

Taylor, J. B. 1979. *Using Computers in Social Agencies*. Beverly Hills: Sage Publications.

Thompson, G. E., and Handelman, I. 1978. *Health Data and Information Management*. Boston: Butterworth.

U.S. Department of Health, Education, and Welfare. National Institutes of Health. National Institute of Mental Health. *A Working Manual of Simple Program Evaluation Techniques for Community Mental Health Centers*. DHEW Publication no. (ADM) 79–404. Washington, D.C.: Government Printing Office.

Vosen, B., and Deeds, S. G. 1981. "Developmental States of Health Education in HMO's." *Health Education Quarterly* 8(4)333–347.

Wolfe, D. (Director of Community Health Education, University of Massachusetts Health Services). 1982. Personal communication.

Analysis

This case presents the health educator in the role of manager. The setting is the health education department of a large organization. The focus of the case is on the development and implementation of a departmental information system that, Zapka states, illustrates how a number of management functions are integrated to achieve a certain purpose.

Implicit to this case is the belief that management is necessary if an organization is to achieve its purpose. This may seem to be a trivial statement that is beyond dispute, but that is only because we are so accustomed to the concept of management. Yet the word *management* is relatively new in the lexicon of organizations. It is a recent construct that is less than 100 years old. For example, it was only after its first 50 years of operation that the Ford Motor Company in the 1940s began to utilize management practices. Ford turned to management only after its share of the new car market had deteriorated to the extent that the firm was in danger of collapsing. Ford was run as an autocracy in which the prevailing belief was that only an owner-entrepreneur and "helpers" were needed to make the company run successfully (Drucker 1974). None of the managerial functions listed by Zapka were allowed to be assumed by subordinates. As Zapka states, a general consensus has now developed as to what these managerial tasks are. However, the question now is, What model of management is best? It is important to note that there continues to be vigorous discussion of how these tasks should be carried out within management models, as the great interest in the so-called Japanese style of management illustrates.

A major issue that emerges from this case is the general relationship of health education to management. Zapka notes that health educators usually don't consider themselves to be managers, even though much of their day-to-day functioning is concerned with carrying out managerial tasks. Perhaps the absence of a managerial identity stems from an incomplete understanding of management. It is possible that many health educators equate management only with control and/or bureaucracy. Interestingly, according to Drucker (1974), bureaucracy is a degenerative disease that management is at risk of developing when it begins to see itself as an end and the organization as the means.

As health educators continue to learn more about management, commonalities will emerge that should lead to greater comfort with the managerial role. Health educators may find more in common with particular management models than they did before. For example, Likert's (1967) System 4 model, which focuses on the building of effective work groups to achieve high performance goals, may be appealing to health educators because of its openness. Japanese management, with its emphasis on the four S's of skills, staff, style, and superordinate goals or guiding concepts may be more attractive to health educators than American management, which traditionally has stressed the three S's of strategy, structure, and systems. However, according to Pascale and Athos (1982), the most successful organizations are those that utilize and integrate all seven S's.

In any event, health educators, at least those who are interested in advancement, will very often find themselves in managerial or administrative positions (Parlette, Glogow, and D'Onofrio 1981). It is important for health educators to assume managerial positions so that they can strengthen the profession internally and gain greater credibility with other professionals. But health educators may not be adequately prepared for management positions. Training in management should be a part of both basic preparation and continuing education. Researchers in role delineation have already recognized this training need, and perhaps their recommendations in this area will be rapidly put to use.

In this case study, we see that Zapka used several procedures worthy of emulation in setting up the departmental information system. For example, a needs assessment was carried out; the existing system was analyzed, and other systems from around the country were reviewed. The effect that implementing the new system had on staff was anticipated; thus attention was directed toward the "people issue." In action here we see planned change that necessitated involving staff in the design and implementation of the system. Every good manager learns early that management, while being production-oriented, still must be people- or process-oriented.

References/Select Resources

Drucker, P. F. 1974. *Management*. New York: Harper & Row.

For anyone interested in understanding contemporary management practice in the United States, this book is the one to consult. Though at first glance this long book may not appear relevant to health educators, a closer look will enable health educators to function better in the organizations in which they are employed.

Likert, R. 1967. *The Human Organization*. New York: McGraw-Hill.

This work by the originator of the Likert scale is a classic statement on organizational behavior. In this book and an earlier one, *New Patterns in Management*, Likert promotes an "interaction influence" system, which emphasizes the use of effective work groups that are linked to one another through supportive relationships.

Parlette, W.; Glogow, E.; and D'Onofrio, C. 1981. "Public Health Administration and Health Education Training Need More Integration." *Health Education Quarterly* 8(2):123–146.

The authors report that many health educators, particularly at the master's and doctoral level, quickly assume administrative positions at or soon after graduation. Therefore health educators should receive more taining in administration, because they function more as managers than as health educators. The authors further state that health education has much to contribute to health administration, which is another reason why training needs to be better integrated.

Pascale, R. T., and Athos, A. G. 1982. *The Art of Japanese Management*. New York: Warner.

The title is somewhat of a misnomer because this book is actually a presentation of the author's model of management that is based on both Japanese and American models. This model, like the one by Likert, could be readily adapted by health educators who have managerial responsibilities.

Discussion Questions

1. What are some of the issues that a health educator as a personnel or human resources manager might have to face?

2. What would be some commonalities and differences in managing in a medical setting versus a commmunity setting?

3. Why is the proper balance of authority and responsibility necessary for a manager to be successful?

4. Develop an outline for staff training on the use of the departmental information system described by Zapka.

5. What difficulties might a health educator encounter in a medical care setting as a result of the interplay between the formal power vested in management and the informal power of the physicians?

PART THREE

Case Studies in Community Settings

HISTORICAL PERSPECTIVE

Community health education, formerly sometimes known as public health education, had a long preprofessional phase before the term *health education* was first proposed in 1919 at a conference called by the Child Health Organization (Rosen 1958). In ancient Greek medicine, the preservation of health, and not just cure, was of prime importance. In the Middle Ages a plethora of books directed at the upper classes were written on the preservation of health.

During the Enlightenment, health education, like so many other areas of inquiry, became increasingly important. The Enlightenment's emphasis on reason and perfectability proved to be a fertile ground for the spread of health information. Early in the nineteenth century a number of periodicals with a health education flavor appeared. In addition, the nineteenth century gave birth to a host of domestic medicine books whose primary audience was women. General periodicals such as almanacs published short tracts on health information.

After Pasteur and Koch ushered in the age of bacteriology, attention was directed toward disease control. Public information campaigns on tuberculosis and diphtheria were early examples of disease-specific community health education programs. At first, health departments were the main source of these information programs, but they were soon supplanted by voluntary associations. According to Rosen (1958), the tuberculosis movement was the trailblazer in community health education. The first tuberculosis exhibit took place in Baltimore in 1904, and traveling exhibits were soon after offered in major cities throughout the United States. Sponsored by the National Association for the Study and Prevention of Tuberculosis, these exhibits used lay people trained by health professionals to bring their health message to the public.

At the same time a vigorous maternal and child health movement commenced. To a great extent it was a product of changes that immigration wrought in American society. As Rosen (1977:47) notes, "Activities concerned with infant health and welfare were aimed . . . at mothers and children in immigrant groups living under poor environmental conditions. The campaign to improve child health must be seen in part as an element in the Americanization movement which had its beginning at the end of the last century, reached its peak during the First World War, and ebbed away during the 1920's."

As this movement "ebbed away," it helped give birth to what today we call community health education and school health education. The latter was the more immediate beneficiary of the maternal and child health movement, because training programs for school health educators began in the 1920s. Eventually, as Nyswander (1980) states, many school health education leaders were to become the early community health education leaders. Among these early leaders, Nyswander herself serves as an important example.

By 1946 a survey found that 460 people were employed as health educators in official and voluntary agencies. Graduate training programs were offered at a number of universities. In 1950 the Society of Public Health Educators was formed as the professional organization for community health educators. This event, in conjunction with graduate training programs, serves as a benchmark in the professionalization of community health education, a process that is still taking place today.

ROLE OF THE COMMUNITY HEALTH EDUCATOR

In recent years there has been considerable discussion on the professional role of the health educator. This role has been the focus of the federally and privately funded Role Delineation Project (National Center for Health Education 1980). The entry-level health educator's responsibilities and functions as defined and verified by this project are the same for all health educators regardless of the setting in which they practice. However, practice in different settings will emphasize one responsibility more than another. In addition, certain strategies will be employed more often in different settings. A strategy often used in community health education is community organization, labeled by Bivins (1979:109) as "an old but reliable health education technique." The knowledge and skills required to do community organization are likely to be applied more often in the community than in other settings.

Nyswander (1980:14), a pioneer in community health education, has listed what she sees as the most important functions of community health educators:

1. Obtaining people's participation on varied operational levels in a program
2. Defining operational objectives
3. Planning the program
4. Determining strategies to bring about change
5. Developing viable working groups
6. Training others
7. Doing evaluation and research

These functions are carried out by the health educator in the community, as will be seen by the cases in Part 3. But they are also functions of health educators in all other settings, as illustrated by the cases in the other parts of this book.

Ross and Mico's (1980:311–312) definition of community organization for health is useful to consider when reading the cases in this part: a "health-education process or method in which the combined efforts of individuals, groups, and organizations are designed to generate, mobilize, coordinate, utilize, and/or redistribute resources to meet unsolved or emergent health needs and problems."

Community organization is the strategy for most of the cases in this part. Either it is the prime one, as in the case studies by Thomas and her colleagues and by Campbell and Williams, or it provides the basis for the use of specific strategies, as in the Rosenberg case on the cervical cytology demonstration project, in Semura's efforts to develop a primary care clinic, and in Santos's work in women's health.

As the study by Thomas, Israel, and Steuart shows, when the emphasis is specifically on community organization with the focus on general skill development, time becomes an extremely important ingredient. Community organizing will rarely take place within the confines of a year. It requires a multiyear commitment, a fact that funding sources have been unwilling to recognize. If the project is limited to a year, the objectives of community organizing will have to be narrowed. For some this constriction is contrary to the spirit of community organization. But when time is limited, difficult choices must be made. The Santos case illustrates how community organization can be a result of individual change. As the individual assumes responsibility for his or her health behavior, self-empowerment can occur, which can lead to social change.

In addition to functioning as community organizers, health educators in the community are often called upon to do training. In Nyswander's (1980) judgment, this has been their most common role. In the Hamrell/Raiser case, the training of public health nurses enabled them to carry out a hypertension control program. In the Lorig/Lauren case, lay volunteers were trained to lead courses for arthritis patients. The training of other health educators is very often the responsibility of health educators in a managerial position, as in the Salisbury case. Training is a generic skill, that is, competent trainers can apply their skills to many content areas and target groups. The skills used in training community members to understand and contribute to the health planning process, as described in the study by Pinkett-Heller and Clark, are readily adaptable to other training situations.

Developing viable working groups is another activity that concerned health educators in these cases. This task, which demands highly skilled professionals (Nyswander 1980), must be carried out early if a community health education effort or program is to be successful. Lorig and Lauren found that they would have to gain the cooperation of the medical community if they were to fullfill their project's potential. The creation of a task force, as described in the Semura case, is a fine example of how the health educator must be both process- and task-oriented. Basic training in health education has often stressed process. Process is indeed important and is one of the main skills of health educators that distinguishes them from other health professionals. It is true that assiduous attention to process helps achieve the task at hand. But trouble occurs when process becomes an end in itself and the task falls by the wayside. Ogasawara, in the effort to change the method of treatment for tuberculosis, worked with a number of groups who were called upon to develop policy. At times process had to be short-circuited; otherwise the task would never have been completed.

Community health educators, like health educators who practice in other settings, are responsible for selecting and implementing strategies to bring about change. The Morehead case provides an example of an innovative strategy, story telling, that was well matched to the target population's culture. The lesson to be learned from this case is that a strategy cannot be selected without attention to the needs and characteristics of the target population as well as to the type of resources that are available. In the same sense, according to Green and his colleagues (1980:105–113), the strategies should be linked to particular diagnostic criteria (e.g., characteristics of the health problem).

In community work, as in all areas of health education, evaluation is a pivotal function. It is pivotal in the sense that (1) it can help tell us what we accomplished, as well as whether the program actually brought about the results, and (2) health education's future as an enduring profession is dependent on the results of program evaluation. As the Windsor case indicates, evaluation in the community is not an easy task, but it can be done if adequate resources are allocated and if planning for evaluation takes place in conjunction with program planning.

REFERENCES

Bivins, E. C. 1979. "Community Organization—An Old but Reliable Health Education Technique." In *The Handbook of Health Education,* edited by P. M. Lazes. Germantown, Md.: Aspen Systems Corp.

Green, L. W.; Kreuter, M. W.; Deeds, S. G.; and Partridge, K. B. 1980. *Health Education Planning: A Diagnostic Approach.* Palo Alto, Calif.: Mayfield.

National Center for Health Education. 1980. "Health Education and Credentialing: The Role Delineation Project." *Focal Points* 3 (July):1–31.

Nyswander, D. V. 1980. "Public Health Education: Sources, Growth and Operational Philosophy." *International Quarterly of Community Health Education* 1(1):5–18.

Rosen, G. 1958. *A History of Public Health.* New York: MD Publications.

Rosen, G. 1977. *Preventive Medicine in the United States, 1900–1975.* New York: Prodist.

Ross, H. S., and Mico, P. R. 1980. *Theory and Practice in Health Education.* Palo Alto, Calif.: Mayfield.

Ross, M. G. 1955. *Community Organization.* New York: Harper.

The Vermont Connection

Marjorie Hamrell, B.S., M.Ed. and Amy Raiser, B.S., M.Ed.

This case will describe a training program in hypertension control for nurses in home health agencies. The program was developed by the program director of the Vermont Heart Association (an adult educator) and the project director of the Hypertension Control Project for the Vermont State Department of Health (a public health nurse).

Background information on the development of the total hypertension control program in the state and on the relationship between the two agencies involved—the Heart Association and the Health Department—will be presented before discussing the training program.

BACKGROUND

Federal public health dollars, particularly in the 1970s, were heavily laden with mandates for the public and private sector to coordinate and integrate programs and services. Coalescence was rarely achieved in an altruistic sense. The favored economic position of the public agency established the direction and role that private agencies would play via subcontract.

Despite this situation, public and private agencies did develop coalitions that carried out effective public health programs. Such a coalition was basic to the training program described in this case. The events that led up to this coalition and the factors that made it possible are discussed in this section.

Marjorie Hamrell is the Director of Health Promotion for the Vermont Department of Health and was formerly Director of the Hypertension Program. Amy Raiser is Director of the Visiting Nurse Association Foster Grandparent Program in Burlington, Vermont, and was formerly Hypertension Program Director of the Vermont Heart Association.

In the 1970s, the U.S. government allocated funds to establish a National High Blood Pressure Detection and Control Program. These funds were appropriated through a block grant known as "314d" monies. Programs under category "314d" of the federal budget (often referred to as "Public Health Revenue Sharing") were lumped into one fund and distributed to each state to use according to the state's discretion. So little money was available that states were frustrated or apathetic in their attempts to institute meaningful programs for hypertension control. This was particularly true in Vermont, a small state where resources have always been limited, both for the funding of public and private programs and in the availability of qualified professionals to develop and implement public health programs.

By 1979, funding levels improved with a substantial increase in the amount targeted for high blood pressure (HBP) control. It was then that both the Vermont Department of Health and the Vermont Heart Association applied for and received federal funding under the newly designated categorical funding for hypertension control. Despite the fact that the Health Department, as the official agency, submitted the master grant and was the recipient of the federal monies, the two agencies wrote their grants independent of each other and without collaboration. When the grants were implemented, it was apparent that the agencies were in conflict. Both were duplicating program activities such as professional education, public education, and community control projects with local home health agencies. Program personnel from both agencies did not differentiate their roles, objectives, or areas of expertise. In short, the Heart Association and the Health Department were in competition.

The Heart Association's project design focused on epidemiology and research, not on education or delivery of service to the community. The Health Department staff was wary of this approach to programming because it fostered a perspective of research versus service. In 1979 this conflict in philosophy encouraged the agency that held the purse strings (the Health Department) to establish control of the direction of the program. The Health Department assumed the leadership role by (1) constructing a plan to define the extent of the hypertension problem in Vermont, (2) establishing parameters for hypertension control, and (3) evaluating the effectiveness of selected interventions.

The approach to hypertension control in Vermont up to 1979 initiated some activities that laid the groundwork for achieving these three tasks. Listed in Table 1, these activities included the initial attempt to introduce hypertension control as a public health concept to the Vermont physicians. This was done through two surveys to determine (1) the physicians' knowledge and practices in the clinical management of patients with HBP, and (2) the potential use of a patient registry.

The State Advisory Council was organized in 1979 with 25 representatives from key organizations as well as other persons interested in hypertension control. An eight-member Executive Committee, in conjunction with project staff, developed a five-year State Plan for hypertension control, approved by the Advisory Council.

Because of the magnitude of the problem, the State Plan called for a long-term approach to hypertension control based on building strong local political support. Strengthening local community resources so that hypertension control efforts would continue when federal funds were no longer available was seen as critical to hypertension control in the state.

Among the key components of the plan were the following:

1. Education of consumers as well as professionals
2. A public information campaign
3. Direct services to the public through community health agencies providing detection, referral, and follow-up services
4. A long-term educational plan for all health professionals (i.e., physicians, nurses, optometrists, dentists, and pharmacists)
5. Primary prevention with selected high-risk populations
6. Primary prevention in industry, schools, and public health pediatric programs

THE COALITION

Federal regulations required an annual application for funds. When the 1980 application was funded, the Advisory Council designated the Heart Association as the agency responsible for developing professional, paraprofessional, and school health education and training programs. The State Department of Health (there are no local health departments in Vermont) was to develop and monitor 13 hypertension control programs in local communities and prepare public education materials. The decision about which agency would assume what role was determined primarily by the agency that controlled the dollars—the public agency—through the Advisory Council. However, the Health Department could not arbitrarily determine that the Heart Association would assume the leadership role for the educational aspects of the State Plan without its concurrence. Subsequent to this decision, the Heart Association hired a new hypertension program director, who had formerly worked at the Vermont Department of Health, where she had a close working relationship with the director of the department's Hypertension Project. This change in actors provided an opportune time for the two organizations to sort out roles and areas of expertise.

As stated earlier, a key component of the State Plan was the development of local capability to carry on hypertension control whether or not federal funds were available. This goal was implemented in part by allocating a portion of available funds for community hypertension control projects. Sixteen local agencies, that is, home health agencies and health centers, each submitted a proposal in response to a request for proposal from the State Department of Health for community projects.

These proposals were rated by the Executive Committee of the Advisory Council. The committee recommended to the Health Department that 13 local agencies be funded to develop community control projects. The department, concurring with

Table 1
Chronology of Activities Initiated in Vermont to Ameliorate Uncontrolled High Blood Pressure, 1970–1981

Year	HBP Activity	Lead Agency	Source of Funds
1970–1974	• Public and professional education	Vermont Heart Association	Public and private
1975–1977	• Industrial screening • Community control projects	Vermont Heart Association	Regional Medical Program funds
1976–1978	• Public and professional education; physician surveys	Vermont Heart Association with money subcontracted from Vermont Health Department	Block grant 314D
1978–1979	• Public and professional education • Community control project	Vermont Heart Association with money subcontracted from Vermont Health Department	Categorical public health money
1979–1981	• State Advisory Council on HBP • State Plan focused on reducing the prevalence of uncontrolled hypertension through detection and educational intervention • Professional public education • 13 community control projects in state plan for HBP control	Vermont Health Department and Vermont Heart Association	Categorical public health money

the committee's recommendations, contracted out 70 percent of the federally allocated funds to these agencies.

These 13 local community agencies included 2 health centers and 11 home health agencies. The education and training needs of the staffs of these agencies provided the vehicle around which the director of the Hypertension Project for the Health Department and the program director for the Heart Association developed a collaborative relationship.

The following set of circumstances made it possible to develop and implement this training program, in spite of the usual constraints of too little time and money.

1. The new program director of the Heart Association (Raiser) had both educational preparation and work experience in training, staff development, and adult education. She had worked as director of the Health Department's Health Education/Risk Reduction Program intended to foster healthy life-styles.
2. The Health Department's project director (Hamrell) had experience with special grants and projects requiring community outreach. In addition, she had been a director of one of the county home health agencies for several years and therefore had credibility with these agencies.
3. Both these directors trusted each other, and each respected the other's professional integrity and ability. This relationship evolved as a result of working together when both were employed at the Health Department.

4. Both directors felt competent in their respective and complementary roles. Each was well known throughout the Vermont public health community.
5. The administration of the Heart Association was eager and willing to cooperate on this project because of its own fiscal constraints and limited funding resources.

THE TRAINING PROGRAM

In January 1981, two directors (Hamrell and Raiser) met with Heart Association and Health Department staff to develop a needs assessment for 22 home health agency and health center staff who were to be responsible for the implementation of the hypertension control projects in their communities. Because we had only one year in which to help local agency staff develop the essential knowledge and skills, and because we had some idea of the needs of this population from previous contact, we also developed a skeletal plan for the training program. We considered 3–4 two-day workshops, tentatively reserved dates and places, and lined up some key faculty. We could always cancel should this format not be useful. But if we waited until the needs assessments were returned, we might not be able to get either the choice site or the faculty we wanted for the workshops.

The needs assessment was mailed the end of January to the staff in the 13 participating agencies. Essentially, it asked staff members to indicate the type of training they felt they needed to implement the HBP control program in their community. Their response confirmed most of what we suspected was needed.

The data from the needs assessment, coupled with our experience with the local agencies, suggested the following needs:

1. Most local agency staff had little (if any) formal training or experience in community organization theory or skills.
2. Most practitioners were not current in their clinical knowledge of hypertension or in detection and control skills.
3. In applying for grant funds, many agency administrators had goals that differed from their staff's, and in some instances from the state's, goals. This issue had to surface during the training program.

With an outline of the content in hand and with a tentative schedule for three workshops, we considered the educational strategies to be used during and between the workshops. Because of the nature of the knowledge and skills that had to be learned and the limited time in which to do this, we decided the strategies selected must maximize the involvement of the learner. Because so much of what had to be learned would be new to the trainees, we needed as many opportunities for reinforcement as possible during the year.

Our plan for the workshops called for a maximum of "doing" and a minimum of lecturing. When a lecture was necessary (e.g., information on the pathophysiology of hypertension), it would be set up with as much interaction as possible between the lecturer and the trainees. If a lecturer told the trainees how to organize a community for hypertension control, they would develop a plan during the workshop. Whenever feasible, the expertise of trainees would be used to do the training (we learn from our peers because we have the same reality).

The activity between workshops would be twofold:

1. Immediately after the workshop, a questionnaire would be distributed for feedback on what was useful and what was not, and on what the trainees wanted for the next workshop. A second questionnaire, one month later, would ask for more detailed information on the tentatively identified needs for the next workshop.
2. The Health Department project director would visit as many of the 13 participating agencies as possible between workshop sessions. Some of these visits were necessary to deal with the project's fiscal issues, but they would be used as well to observe how the agencies were progressing with plans for hypertension control, issues of concern to individual staff, and so on.

The between-sessions strategy allowed for reinforcing the training given at the workshops and for getting from the trainees some feedback that could be fed into the planning for the next session.

Thus the "curriculum" for the three workshops would be developed sequentially.

Although we were both well known in, and felt respected by, the Vermont public health community, we knew that extra credibility wouldn't hurt. In fact, given the short time for the training, we really needed as much credibility as we could muster to get us started. So, to the extent possible, we recruited "names," who were of course competent, to deal with the clinical issues. We also recruited a health education consultant both to help with the workshop sessions and to support us in the planning and implementation of the training program. This consultant had worked with the State Health Department and was therefore perceived as credible by the Vermont public health community.

We planned the first workshop for March and prayed that the Vermont weather would cooperate. We could not afford to wait till April if we were going to get three workshops in before the Thanksgiving and Christmas holidays.

IMPLEMENTATION

In the initial two-day session in March 1981, didactic information about the management of HBP patients was coupled with approaches for community organization. Experts in hypertension—the physiology of HBP, drug management, and alternative therapies—presented current information. The format allowed participants to question and interact with the experts.

For the community organization session, an important strategy was the requirement that all agency administrators attend the first day's session with their staff so that the agency staff could leave with a plan for organizing their community.

Most agencies did use community organization strategies developed during the workshop. These proved to be critical to the effectiveness of the hypertension control program. Among the strategies were the following:

1. Contacting (by letter, phone, or in person) all community-based physicians to share information about and enlist support for the impending program
2. Approaching groups that were already involved with some aspect of HBP control (e.g., the Lions Club, which operates a mobile van that provides screening for chronic health conditions such as glaucoma and hypertension)
3. Enlisting support from agency board members
4. Holding public meetings to describe plans for control of hypertension
5. Inviting every local physician to the agency office to learn about the project's plans for local hypertension control

Community organization theory presented during the initial training session emphasized the need for the active involvement of physicians to achieve hypertension control in local communities. Two local agency administrators supported extensive orientation of physicians through direct communication with them. Physicians were contacted with the express purpose of discussing hypertension as a public health problem, the community control project, the role of the home health agency, and the physician's role. They were asked for their cooperation, that is, acceptance of referrals and notification of confirmation of screening findings. Physicians' suggestions for the program were actively solicited.

The other administrators employed the strategy of proving themselves before contacting the physician. They did this by "backing into the physician's practice"; that is, they obtained effective screening—minimal or no false positives—and sent the physician new patients. Having established competency and good will, these agency administrators felt the physicians would be more likely to cooperate with them.

Getting in touch with physicians individually facilitated referral and follow-up of patients and in many cases led to eventual referral back to the project staff for ongoing patient and family education. There was thus a good follow-up of the earlier (1965–1978) surveys of physicians.

A month after the first training session, a questionnaire was sent to all participants, asking what aspects of the training had been useful or not so useful, and what areas they felt needed continued development and expansion. A month later, another, more specific questionnaire was sent. In addition to this written feedback from the trainees, the Health Department's NBP project director began the process of official "site visits," enabling one-to-one feedback and observation of individual community projects. By carefully examining what staff members had accomplished, listening to what they said they needed, and reviewing the questionnaires, we planned a second training series for June. The site visits also provided a mechanism for fostering continued communication among the state program staff and the staff of the community health agencies.

The second training session for community control staff focused on the areas they identified as most needed: (1) skill development in patient and family education strategies, and (2) skills to improve program management (referral and tracking systems, etc.). The format of the session gave the staff frequent opportunities to share their experiences in implementing programs. A few members of the community agency staff served as "faculty." Presentations on referral and tracking systems were made by staff who had firsthand, recent experience in developing and implementing a tracking system. This strategy actively involved the trainees in the learning process and enhanced group camaraderie.

The health education consultant who participated in the first session returned for the second, as did staff from the Health Department and Heart Association. Participants thought that the continuity of staffing for both the trainees and the workshop staff enhanced the training process.

During the second training session it was clear that although staff members had absorbed and used much of the information presented during the first session, they needed to hear certain things a second and even a third time before they were ready to use some of the information. They required repeated opportunities to try out their skills before further implementing the projects. The sequential nature of the training allowed time for this.

The "processes" used for determining the content of the third session were similar to those used between the first and second sessions. The state project director, during summer site visits, recognized the need for staff to refine their skills in counseling patients and families. Unlike public health nurses, who are familiar with the home visit and experienced in one-to-one counseling over a prolonged period, staff implementing hypertension control programs see numbers of people, often those with serious medical and psychosocial problems, but there is little or no time to counsel. After six months into the development of a community control program, a substantial number of hypertensives had been identified. The most difficult aspect of a community control program—helping those identified as hypertensive reach normotensive status—requires good counseling skills.

In Vermont the community control projects function as adjuncts to regular medical care. The nurse tracks HBP patients, ensuring that each reaches medical care, and then keeps in touch with them to offer support for and education about lifestyle changes and the prescribed HBP medical regimen. Many physicians refer patients and family members back to community control staff for follow-up once the diagnostic work-up is completed.

The third training session focused on development of counseling skills. One objective was to provide emotional support for community staff members so that they would be more effective and skillful in counseling clients. An expert in one-to-one counseling was hired to facilitate this session. As in other sessions, participants had an opportunity to share positive and negative concerns about their local programs, and some served as "faculty."

EVALUATION

Each training session was evaluated as described earlier. The evaluation of the project's goal—that is, continuation of hypertension control activities in communities when federal funds terminate—cannot be done at this time. Federal funds terminated in 1982.

We do know the following:

1. All but 2 of 13 agencies implemented a community HBP control project of some type after one year. The two that did not succeed had not participated in the training. Attendance at training sessions was not mandatory as a condition for receiving a grant.
2. By spring 1982, 11 communities that had developed a hypertension control project continued project activities (i.e., screening, follow-up, referral, education), in spite of continued reductions in funding of all community control projects.

We have learned a number of valuable lessons through the training program:

1. Although 13 community agencies were funded in 1981, each received different amounts of money varying from $1,200 to $15,000. In retrospect the five agencies that were funded at a *minimal* level accomplished detection but did not have the resources or the administrative support for referral and follow-up. Resources could have been better utilized by funding fewer agencies at a higher level.
2. Volunteer/official partnership can work and work well. A close working relationship among staff members is essential for effective programming.
3. A theoretical framework for the training plan was a critical ingredient in our understanding of why we were doing what we were doing.
4. Task-oriented persons could not extrapolate the concepts of community organization provided in the training sessions and were not able to use a process orientation for problem solving.

That fourth item serves as a good reminder of what *not* to do. One small agency became so committed to the concept of community organization that agency staff spent 8 of the 12 months of the contract organizing the community. To secure the most fundamental support for its program, this agency developed an elaborate process for contacting key physician providers and community groups. Little time was left for hypertension control activities!

Analysis

This case focuses on a collaborative relationship between a public health nurse in an official agency and an adult educator in a voluntary agency. Their task was to plan and implement, in one year, a program that would give the staff of home health agencies the knowledge and the skills to develop a community control program for hypertension. "Community control" means the development of a system for the detection, referral, and follow-up of persons with hypertension. It requires developing support from physicians and other community resources that can contribute to or are interested in hypertension control. The needs assessment showed that the trainees had no community organization skills and that many had not updated their clinical knowledge or skills in hypertension. The task was formidable.

The planners couldn't judge the motivation of the participants. They had to assume they came to learn, and plan accordingly. They based their plan on the following principles of learning/social change: Participation enhances learning; learning (behavior change) is the result of experience; repetition strengthens learning; support at the home base is necessary for the use of a new knowledge or skill.

There was a conscious effort to set up the methodologies during the training session so as to involve the participants. The three workshops were held several months apart to allow for experience with the new skills and knowledge. Agency administrators were requested to attend the first session so that they would understand the needs of the program and support their staff in trying to meet those needs. Each workshop reinforced what had been covered in the previous workshop; the site visits of the State Department of Health's hypertension coordinator provided additional reinforcement. Written and verbal feedback from the trainees keep the training in line with their needs. It is not surprising that staff from 11 of the 13 agencies attended all three workshops. Their needs were being met.

One year is an unreasonably short time in which to expect any group to move from having no or very limited knowledge or skill to having sufficient competency and confidence to then manage on their own with minimal or no help. The training program did move the trainees well along to a good degree of competency in one year. Two factors contributed to making this possible. First, the planners had good interpersonal relations. They already knew and liked each other and had a mutual respect for their professional competence. Therefore time was not wasted in mending egos or in fighting turf battles. Second, the planners knew the target population. They did not have to spend time getting acquainted. So they could do a good bit of preplanning before receiving the needs assessment. Although it is not ideal to make plans before having the data from the needs assessment, in this case it was necessary because of the time constraint.

Further, one formal needs assessment is unlikely to provide all the information needed about a target population to adequately prepare a training program for its members. A multitiered needs assessment such as is described in the Falck case (p. 362) can provide a much more adequate view of a target population. But it is not always possible to do an in-depth needs assessment. The pattern described in this case works: that is, do a needs assessment, work with the target population, and *listen to what these people tell you they need*; and then feed this information back into the program. A needs assessment is an ongoing activity; one never stops learning about a target population (Gilmore 1977; Steadham 1980).

The method of funding, one year at a time, placed severe constraints on long-range planning for hypertension control. The funds were expected to be available for three to five years, but the state had to apply for funds every year. The state in turn issued requests for proposals to local agencies for only one year. Very little of long-term value can be accomplished in one year for a problem as complex as hypertension; agencies did try to plan as though they would be refunded, but they were never sure. There was no guarantee that in the following year staff members would still have their jobs or that agencies could continue to offer a service. Such an unstable environment is not conducive to the kind of long-range planning that hypertension control requires.

From an educational perspective, the time constraint is a disaster. Hamrell and Raiser did develop a good training program; the agencies did make excellent beginnings in establishing sound hypertension control programs in their communities. But one year is not enough time for staff to change established practices and to learn new practices. Nor is it enough time for the community to become accustomed to and accept staff in their new role. Education (change) takes time, as the Robinson (p. 68) and Campbell/Williams (p. 288) cases illustrate.

This case demonstrates that good interpersonal relations between staff members is a key ingredient in collaboration between or among agencies, both official and voluntary. Agencies do not necessarily work together in planning and/or implementing programs for a given public health problem.

In this case, the two staff members happened to know, like, and respect each other. Suppose they hadn't gotten along? Would there have been competing training programs or turf battles over who trained whom? Sad to say, these situations do occur more often than we'd like to think. Cooperation among all available resources is essential to effectively deal with today's complex public health problems. It is people who cooperate, not agencies. The lack of understanding of how to effectively work together with staff of other agencies speaks poorly for the "professional" training of the personnel staffing these agencies.

References/Select Resources

Gilmore, G. D. 1977. "Need Assessment Process for Community Health Education." *International Journal of Health Education* 20(3):164–173.

This article offers a clear and concise description of the major methods of needs assessment. Very readable but not simplistic, it should be in the files of every health educator.

Kidd, J. R. 1977. *How Adults Learn* New York: Association Press.

This volume focuses on the adult learner's capacity to learn. It also offers useful information on the learning process. The chapter on learning theories is comprehensive and easy to understand, an excellent resource for the beginner. The same is true for the chapter on the teacher's role. This book is recommended reading for all health educators who have responsibility for working with adults.

Lynton, R. P., and Pareek, U. 1978. *Training for Development*. West Hartford, Conn.: Kumarian Press.

This book should be part of every health educator's professional library. Although it is primarily directed at those responsible for developing training programs, the material presented is applicable to anyone faced with developing a program for the public, special groups, or other professionals. In their study, Hamrell and Raiser illustrate the application of the training process, including the pre- and posttraining phases that the authors discuss.

Steadham, S. V. 1980. "Learning to Select a Needs Assessment Strategy." *Training and Development Journal* 34(1):56–61.

Steadham gives criteria for selecting the right needs assessment method and identifies the advantages and disadvantages of nine basic assessment methods. He provides a checklist of criteria—a handy reference. This is a very useful article for the health educator.

Discussion Questions

1. Assume you are the educator on the Heart Association Staff. You've just taken the job and have been told by the agency executive that you are responsible for developing the educational program for hypertension with the Health Department for staff of community health agencies. List your first five activities by rank.

2. Suggest three or four ways in which you could try to develop a working relationship with the staff member of another agency with whom you must work but whom you don't like very much.

3. Assume funding terminated after the first year of the program described in this case. Yet a number of agency staff are interested in continuing their training.

They can reserve two days a year; your resources are limited to your time, to materials you can beg, borrow, or steal, and to people who might volunteer a few hours. Describe how you would use these resources to help the agency staff improve their knowledge and skills for community control of hypertension.

4. Write a letter to the funding agency explaining why one-year funding is unsatisfactory for developing long-term community hypertension control programs.

5. What are the advantages and disadvantages of a private, volunteer sector in the health field?

The Practice of Health Education with a Chicano Population

Yolanda Santos, M.S.W.

INTRODUCTION

This case study focuses on a health education conference in a Mexican American/Chicano community utilizing the innovative pedagogical methodology developed by Paulo Freire (Freire 1975). The Women's Health Conference, sponsored by the Barrio Education Project, Inc. (BEP), was held in San Antonio, Texas, on April 11–12, 1981. It demonstrated the applicability of this methodology to a target population that historically had not been reached by traditional health education strategies.

Organized as a nonprofit, community-based organization, the BEP has as its primary goal the self-empowerment of economically disadvantaged women as a means of maximizing their human potential. One of its unique attributes is that it is a project totally centered on the needs of women. The board of directors, staff and program participants are all bilingual/bicultural women who are familiar with the Chicano life experience. (It is beyond the scope of this article to enter into the philosophical and political distinctions among the Chicano, Mexican American, and Hispanic people. Throughout this article the three terms are used interchangeably.) Illiteracy, unemployment, and poor health care services are a reality of life in the Chicano barrio. Poverty, low self-esteem, feelings of alienation, isolation, and a sense of powerlessness are outcomes of these social factors. To effectively intervene in the Chicano community, innovative strategies need to be employed. Since its inception, the BEP has incorporated Freire's philosophy and methodology of *concientización* (critical consciousness) for creating social change in the community. The staff has worked closely with the Institute of Cultural Action in Geneva that Freire was instrumental in organizing. The institute has provided technical assistance around the world to community groups focused on creating social change through a process of sociocultural transformation. A working relationship between the BEP and the institute has been maintained since 1975.

The pedagogical process of *concientización* centers on awareness, at both the community level and the personal level. The initial phase involves a process of reflection upon aspects of community reality (e.g., health problems, drug problems, literacy problems). The next phase looks behind these identified problems to their roots. This is followed by a process of examining the implications and consequences of these issues. The final phase of this process is the development of a plan of action for dealing with the problems.

The primary difference between Freire's approach and those of other social action theorists and practitioners is its elimination of the asymmetrical aspects of the leader's role. The process of *concientización* requires total involvement by participants. The methodology is a step-by-step process in which the participants set the theme for instruction/learning. Discussions are initiated through the use of visual aids that frequently depict universal situations. The crucial element of learning stressed in this program is to involve the participants in designing the learning activities. The dialoguing process between teacher and learner is one based on equality and mutual sharing. This approach is experiential; it replaces the hierarchical

---

Yolanda Santos is a doctoral candidate in the University of Texas School of Public Health in Houston, Texas.

competitive learning structure with a more cooperative mutual learning process. The outcome is one of self-empowerment. This pedagogical approach is integral in all BEP programs and activities.

Utilizing Freire's philosophy of education for critical consciousness, the BEP has conceptualized a bilingual/bicultural modality for assisting the community to attain self-efficacy through utilization of the pedagogical approach. The BEP has developed a program motif consisting of four interrelated components: (1) literacy, (2) cultural arts, (3) health, and (4) advocacy. The initial program developed in 1975 was the Spanish Literacy Program. Through a community survey conducted by the first board of directors, an unmet community need was identified—a desire for basic literary classes in Spanish. The classes always have been limited to 15 students because of the imperative nature of total participation. To date, 75 barrio residents have completed the 45-hour program. The classes have had a phenomenal attendance rate. The dialoguing that occurs in the class is a strategy that enables people to move toward liberation and change. For many participants this is their first experience in a shared interactional forum. The learning process fosters self-confidence and self-esteem.

The Cultural Arts Component of the BEP is primarily represented by Teatro del Pueblo, a community-based theatre group. Teatro is used as a vehicle for developing a sense of cultural awareness. The plays and skits depict the life experiences of *la familia* (the family) and the community that are inherent in the Chicano culture. The utilization of Teatro as a pedagogical teaching/learning tool has been very effective in creating critical consciousness in a variety of the agency's activities. Additionally, the BEP is involved in a Folk Arts Project that focuses on researching and documenting indigenous folk arts in order to preserve these aspects of *la cultura Chicana* (Chicano culture). During July 1980, the BEP organized and sponsored the Feria de Artes Hispanas (Hispanic Arts Festival), a tribute to community art groups and artists.

Health promotion has been a top priority for the BEP since its inception. The Health Component provides community-based classes in preparing economically disadvantaged Chicanas for childbirth. Utilizing the pedagogical methodology, classes provide needed information on the psychological and physiological aspects of conception, pregnancy, and childbirth to young Chicano couples. The classes adopt aspects of the Lamaze method and prepare the expectant mother and her partner for the birth. The BEP has developed a Trainer's Manual for the Preparing for Childbirth Program (PCP), incorporating the pedagogical approach. Average class enrollment is eight couples. The majority of new participants are recruited into the program through a network of prior PCP participants, although referrals are accepted from the Bexar County Hospital District. Since the PCP's inception in 1975, over 650 couples have been trained. Breast feeding is the preferred practice of the mothers who have participated in the PCP, with 90 percent reporting this practice.

The Advocacy Component, the BEP's most recent segment, provides technical assistance and initiates research efforts aimed at developing leadership capabilities among Chicana women. It offers workshops for women focused on developing self-esteem and self-empowerment. The institute utilizes Freire's process-oriented pedagogical approach as a means of enhancing personal growth. Strong emphasis is placed on developing social support systems.

This cursory view of the BEP was presented to create an awareness of the overall diversity of its programs. Its uniqueness lies in its philosophy and approach to creating social change in the community. The Women's Health Conference exemplifies an attempt to utilize the pedagogical approach to discuss relevant health problems and to promote personal responsibility for health maintenance.

WOMEN'S CONFERENCE

PLANNING PHASE

Because of its six-year history of community involvement, the BEP was knowledgeable about the dire need for health promotion activities geared for Chicanas. In San Antonio, accessibility to health care and the lack of bilingual/bicultural health promotion programs has created a serious gap in meeting the health needs of these Chicanas. In attempting to fill this void, the BEP board of directors approached the Ms. Foundation, devoted entirely to assisting women's activist self-help projects, for funding of a Women's Health Conference. The Ms. Foundation proposal requested funding for a two-day bilingual/bicultural health promotion conference on (1) the mystique of health care providers and systems; (2) analysis of pending legislation, with emphasis on the Hyde Amendment (anti-abortion); (3) folklore, myth, and legend and their effects on health care choices; (4) self-examination, self-advocacy, and the well woman; and (5) reproductive rights and choices.

This proposal was funded in early 1981. The initial phase of planning involved a series of informal *platicas* (mutual dialoguing) held by various board members with women in the Edgewood community, a predominantly Mexican American community in the westside of San Antonio. The BEP is located within the Edgewood Independent School District (EISD), one of the most economically depressed districts in Texas. The 8, two-hour informal *platicas*, along with input from health professionals, helped crystalize not only the most relevant discussion topics but also the approach best suited for the conference. Since many of the women were not accustomed to the participatory structure of the pedagogical approach, it was recognized that the strategy of encouraging participants to use *chistes, dichos y cuentos* (jokes, proverbs, and short stories) when sharing their experiences would facilitate communication. The need for day care services during the conference was clearly identified.

With the initial phase of planning accomplished, the board of directors and the BEP staff concentrated on the next six phases of planning. Specifically, these included:

1. Developing the specific objective, goals, and format of the conference, given the input provided by the community
2. Reviewing the methodology of the *concientización* process that would be utilized throughout the conference
3. Reviewing available health and mental health educational materials to find those most appropriate for the conference participants
4. Identifying resource persons in various health fields who were bilingual/bicultural and sensitive to the needs and problems encountered by Chicanas within the health care system
5. Delineating strategies for creating community awareness of the upcoming conference to ensure attendance of 100 women
6. Developing an evaluation component for the conference

IMPLEMENTATION PHASE

On April 11–12, 1981, the BEP held its First Women's Health Conference at Gus Garcia Junior High School in the EISD. The conference was titled "Nuestro Bienestar: Reflejos, Conceptos y Perspectivas" (Our Well-Being: Reflections, Concepts, and Perspectives). The objectives of this conference were cogently expressed in Spanish:

1. *Ampliar el conocimiento de todas sobre nuestro cuerpo para mantenernos saludables* (to amplify everyone's knowledge of their own body for the maintenance of health)
2. *Presentar una oportunidad para refleccionar sobre los aspectos culturales, educativos, legislativos y medicos que nos afectan* (to provide the opportunity for reflection on aspects of culture, education, legislation, and medicine that affect us)
3. *Dar la oportunidad a mujeres de platicar, preguntar, escuchar y compartir con nuevas amigas sus ideas, datos, problemas, soluciones y opiniones sobre nuestra salud* (to provide an opportunity for women to speak, question, listen, and share with new friends their ideas, data, problems, solutions, and opinions about their health)
4. *Iniciar un dialogo para el desarrollo de una red de unidad que activamente promueva el bienestar de la mujer* (to initiate dialogue for development of a network of unity that will actively promote the well-being of women)

To attain these goals, the conference harnessed the key elements of the pedagogical approach. The conference was initiated by an Opening Session led by the board of directors and executive directoress, who delineated the process and philosophy of *concientización*. Utilizing the *platica* format, the speakers discussed the learning experiences that the conference hoped to promote. The role of the "experts" was defined as that of facilitators interacting as equals with participants. All activities utilized the *platica* format, which helps facilitate sharing and more open communication. It was a format that effectively removed communication barriers because it encouraged people to trust and risk. The final presentation of the Opening Session was titled "Todas Somos Importantes" (We Are All Important), which set the tone for the two-day learning experience.

The conference format employed an integrative approach for presenting a broad array of topics. Although the conference was designed to use a concurrent workshop format, participants requested that this structure be modified because there was not sufficient time for repetition of workshops. The participants expressed their desire to maximize the opportunities for learning because a similar conference was not projected in the near future. The conference planners responded positively to the initiative demonstrated by the participants, combining the concurrent workshops into single sessions. The flexibility and responsiveness of the conference planners to the expressed needs and assertiveness of the participants created a sense of group cohesiveness that contributed to the learning environment. Both days concluded with a session titled "Platicas entre Mujeres" (Mutual Dialoguing among Women), which provided a means of synthesizing the learning experiences of each day. It also provided a milieu not only for the interchange of information but also for the sharing of personal life experiences. The use of jokes, proverbs, and short stories to facilitate interpersonal interaction enhanced the learning experiences of all participants. The informal group structure that developed encouraged women to share personal experiences related to employment discrimination, family life-styles, and poverty. The flowchart of Figure 1 provides an overview of the topics discussed during the conference.

PARTICIPANTS

Extensive use had been made of the mass media and conference posters to create awareness of the conference. No registration fee was charged. The conference goal of involving 100 women, representing health providers and consumers, included social service workers, teachers' aides, bank tellers, health and mental health workers, secretaries, and child welfare workers. Also represented were community organizers, students, elected officials, and faculty members. A number of the participants were not employed outside the home. For some of the women, this was their first experience in participating in a community health promotion activity. From the personal sharing of life experiences that occurred throughout the conference, it became evident that the majority of the women were single parents. Many spoke of marriage at an early age. The participants were predominantly in their early thirties and life-long residents of San Antonio. Participants were bilingual; they demonstrated a consistent style of language switching, especially when sharing personal feelings.

A registration roster was compiled that included the participant's name, address, phone number, and areas of special concern and/or community involvement. Copies of this roster were mailed to all participants shortly after the conference. It served as an initial organizing tool from which conference participants were able to organize a voluntary women's network to follow up on issues identified during the conference.

This networking effort utilized the principles and methodology of Freire's pedagogical process inasmuch as the network organized around issues selected by the women and used a rotation of facilitators rather than elected officers to organize ongoing meetings. Networking was envisioned not only as a vehicle for sharing information but, more important, as a mechanism to facilitate teaching women the skills needed for planning, organizing, and expediting additional "special focus" conferences. The network organizing effort that evolved from the Women's Health Conference later was incorporated into the BEP's Advocacy Component.

EVALUATION

The evaluation of the Women's Health Conference was obtained from evaluation sheets that were distributed each day and from the *platica* sessions at the close of each day. There was a 50 percent response rate on the written evaluation. The written and verbal feedback was positive, with participants giving high ratings to the content as well as the process of the conference. The workshops the women selected as most informative and beneficial were (1) breast cancer self-examination, (2) stress management, (3) abused women and children, (4) needs of special children, and (5) legislation affecting women. The main focus of evaluative re-

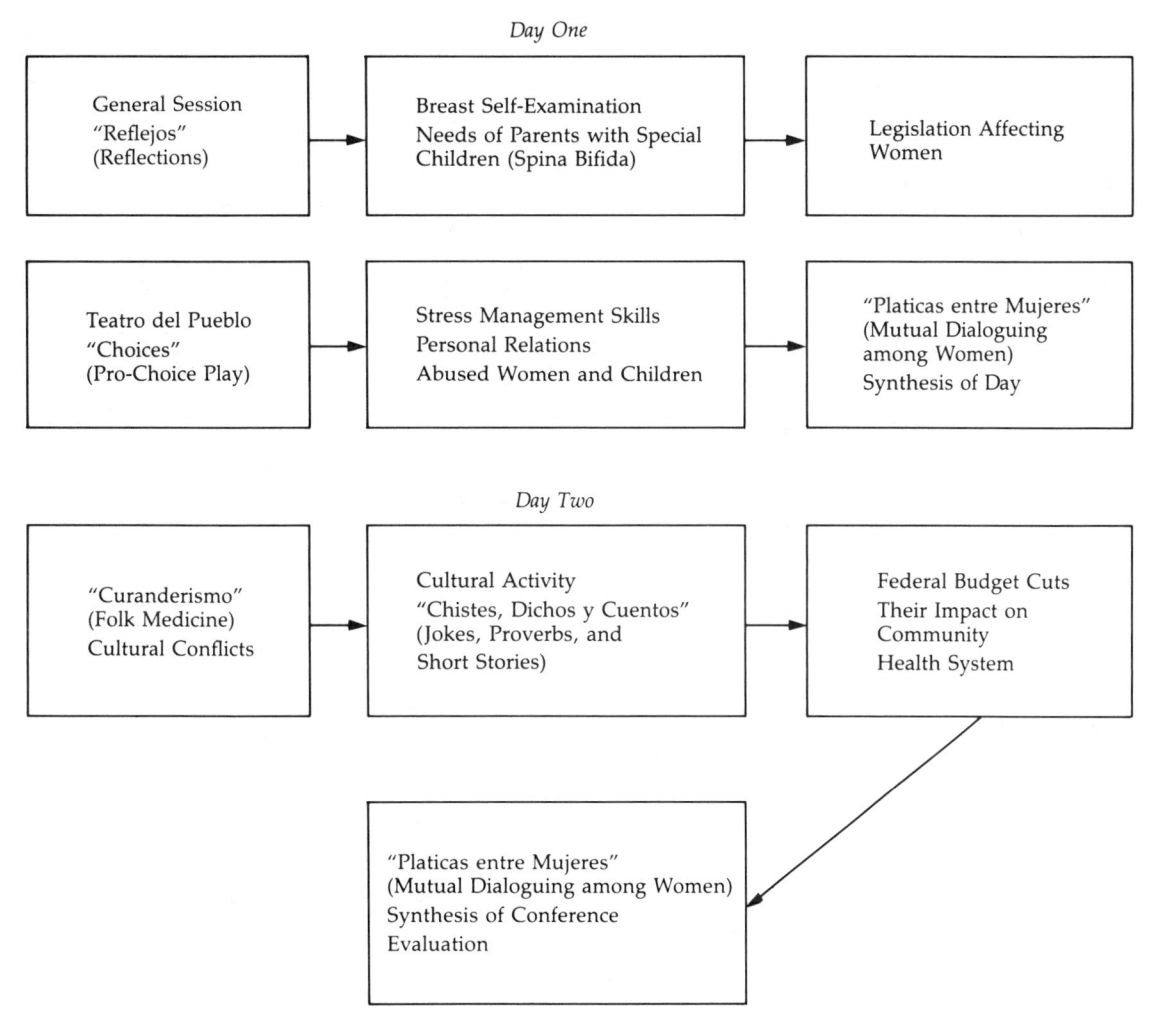

Figure 1
Overview of the Women's Health Conference

Day One

- General Session "Reflejos" (Reflections) → Breast Self-Examination / Needs of Parents with Special Children (Spina Bifida) → Legislation Affecting Women
- Teatro del Pueblo "Choices" (Pro-Choice Play) → Stress Management Skills / Personal Relations / Abused Women and Children → "Platicas entre Mujeres" (Mutual Dialoguing among Women) / Synthesis of Day

Day Two

- "Curanderismo" (Folk Medicine) / Cultural Conflicts → Cultural Activity "Chistes, Dichos y Cuentos" (Jokes, Proverbs, and Short Stories) → Federal Budget Cuts / Their Impact on Community Health System → "Platicas entre Mujeres" (Mutual Dialoguing among Women) / Synthesis of Conference / Evaluation

marks related to the conference's format. Participants expressed approval of the informal group interactional structure, stating that it provided a forum in which women could openly express their opinions on issues in a supportive milieu.

Utilizing this methodology for health education provided an opportunity for learning to occur simultaneously but at distinct levels, according to the individual's needs. For some participants, the conference provided a setting for becoming aware of community problems with which they were unfamiliar. For others, it provided a linkage with new resource persons in the community who were involved in issues of mutual interests. The *platica* sessions provided an assessment of the appropriateness of using jokes, proverbs, and short stories for enhancing communication. The level of interaction that was evident throughout the conference created a spirit of unity that enhanced the learning experience. The recommendations for future workshops reflected the participants' awareness of the seriousness of community problems and issues. They recommended workshops on (1) rape, (2) mental health, (3) self-esteem, (4) early detection screening, (5) ways that Mexican American women can deal with pressures of society, and (6) ways to get involved in community-oriented activities. The suggestions for improving any further conferences centered on use of more bilingual visual aids and the inclusion of more women.

COMMENTARY

This case study has been presented to demonstrate that often innovative health education strategies must be used to reach a specific target population such as economically deprived Chicana women. Traditional health education/health promotion techniques that fail to involve the learners in defining the problem from their own value system result in programs that are culturally and linguistically inappropriate for Chicano client groups. The BEP's utilization of the Freire philosophy and methodology has created a modality for structuring learning so that the self-efficacy of the learner is reinforced and the result is self-investment in the learning process. Its versatility across all BEP program components demonstrates its usefulness as an intervention strategy that can promote personal growth while creating needed social change. It is especially applicable in teaching modification of health behavior in order to enhance healthy life-style practices.

In relation to health promotion, the learning process suggested by the process of *concientización* is that the learner assumes self-responsibility for negative health behavior. The resulting changes in health behavior are outcomes of a self-appraisal process that originates from a plan of action focused on self-empowerment. The potential for long-term modification of unhealthy life-styles practices makes the pedagogical approach to health education/health promotion a powerful strategy, especially because of its appropriateness for hard-to-reach target populations and its emphasis on social change.

This case study exemplifies the potential of using the pedagogical approach in health promotion. To assess its viability as a nontraditional model for health promotion with hard-to-reach populations, additional attention must be given to the development of programs with comprehensive evaluation components. Its potential for improving the health status of communities that have not responded to other strategies makes this a methodology worthy of pursuit.

REFERENCE

Freire, P. 1975. *Pedagogy of the Oppressed*. Middlesex, Harmondsworth, England: Penguin.

Analysis

This case documents the planning and implementation of a Women's Health Conference by a community-based organization for a Chicano population. The conference was one component of a broad-based program that included literacy, cultural arts, health, and advocacy. The program's Health Component included the provision of childbirth education classes for low-income women. All components of the program were directed toward creating social change in the community. Santos was a community organizer and program planner.

The Barrio Education Project operates under a well-defined theory based on the work of Paulo Freire, the noted third-world educator (Freire 1975). As did John Dewey and later Jerome Bruner, Freire emphasizes the participation of the learner in education. But he openly defines education as either a tool of oppression or a liberating force that will lead to social change, depending on who is controlling the system. Freire, like Dewey, sees education as a means to an end, but his emphasis is on the community rather than the individual. Freire's theory of *conscientización*, as Santos describes it, is the process by which individuals develop a positive self-concept and a sense of power to change their world.

Community organization provided the strategic base for this case, although the steps taken in organizing are not fully described. Organizing took place during as well as before the conference. The roster of participants was used to develop a voluntary network to follow up on issues. This networking process was also grounded on principles developed by Freire. Group process was prominently used throughout the conference. Apparently, for the most part, informal group procedures were employed rather than more formal methods.

A number of interesting procedures were imbedded in the strategies used in this case. For example, conference participants were encouraged to tell jokes and short stories to overcome communication barriers. Workshop organizers were able to modify the workshop to meet the immediate needs of the participants. It is obviously important to plan workshops and conferences so that they function smoothly, with the roles of the convenors well defined and executed. Flexibility must also be a planning consideration, because circumstances can always change when people gather. It should be noted, however, that if planning includes an adequate needs assessment, there is less likelihood of unanticipated occurrences.

Implicit in this case is an issue that has generated considerable discussion within the profession in the last few years. The issue comes to the fore in Santos's statement that "the learning process suggested by the process of *conscientización* is that the learner assumes self-responsibility for negative health behavior." Some within and outside the profession have stated that health educators who emphasize total self-responsibility for health behavior are engaging in victim blaming because, it is asserted, individual behavior is more a function of social and economic conditions than of individual volition (Brown and Margo 1978; Crawford 1977, 1978). The individual-change strategists have not been as articulate as their antagonists, but their arguments are basically the following: Health educators can ill afford to concentrate their meager resources on social change; individual behavior change holds out the greatest hope of establishing health education on a firm scientific footing; and at present the chances of success at the individual level are greater than at the social change level.

Although the Santos case is concerned with self-responsibility, we see a clear attempt to join social change concerns with individual change strategies. As the learner assumes responsibility for negative health behavior, self-empowerment can also occur, which can have far-reaching positive effects on the community.

References/Select Resources

Brown, E. R., and Margo, G. E. 1978. "Health Education: Can the Reformers Be Reformed?" *International Journal of Health Services* 8(1):3–26.
Crawford, R. 1977. "You Are Dangerous to Your Health: The Ideology and Politics of Victim Blaming." *International Journal of Health Sciences* 7(4):663–680.
Crawford, R. 1978. "Sickness as Sin." *Health/Pac Bulletin* 80 (January–February):10–16.

These three papers have generated considerable controversy among health educators because they call into question the fundamental practice of many health educators who work primarily with individuals to change health behavior. The authors assert that more attention needs to be directed at socioeconomic factors that are determinants of health and health behavior. To do otherwise would be to engage in victim blaming. All new professionals should consider this issue because it determines how many health educators view themselves professionally.

Freire, P. 1975. *Pedagogy of the Oppressed.* Middlesex, Harmondsworth, England: Penguin.

This very influential book, which has been published throughout the world, has changed the way many people view education. As we noted earlier, Freire was one of the first to clearly explore the political implications of education. His approach to education, with its emphasis on participation and empowerment of the learner, is very compatible with the view many health educators have of their role as community organizers.

Srinivasan, L. 1977. *Perspectives on Nonformal Adult Learning.* New York: World Education.

This short book brings together much of the contemporary thought on nonformal education, that is, education that takes place outside a school system. Most program examples are drawn from international settings. The principles of adult education described are based on the work of Freire, Ivan Illich, Carl Rogers, Abraham Maslow, Jerome Bruner, B. F. Skinner, and Malcolm Knowles. Srinivasan presents a clear exposition of their work and its relevance to nonformal education. Although Santos in her case emphasizes the work of Freire only as a theoretical basis, we see through Srinivasan how many others have contributed to the development of nonformal education.

Discussion Questions

1. The conference was evaluated immediately after its conclusion. How would you evaluate its long-term impact?

2. What are some of the benefits of conducting a health program as part of a broader community program?

3. How would you collect community needs assessment data in planning for a similar conference? What would you want to know?

4. In planning *any* conference, what are some of the factors you need to be concerned with?

5. Describe five ice-breaking exercises that are suitable for workshops with different population groups. Try to devise some exercises yourself.

Telling Stories of Health

Jean E. Morehead, D.Sc.

INTRODUCTION

On a global basis, diarrheal dehydration kills more children under the age of five years than any other disease. The majority of these deaths are preventable! A mother's kitchen even in rural or poor sections of a developing country usually can provide the ingredients for the oral rehydration drink to save these young lives (Johns Hopkins University 1980). Teaching by the "success story" is proving to be an effective tool in enabling mothers and families to learn how to prevent and treat such common illnesses as diarrhea. The "success story" is proving to be an effective educational tool in developing countries in community-based primary health care programs.

CASE STUDY

The clouds sit poised on the horizon like a long white flock of birds, as if some unseen hand holds them against their will. Mari has watched their motionless flight all afternoon, longing for the wetness of cooling rain. As she walks, dust swirls up around her ankles, leaving a little trail of brown smoke to settle slowly behind her in the hot still air.

Mari does not truly mind the heat. She is anticipating the fun of tonight and tomorrow, when there will be gathering friends. "There'll be ten of us," she muses, "two from each small village. It's only been a short time since we've walked this path

---

Jean E. Morehead is Vice President of Child Care U.S.A., Inc.

to our central clinic but it seems like ages—so much catching up to do!"

Mari's mind drifts back to the days when she was first chosen by her village health committee to be a health worker. "What did it feel like when I was first chosen?" she asks herself. "What was it like to fear the new, to be afraid to learn the different, to trust what I hadn't always known. . . ?

"In those days fear kept whispering that my own knowledge was different from what they would require me to learn at the clinic. 'Women knowledge' has always been a deep inner part of me. Long before I became a health worker I knew the special gift of trust the village women gave each time they asked me to sit with them during their special hours. My hands have grown sure, like grandmother's, moving gently to ease the pain in the eyes of the little one who will soon be a new mother."

Mari's thoughts softly whisper, "To help ease pain is to remember beloved grandmother, to feel her beside me gently stroking and soothing a feverish forehead. To live without sharing her special ways could not be!"

Tears come to Mari's eyes as she thinks of her little, bent grandmother. "How many times when I was a child, grandmother invited me along to walk the dusty path to a neighbor's house, holding high the large black umbrella to keep the sun's hot rays from the precious healing herbs. Yes, to heal is the gift; the gift of her life passed on to me as a treasured bowl of cool water, to share with others."

Lost in thought, Mari walks on as the late sun quietly drops behind the clouds, spreading twilight over the heat of the day. The refreshing coolness awakens Mari to the soft sound of her own sandals padding the grassless path without conscious command. Looking down, she smiles, realizing that her feet and this path are now old friends. Mari quickens her pace as she feels darkness approaching. "Tomorrow will be my first day of being the new supervisor. Grandmother would have been so proud!"

With excited anticipation Mari once again thinks over tomorrow's schedule. "All the health workers will sit down together, the new with the old. We will begin our time by sharing what has gone on in our villages since we were last together two weeks ago. Each worker will tell about the families she is caring for, their illnesses, and what she has done to help the sick. We'll talk about who has died. We will support each other as we discuss how each illness and death might have been prevented. We are a team trying to learn together.

"After hearing and sharing each worker's experience we'll learn a 'success story.' It's best to start with newcomers on a story about the sickness they are going to find often in these next days. Diarrhea kills so many little ones, especially in villages where there have never been health workers."

Mari goes over in her mind what she will say. Yes, she will talk about Nita. Silently she rehearses her story.

A STORY ABOUT THE BEST TREATMENT OF DIARRHEA

"Once there was a woman named Nita who lived with her husband and two children by the side of a path in a village. Many people walked that path on the way to the stream to wash their clothes. Two of Nita's children had died of diarrhea. Her remaining two children had runny stools and were so weak they didn't want to play. Nita and her husband also had many runny stools and felt very weak. No one in the village had a latrine. People defecated behind their houses or along the path in the bush.

"One day Nita was at the stream washing her clothes. She felt so tired. Her children were lying under a nearby tree. She was frightened when she saw that they hadn't gotten up to play with the other children, but were simply lying there watching.

"Wanite, a young woman, who is a health worker, came by and stopped to sit under the tree. She spoke gently to Nita and inquired about her two children. Nita told her that they seemed to be getting more tired every day. They were having many runny stools and losing weight. Wanite asked if they used a latrine for defecating.[1] Nita said they did not have one. Wanite said that when people go out in the bush or behind their houses to defecate, little germs, too small to see with the eyes alone, are in the stools and cause sickness. When someone with diarrhea defecates on the ground, the flies or animals come and walk over it and take these germs on their feet into the homes and on to food. Children also play on the ground and put their hands into their mouths, and these little germs get inside their bodies. This is why children often get sick with diarrhea.

"The health worker told Nita that defecating and urinating in a latrine would help to keep those germs away from her children and her family. When Nita or her family were out walking in the bush, their feces should be buried so that the flies and animals cannot spread the germs. Each person's hands should be washed after defecating and before eating. Food should be covered to keep away the flies.

"Wanite looked at Nita's children and noticed that the baby's head had a sunken soft spot. Their eyes were sunken too and had no tears. She also pinched the skin on their bellies and saw that the skin did not quickly spring back to normal, showing that they were dehydrated. 'You must make the sugar-salt drink for diarrhea and give it to the children as soon as you can!'

"'Use a large bottle and wash it with very hot water. Fill the bottle with boiled water or use the cleanest water available. Add four big spoons of sugar and a pinch of salt.[2] Because too much salt can be harmful, always taste the drink first. If it's saltier than your tears, throw it away and make some new drink.' Nita's baby was still nursing, and Wanite told her to give the child the drink and continue to put it to the breast.

"'If there is fever, or blood in the stool, or if the diarrhea does not stop in two days, take the child to the clinic immediately,' said Wanite. 'You can use this sugar-salt drink for older children and adults too when they get diarrhea,' Wanite told her.

"Nita went home and made the sugar-salt drink

as Wanite had taught her and fed it to her children. Each child drank several bottles of this drink before they got better. Nita and her husband dug a latrine and the whole family used it. They covered their food from the flies and began to wash their hands after defecating and before eating. Soon they noticed they did not have a lot of diarrhea the way they used to. If any of them did get diarrhea, they began right away to make the sugar-salt drink. Nita was very thankful to Wanite for bringing her this health teaching. She now could watch her children happily playing with the other children whenever she went to wash her clothes at the stream."

THE END

When Mari finishes telling the diarrhea success story, she will ask the health workers these questions to see what they have learned:

1. "What caused Nita's two children to die?"
2. "Where did they get this disease?"
3. "How can it be prevented?"
4. "How does one prepare the diarrhea treatment drink at home?"

Now Mari will take some steps to make sure that everyone will remember the story very well.

- Mari will choose one person to repeat the story aloud. (Everyone in the group will listen to see if anything is left out and to help fill in the details.)
- Mari will then divide the class into small groups. Each person will tell the same story to his or her small group until all have had a chance.
- Each small group will now create a drama illustrating the story, using the members of the group as actors.
- The class will reassemble and each group will present its own drama. All the other health workers will evaluate the performance of each small group and may decide to choose the best drama to be presented at the village school next week or at community gatherings of various kinds.
- Songs and riddles about the diarrhea treatment story will be made up by the health workers. The group will sing and dance to these chant-like songs. (Other health stories may be retold for review.)
- Each health worker will know the diarrhea treatment story by heart and will try to share it with as many villagers as possible—in homes, at events, on wash days, in the marketplace.

After the storytelling time, the health workers will open their medical kits to recheck their needs for refills of simple drugs. These workers know what to do to prevent and treat most common illnesses in the community. They also know when to refer the more complicated cases to the central clinic.

Mari is pleased with her health worker's learning. She is eager to see them grow in self-confidence. "Tomorrow will indeed be a good day," she affirms. "Yes, grandmother would have been proud!"

DISCUSSION

GOAL OF STORY

The goal of the "success story" is to help families learn *what to do* to become and stay healthy (Werner and Bower 1982). If one is teaching, for example, about malaria, this is neither the time nor the setting for such nonessentials as the life cycle of the mosquito (i.e., the sporozoite, etc.). The questions are: What *action* does one need to take to prevent malaria? If one contracts the disease, what are the symptoms? What can be done to treat it? Nothing more—but nothing less!

The noted linguists Drs. Tom and Betty Sue Brewster (Pasadena, California) have coined the concept of "power texts" and stories in language acquisition. The same concept applies to acquisition of health learning through stories.

Stories must be clear and practical, giving the listeners the "power tools" to know what to do, how to take action to prevent and treat disease. A health lecture or story, even if accurate, is insipid or powerless if the listeners don't know what specific action to take to help themselves and to learn more about health.

EMPHASIS ON PREVENTION

The emphasis of every story must be on how to prevent the disease. The storyteller multiplies the story's impact on the community's health by emphasizing prevention. The "treatment trap" is a working mode in which a medical facility places priority on repairing lives and then simply sends people out once again into the same community to be redamaged.

Dr. Mary Annel, an M.D. in the Rural Health Promoter's Program, Huehuetenango, Guatemala, has said: "You can be either a sopper up of water—or a turner-off of the faucet. I wanted in my health care work to try to turn off the faucet" (Annel 1981). Thus, she emphasizes prevention.

PRIORITY AND AUTHORSHIP OF STORIES

There is a priority to the subject of stories. The most prevalent serious illnesses become the topics for the first stories. The stories are most likely to be effective if they have been made up by nationals who live in the local setting and therefore understand the nuances of the culture. There is growing evidence of the effective impact on health of appropriate "success stories." Dr. David Hilton, an M.D. who served as medical consultant in the Lardin Gabas Rural Health Program in Nigeria (where all health teaching is done by stories), has documented successful programs (Hilton 1980).

MODELING

It cannot be emphasized too strongly that students will teach by emulating the way they themselves have been taught. One does an immense disservice to the "success story" method by talking about how one should do the storytelling. The method is always taught simply by doing it, including the dramatization. Analysis and discussion about why or how it works come later—if appropriate to the teaching setting.

Note that in this case study, Mari simply began by telling the story about diarrhea. The story was followed by just a few brief but key questions. A group member then retold the story, and the group itself listened to help fill in any details that had inadvertently been left out. Later, small groups formed and each person told the story. Dramatization, a key element, then followed. Health workers thus trained were prepared to actively share this story with the villagers.

WHY A STORY

Those who have had the experience of attempting to teach health lessons to a group of mothers with small children in a clinic or village setting in a developing country have rapidly become sensitized to the monumental challenge of health education and enablement. Such mothers have often walked a fair distance to the clinic and thus are tired, hot, and often anxious. Rarely is a mother there simply for a well-child clinic. The scene is usually one of movement, noise, and minor chaos. But let a good storyteller begin a tale and the hubbub begins to quiet down and be muted as attention is focused on the plight of the person in the vignette. Nothing grips an audience like a good story.

Stories require no expensive equipment on the field to maintain. One often finds rain-soaked flip charts, projectors that fail as electricity goes off or parts break down, and literature that has been destroyed by rodents. Stories are always readily available. You can't lose them or leave them behind by mistake!

In the clinic setting, the "success story" is used both on a one-to-one and on a group basis. But far more important are the stories that are spread in home visitations by the health workers as well as in community gatherings, school classrooms, churches, and the like. Children should not be overlooked; they can learn storytelling, too,. They are effective spreaders of health learning in their families and in the community.

The family that is in the midst of wrestling with an illness is searching for an answer. But far too often the mother brings a sick child or other sick person to a medical setting only to be accosted with the fact that she did not take proper health measures. She is made to feel guilty. When confronted like this, her defenses immediately go up. Walls are erected and the openness of learning is now gone. Survival of human dignity is in question. There is an irreparable loss of an opportunity for health education and enablement.

The "success story" can present the same truth in a format that is nonaccusatory. The listener hears about both the plight of the victim and the solution. A woman, for instance, sees that the situation may be similar to her present circumstances and can choose to apply the same action. "What worked for her may just work for me!" The solution is her own, not one thrust on her from outside. "Success stories" are thus stories of peers who battle with the very same problems facing the listener. The solutions seem possible. They have a way of ringing true.

THE COMMUNITY HEALTH WORKER AS STORYTELLER

Over the past ten years there has appeared a growing body of literature dealing with various methodologies in training community-based primary health care workers. But such literature has recently begun to emphasize the finding that these educational training tools are only as effective and strong as the system in which they are being utilized.

The "success story" in this case study was set on a foundation that gave it the greatest possible chance for succeeding as an effective educational and health enablement tool. What are some of the key foundational factors?

1. The health worker who will tell the story is a community member, an insider. The worker has been chosen by a village health committee, that is, a by consensus of the community and therefore is known by the community. He or she has earned the right to learn more of health and has the obligation to share it with the community. Consider the impact on our health system if all levels of health professionals were to prove their concern and commitment to a community before they were chosen, by consensus, to be allowed to *learn* (i.e., to attend medical or nursing schools) and later to have the responsibility to *share* this learning with the community.

2. Mari, the health worker, has a high motivation to learn. She has a background of following in her grandmother's footsteps and a very real pride in her heritage of serving others. The storytelling method integrates new knowledge with what she already knows. It does not denigrate the old.

3. Mari may or may not be literate. This is not of great importance to her health ministry. It certainly is not a stumbling block to her storytelling abilities!

In the Comprehensive Rural Health Project of Jamkhed, India, directed by Drs. Rajanikant and Mabelle Arole (Arole and Arole 1975), the health workers themselves have increasingly wanted to become literate. They have sought out others who would teach them to read and write.

4. In this case study the setting for the initial health workers' training and for the refresher meetings is within walking distance of the health workers' villages. Thus bad weather is less likely to prevent such gatherings than if they were at distances necessitating vehicles.

Such proximity is important to continuing education and to supervisory guidance. All education should be a "learn as you go" type of growth process. Weekly meetings are ideal; one day every two weeks is realistic. If greater blocks of time are allowed to stretch between gatherings, a critical opportunity is lost both for ongoing education and for supervision and accountability. The priority and time emphasis given to continuing education may well be one of the key indicators of a well-functioning community-based primary health care system.

5. The health worker is operating in all three enablement modes simultaneously: curative, preventive, and promotive. He or she is being enabled to recognize common illnesses and treat with simple effective drugs. Eighty-five to 90 percent of the community's illnesses will be handled at this level. He or she will refer the other illnesses (approximately 10 percent) that necessitate clinic- or hospital-based treatment to the appropriate setting. Thus the educator is one who simultaneously enables and treats. There is not the artificial dichotomy we usually see: an educator who is not allowed to heal, and a healer who has no time for educating.

6. The primary goal of Mari, as a health worker, is to *share* her knowledge as widely as possible and to multiply herself. She is not a hoarder of her storehouse of healthful knowledge; rather, she is an *enabler* of the people in the community. She attempts to call forth from within her people the great depth of potential resources that they possess to grow to be healthy. This goal is emphasized in every

training session. It is truly worthy of emulation by health professionals in our own Western health care system as well.

SUMMARY

Simple health stories that help people learn what actions to take to become healthier are being used as effective health education tools in developing countries. Such stories build on the age-old traditions of oral learning processes found in numerous cultures.

Local health workers make up stories about the most prevalent serious illnesses, emphasizing how these diseases can be prevented. In a single story the listener hears about a health problem he knows all too well plus a solution that a peer has found to work. The new health knowledge and actions are imparted in a nonaccusatory format, allowing the listener to make the identification with both the problem and the solution.

Such stories are most effective when used in a people-enhancing health care system. That is, the "success story" neatly doubles its success when it does not denigrate traditional health practices but builds upon them whenever possible; the storyteller is a member of the community, not an outsider; when she or he is given the opportunity to be both a healer and an educator; when continuing education and supportive supervisory guidance are emphasized in the setting; and when the ultimate goal of the health system is to equip people to share health knowledge, thus multiplying the number of storytellers who are enabling people to live a healthier life.

NOTES

1. Common local words are used for these body functions.
2. 1 liter water, 4 tablespoons sugar, ½ teaspoon salt. If available, ½ cup orange juice and ½ teaspoon baking soda can be added.

REFERENCES

Annel, M. V. (Director, Health Promoters Program, Jacaltenango, Huehuetenango, Guatemala). 1981. Personal communication.

Arole, M., and Arole, R. 1975. "A Comprehensive Rural Health Project in Jamkhed (India)." In *Health by the People*, edited by Kenneth W. Newell. Geneva: World Health Organization.

Hilton, D. 1980. *Health Teaching for West Africa: Stories, Drama, Song*. Wheaton, Ill.: M.A.P. International.

Johns Hopkins University. 1980. "Oral Rehydration Therapy (ORT) for Childhood Diarrhea." *Population Reports*, ser. L, no. 2.

Werner, D., and Bower, B. 1982. *Helping Health Workers Learn*. Palo Alto, Calif.: Hesperian Foundation.

RECOMMENDED RESOURCE

Christian Medical Commission. 1977. "Rural Basic Health Services: The Lardin Gabas Way." *Contact* (Geneva), no. 41.

Analysis

This case tells of the experiences of a health educator in a foreign country. As you began reading this study, you probably thought it would relate strange but interesting events among people having different customs from your own. Some differences are to be expected. But the essence of the case is that basic principles of education and human relations are the same for this case as for any educational program in the United States. Although customs, language, resources, and barriers may require some modification of the basics, the theories and principles of education are universal.

The theoretical basis for the health stories and their use as an educational method is well founded in modeling theory (Bandura 1977). As this case illustrates, the use of observation for modeling is efficient because people learn what to do from visual examples before trying the behavior themselves (p. 22). Bandura has categorized four processes of observational learning: attentional, retention, motor-reproduction, and motivational processes (p. 23). Morehead utilized each of those processes in the storytelling method. For example, the use of motivational processes, defined by Bandura as external and vicarious self-reinforcement, is illustrated by the case as follows: The story was told by everyone in turn; it was acted out by each group, and it was again presented to the communities through a skit or reenactment.

Storytelling is a method of education. That is, it is a tool just as films, lectures, slides, posters, and discussion are tools. The method of instruction should be selected according to the objective domain: cognitive, affective, or psychomotor. However, in selecting a method, the educator must keep in mind the barriers to its use. As Morehead notes, audiovisual aids are good instructional tools. But a film cannot be shown if there is no electricity for the projector.

Diffusion of innovation offers the best theoretical fit for the diffusion of the new health practice through the communities served by the native health educators. In adoption-diffusion theory, it is emphasized that people may be reluctant to adopt a new practice unless they see its advantage. This factor was accounted for by the *success* part of the story: the children and the family got well. The main characters of the story represent innovators or early adopters (Rogers 1983) who benefited from the new practice.

The process-content-action method described by Reynolds (1973) is also a method for training field-workers to develop skills of problem solving in their local villages. This method was first used extensively in training family planning workers in Bangladesh, but it may be adapted elsewhere. It emphasizes reenactment of actual field experience and small discussion groups.

Morehead does not explicitly describe the professional operating style of the educator. But it is evident from the story and from the care given to respect local customs that the educator was a person who (by her personality and her actions) did nothing knowingly or accidentally to antagonize the people. We could hardly see her behaving as an "ugly American."

This case raises basic issues for any health educator beginning to work with a new population. Even though we may think we know the culture and the people well, we must do an assessment and continue to be aware of local beliefs, customs, and past experiences with health and disease. It is necessary to respect the old while adding the new. This need is relevant in all of medicine and public health. Because something is old does not mean it is not good. Because a method is new does not mean it is better than the old way.

The role of the health worker in this case differs from the one currently customary in the United States. But the blending of educator-treater-healer is a concept that is growing in the United States as the philosophy of holistic health gains acceptance.

References/Select Resources

Bandura, A. 1977. *Social Learning Theory.* Englewood Cliffs, N.J.: Prentice-Hall.
The author suggests that the traditional psychological theories about human behavior are not adequate to explain or predict human behavior. These theories hold that human behavior is

the result of motivation from within the individual. In contrast, Bandura's theory holds that human behavior is motivated in part by forces outside the individual. In its simplest form this theory, which is applied in the Morehead case, deals with the concept of modeling, one familiar to most educators. This means that people learn from what they see and feel in their environment. Social learning theory does not hold that people automatically respond to external stimuli but rather that they are influenced by it and that "they select, organize and transform the stimuli that impinge upon them." Bandura runs a middle course in defining the causes of human behavior. It is neither totally within the power of the individual to do as he or she pleases, nor is it totally within the power of the environment to influence the individual. There is a continuous interaction between the two. Bandura says, "Both people and their environment are reciprocal determinants of each other." The material in this book is presented clearly and concisely. Bandura's description of learning through modeling will help you understand how that process was applied in this case.

Reynolds, R. 1973. "Process, Content, Action: Training Family Planning Workers as Agents of Social Change." *International Journal of Health Education* 16(2):126–135.

This article supports the training method employed in this case. Reynolds points out that using real situations as the "content" for training provides the necessary reality base and allows for immediate transference of the learning to the trainees' work. He suggests that family planning workers with varying status be brought into the program for training. From the perspective of training, this is a sound idea. But this concept is difficult to implement, especially in a culture in which the right to a status is a long-standing custom.

Rogers, E. M. 1983. *Diffusion of Innovations.* 3d ed. New York: Free Press.

In his first publication on diffusion in 1962, Rogers reported on 405 studies, whereas for this edition, he reviewed 3,085 studies—an indication of the tremendous increase in diffusion research.

Rogers has now extended diffusion theory to include factors that antecede and follow the adoption process, giving rise to new questions. For example: Where did the diffusion come from? Which comes first, the need or the innovation? What kinds of problems are encountered, and how are they solved as the innovation is implemented? The Morehead case offers a classic example of the application of Rogers's diffusion theory and principles.

Srinivasan, L. 1977. *Perspective on Nonformal Adult Learning.* New York: World Education.

This short book brings together much of the contemporary thought on nonformal education, that is, education that takes place outside a school system. Most program examples are drawn from international settings. The principles of adult education described in the book are based on the work of Paulo Freire, Ivan Ilich, Carl Rogers, Abraham Maslow, Jerome Bruner, B. F. Skinner and Malcolm Knowles. Srinivasan presents a clear exposition of their work and its relevance to nonformal education. The Morehead case demonstrates many of the principles drawn together by Srinivasan. Although both Srinivasan and Morehead are concerned with programming outside the United States, it is important to consider how nonformal education methods for health education can be applied in this country.

Discussion Questions

1. Is the success-story method currently used in any health instruction in the United States? If so, give examples.

2. Can you compare the storytelling that captures the rural audience in this case to any similar storytelling that appeals to large audiences in the United States

today? What group of people seem to be most interested in the storytelling approach? Why do you think there is such strong appeal in any culture for storytelling?

3. What additional principles of learning do you see in the case, either in the in-service training sessions or in the use of the story method with the public?

4. What role do you think the foreign consultant in health education should play in rural areas such as the one described in this case?

5. How might the PRECEDE model be used in a situation like the one in this case?

Arthritis Self-Management; or, The Chocolate-Chip Cookie Caper

Kate R. Lorig, R.N., Dr.P.H., and Janette Laurin, M.P.H.

All health education projects must have a beginning. This beginning often sets the course for the whole project, as was true for the Arthritis Self-Management (ASM) study. The Stanford Arthritis Center (SAC) had been funded by the National Institutes of Health to study the outcomes of arthritis patient education. To accomplish this analysis, a health education doctoral student was hired. Thus the ASM project was created out of the combined needs of a school of medicine to comply with a funded study and the needs of a doctoral student to complete research for a dissertation. The combination of these two needs produced the strong research emphasis of the ASM project.

The purpose of the ASM project was to determine if community patient education regarding arthritis could change self-management behaviors such as walking, arthritis exercise, and relaxation. More important, would such education affect such measures of health status as pain and disability? We also wished to test the cost-effectiveness of education by determining if it was possible to reduce the frequency of outpatient visits for arthritis.

The setting for the original project was several communities located about 40 miles south of San Francisco. These communities are predominantly white and middle and upper-middle class. Because of the proximity of Stanford University and the large semiconductor industry, the population tends to have a high educational level. The ASM course was designed for anyone over the age of 18 with any type of arthritis. Although there were no other formal criteria for attendance, we found the program to be most successful with people who had at least a fifth-grade reading level. Participants ranged in age from 19 to 92. Seventy-five percent had osteoarthritis, 12 percent had rheumatoid arthritis, and 13 percent had other types of arthritis. The mean age was 67 and the mean educational level was 14.5 years.

PHASE 1: NEEDS ASSESSMENT

The needs assessment phase of five months was a time to learn about arthritis and about the people who would be involved in the ASM study. In all, five separate needs assessments were conducted, which, when considered together, form a stakeholders analysis (Ratcliffe 1981). Such an analysis consists of getting information from all interested parties, or stakeholders, before implementing a program.

In the first part of the needs assessment, eight patients chosen by Stanford rheumatologists were visited in their homes, and in-depth, nonstructured interviews were conducted to determine how arthritis patients live in the community and how they perceive the effects of the disease on their daily lives. The single most important outcome of these interviews was that patients wished to be separated from their disease. For this reason, we started talking of "people with arthritis" instead of "arthritis patients" or "arthritics."

The second part of the needs assessment involved having 100 people with arthritis who attended a senior citizens' forum on arthritis fill out a questionnaire that contained three queries:

Kate R. Lorig and Janette Laurin are researchers at the Stanford Arthritis Center at the Stanford University Medical Center in Palo Alto, California.

This work was supported by NIH Grant 20610-05 and an Arthritis Foundation Fellowship.

1. What do you think of when you hear the word *arthritis*?
2. What things do you do that make your arthritis better?
3. What things make your arthritis worse?

These three questions were aimed at determining the salient, or most important, beliefs of patients about their disease (Miller 1956; Fishbein and Ajzen 1976). From these questions, it was very clear that the number one concern of patients was pain, followed a distant second by disability, and then by a variety of emotional problems that were grouped as fear and depression. Disfigurement, surprisingly, was fourth and far down on the list of concerns (Lorig and Cox 1980).

A third assessment was done by giving a questionnaire to 50 rheumatologists attending the Western Regional American Rheumatism Association Meetings. There were five questions:

1. What do you think of when you think of arthritis?
2. What can patients do to help their arthritis?
3. What do patients do that makes their arthritis worse?
4. What do patients think makes their arthritis better?
5. What do patients think makes their arthritis worse?

The outcome of this assessment was that physicians and patients agree very closely on what one can do that makes the disease better or worse. However, what physicians think patients believe and what patients actually believe are very different. In almost all cases, physicians have underestimated the patients' ability to know how to treat their illness.

The fourth assessment was conducted by interviewing a variety of physicians, nurses, occupational therapists, physical therapists, and social workers who had worked with people with arthritis. These people, some of whom had been very active in arthritis patient education, were chosen because they were known for their interest in arthritis or they were recommended by others in the field. From these professionals, we gained the "conventional wisdom" about arthritis patient education. In addition, several professionals felt that any educational intervention must be cost-effective and should not decrease patient satisfaction with the physician.

The final assessment was a literature search of models of arthritis patient education and of information on evaluation of arthritis patient education and, most important, on the effectiveness of the various treatment modalities taught in patient education.

From these assessments came three basic assumptions upon which the ASM program was built:

1. People with arthritis can learn the general principles of arthritis management, including the use of drugs.
2. Knowledgeable patients practicing self-care would experience improved functional outcomes, less pain, and reduced health care costs.
3. There was a need to provide education for large numbers of patients and to have an easily replicable low-cost program. Thus, lay persons would be used as patient educators. (Lay leaders were used because we were trying to develop a model for nationwide use and it was questionable if enough professional time would be available.)

PHASE 2: WRITING THE ASM COURSE

Having completed a series of assessments, it was time to start developing the ASM educational intervention. The course had to meet several criteria.

First, it needed to have a rationale built on theory. This rationale was supplied from a variety of sources. The self-care movement supplied a historical rationale (Risse, Numbers, and Leaville 1977). The interactionist movement headed by Kelly (1955), Bateson (1979), and others supplied a communications framework. This framework states that people act on the basis of their personal constructs of reality. To a great extent, these constructs are built on past experience. Thus, for any individual, the base of reality is his or her perceptions. To change behaviors, one often has to change individual perceptions. The ASM course changes these perceptions by exposing the individual to many new ideas about arthritis. These include seeing successful people with arthritis who act as group leaders, talking with classmates, and utilizing a book that emphasizes arthritis self-management. Most important, the course is taught in an atmosphere that encourages the exploration of new ideas.

The work of Fries and Crapo (1981) on vitality and aging supplied a life-style rationale. This work argues that the human life span is not infinite and probably cannot be expanded much beyond 80–85 years. However, a healthy life-style can help maintain vitality until near the time of death and shorten the number of years of decline that are often experienced by older persons.

The Whorf–Sapir hypothesis (Whorf 1956) supplied a linguistic framework. This hypothesis demonstrates how one's reality is largely formed by one's language. We cannot think abstract thoughts without the use of words. The language we use frames the way we think. It is for this reason that the word *patient* is seldom used by the ASM project. Rather, we talk of participants or people with arthritis. Because of the Whorf-Sapir hypothesis, there is a conscious attempt throughout the ASM course to reinforce the normality, rather than the illness, of people with arthritis.

Work by others (e.g., Nuckolls, Cassel, and Kaplan 1972; Syme and Berkman 1976; Berkman and Syme 1979) supplied the social network aspects of the ASM project. These epidemiological studies determined that people with strong social support networks suffered less mortality and morbidity than did loners. The ASM course attempts to build a social support network by asking participants to bring a significant other to classes. In addition, networking is encouraged among class members through the use of many paired and small-group exercises.

One of the strengths of health education is the ability to borrow theories from a variety of fields and then to mix and match them into a new creation. The ASM course does not have one overriding theory, but rather, each portion is supported by appropriate theories.

Second, the course needed arthritis content that was determined by two criteria: (1) Treatments that were included had to have been shown effective on the basis of clinical trials or other experimental evidence; and (2) content had to be such that it could be taught safely by nonhealth professionals. Using these criteria, we decided that ASM content would include basic pathophysiology of osteoarthritis and rheumatoid arthritis, design of exercise programs, relaxation techniques, overview of medications, joint protection, nutrition, physician/patient communications, ways to make judgments about nontraditional treatments, and problem solving.

Third, the ASM course needed process. The criteria for choosing processes were the same as those for choosing content. Thus the three processes that were mixed and matched throughout the course were brainstorming, lecture/discussion, and demonstration/return demonstration. These were integrated into an experiential learning model based on adult learning theory (Knowles 1960).

The theory, content, and process were finally melded into the *Arthritis Self-Management Leaders' Manual* (Lorig 1981), which is a minute-to-minute protocol of all ASM content and process. To supplement this manual, a book containing all the course content was written for patients (Lorig and Fries 1980). In this way, if the leaders left something out or in some way went astray, the course participants always had access to accurate information. The book also acted as reinforcement after the course was over.

PHASE 3: RECRUITING

So far in our planning we had heeded health education tradition. The next step was to find course leaders. To recruit group leaders, we made announcements at senior citizens' meetings on arthritis and in the newsletter of a local health center. On the day of leader orientation, 17 people appeared, and 14 stayed to become our first ASM leaders. These 14 ranged in age from early twenties to late seventies and participated in 20 hours of training. All additional leaders have been recruited by word of mouth. More than 100 persons, ages 19 to 82, have been trained and have taught ASM courses. Approximately 25 percent of the leaders are active or retired health professionals. Of the other 75 percent, most but not all have some college education. Sixty percent of the leaders have some form of arthritis. Leaders teach their first course as volunteers and thereafter are paid $100 for teaching each course. The money to pay leaders is collected by charging class participants a small fee. In addition, leaders have been paid through arrangements with local community colleges and from small Arthritis Foundation grants.

During the leaders' training, we also advertised the courses in local papers and on the radio. All announcements were free public-service variety spots. More by luck than design, we hit upon a recruitment technique that was to find us over 2,000 participants in the next three years. Unlike most studies, in which physicians are asked for referrals, we recruited the public through use of mass media. As part of the application, the patients were asked to secure signed permission from their physicians. In three years we have received fewer than 25 patients directly referred by their physicians but have had more than 300 physicians sign consent forms.

PHASE 4: THE COURSES

Finally, time came to start the 12-hour courses that were to be held once weekly in various sites throughout the community. Although we believed that lay people could teach complicated arthritis content, no one was really sure if this was so or if they would be acceptable to the course participants. Two weeks after the first class, we had a potluck, the first of many, for the leaders and some professionals from the Stanford Arthritis Center. The leaders were asking the director of the center, a well-respected rheumatologist, many questions that had come up in their classes. The physician offered to go to each course (seven were taking place) and give a talk. During the evening, many leaders told me that although they liked and respected the rheumatologist, they thought they could answer the questions and conduct the ASM course without help. A few weeks later the first courses ended with rave reviews from the participants and a 75-person waiting list for the next courses. The crisis had passed, leaders had enough confidence in themselves to teach, the medical community had not objected to the leaders, and participants had found them more than acceptable.

Of course, there were problems. Leaders were locked out of sites in the rain or the bathrooms were locked. We learned early the value of always having keys to everything. We were not prepared to deal with the 400–500 participants who took courses; yet somehow we had to expand almost daily with no money or space. Thankfully, there always seemed to be volunteers or field students who were willing to do strange tasks at strange hours to make the program work. One wonderful woman with years of organizational experience set up our record system, which is still in use. Students typed, answered phones, coded questionnaires, and did more copying and addressing of envelopes than any of us care to remember. Leaders became active in finding sites for the courses—sites that ranged from churches, senior centers, and apartment complexes to the training room at Sears in a large regional shopping center.

PHASE 5: THE RESEARCH

The reason for all this activity was to determine the effectiveness of arthritis patient education. This objective added a new layer of complexity. All applicants for the course were randomized. The controls were asked to wait four months before taking the course. Everyone, controls and participants alike, filled out questionnaires at the start of the program and at 4, 8, and 20 months. These were not short questionnaires but rather 15 pages long, requiring about half an hour to complete. None of us enjoyed calling the controls to explain that they would have to wait for classes but still needed to fill out all our forms. We were surprised, however, at the willingness of the public to participate in research. When it was explained, there was little resistance. Initially 90 percent of the applicants completed our questionnaires, and nearly 70 percent completed the final questionnaire 20 months later.

PHASE 6: WHAT WE LEARNED

From research on our first 300 people with arthritis, we learned that participants in the ASM course increased their knowledge, practiced more arthritis exercise and relaxation, walked more, had less pain, and saw physicians less than people who had not taken the course. In addition, they had not changed their level of satisfaction with their physicians. This finding was important, because many physicians feared that patient education would be harmful to the physician/patient relationship (Linn and Lewis 1979).

Despite all the positive findings, however, there was a problem. Although we had been successful in changing knowledge, behaviors, and health outcomes, there were no statistical associations. A basic assumption of patient education is that changes in health behavior result in changes in health status. But though the ASM course changed both behaviors and health status, these were not statistically associated. The people with increased beneficial behaviors were not necessarily those with the best health outcomes. In other words, the ASM course was beneficial, but we still don't know why. In view of these findings, it is time to start a new study.

PHASE 7: DISSEMINATION

One problem with most health education programs is that once they are over, they are never repeated. Thus they tend to benefit a relatively few people. The ASM program was started with the idea that it could be easily replicated. That was why the protocol was well documented and lay persons were used as instructors.

The chance for dissemination came when the Arthritis Foundation asked to test the program in 20 of their 74 chapters. To facilitate this testing, in the summer of 1981 staff or volunteers from the selected chapters spent a week at Stanford learning about the ASM course and how to institute it in their own areas.

This week-long training session brought a whole new set of problems. Many participants did not feel that lay persons could safely teach the course. The physical therapists were especially concerned about the exercise section, which they felt might be harmful. Some people felt that the program would be too expensive or would take too much time to administer.

Before beginning the national training, we were aware that there would be resistance. To help overcome it, several very influential persons within the Arthritis Foundation were invited to the training. These included two of five regional vice-presidents and the past and present presidents of the Arthritis Health Professionals Association. These opinion leaders helped in meeting objections and in changing early dissension in training to cooperation.

An indication of the success of the training is that 17 of the 20 participants returned to give the ASM course in their own cities. Several have trained lay leaders. It is hoped that ASM will become established as an ongoing function of the Arthritis Foundation.

Let us now examine two additional factors—why some things didn't work and why other things did.

THINGS THAT DIDN'T WORK— THE PROBLEMS

LEADERS WHO COULDN'T OR SHOULDN'T LEAD

We had several leaders who completed training but should not have taught. One could only talk, not listen. Another was an alcoholic, and a third continued to teach her own opinions and disregard the protocol. In each case we tried to correct the problems by having the problem leaders teach with strong leaders. But finally we just did not ask the problem people to teach future courses.

TEACHING THE COURSE IN MINORITY COMMUNITIES

Twice we attempted to teach the ASM course in minority communities. Although we trained minority leaders and made several changes in the course, it was never successful. Recruitment in both communities was poor and course attendance was quite low. The lesson from this experience is not to try to force a health education program on a community for which it was not designed. We recently conducted a new needs assessment, wrote new materials, and presented a successful, culturally specific course in a Latino community.

WHY THINGS WORKED— THE LITTLE THINGS COUNT

PHYSICIANS ARE NOT THE ENEMY

All too often in health education we openly or not so openly treat physicians as though they were the enemy. From the beginning, ASM has had the strong support of physicians. It was based in a major medical school. Doctors were consulted at all phases of the project. Because they supported the program, it was accepted throughout the local community and the national rheumatological community.

CHOCOLATE CHIP COOKIES—THE SECRET INGREDIENT

It started with the first meeting of group leaders. I made chocolate chip cookies as refreshments. They were such a success that they have become a tradition at all meetings of group leaders and are often served during classes. They were even served the first evening of our national training program. Those close to the ASM project have renamed it the "Chocolate-Chip Cookie Caper."

Although we cannot identify the mysterious ingredient, it is our feeling that chocolate chip cookies are a symbol of caring and stability—or maybe they really do provide the theoretical base of the ASM study.

REFERENCES

Bateson, G. 1979. *Mind and Nature*. New York: Dutton.

Berkman, L. F., and Syme, S. L. 1979. "Social Networks, Host Resistance, and Mortality: A Nine-Year Follow-up Study of Alameda County Residents." *American Journal of Epidemiology*, 109:186–204.

Fishbein, M., and Ajzen, I. 1976. *Belief, Attitude, Intention and Behavior: An Introduction to Theory and Research*. Reading, Mass.: Addison-Wesley.

Fries, J. F., and Crapo, L. 1981. *Vitality and Aging*. San Francisco: Freeman.

Kelly, G. 1955. *The Psychology of Personal Constructs*. New York: Norton.

Knowles, M., ed. 1960. *Handbook of Adult Education in the United States*. Washington, D.C.: Adult Education Association of the U.S.A.

Linn, L. S., and Lewis, C. E. 1979. "Attitudes toward Self-Care among Practicing Physicians." *Medical Care* 17(2):183–190.

Lorig, K. 1981. *Arthritis Self-Management Leaders' Manual*. Atlanta: Arthritis Foundation.

Lorig, K., and Cox, T. 1980. "Beliefs about Arthritis: A Needs Assessment and Comparison of the Perceptions of Rheumatologists and Patients." Paper presented at the Arthritis Health Professionals Meeting, Atlanta.

Lorig, K., and Fries, J. F. 1980. *The Arthritis Helpbook: What You Can Do for Your Arthritis*. Reading, Mass.: Addison-Wesley.

Miller, G. 1956. "The Magical Number Seven, Plus or Minus Two: Some Limits on Our Capacity for Processing Information." *Psychological Review* 63:81–97.

Nuckolls, K. B.; Cassel, J.; and Kaplan, B. H. 1972. "Psychological Assets, Life Crisis, and the Prognosis of Pregnancy." *American Journal of Epidemiology* 95:431–441.

Ratcliffe, J. 1981. "Qualitative Evaluation Research: New Paradigms for Old." California Journal of Teacher Education 8:27–42.

Risse, R.; Numbers, R. L.; and Leaville, J. W., eds. 1977. *Medicine without Doctors*. New York: Science History Publications.

Syme, S. L., and Berkman, L. F. 1976. "Social Class, Susceptibility and Sickness." *American Journal of Epidemiology* 104:1–8.

Whorf, B. L. 1956. *Language, Thought, and Reality*. Cambridge: MIT Press.

Analysis

This case documents the development and implementation of an arthritis self-management course. The health educator's primary task was to develop the course and evaluate its impact; her role was that of planner and researcher. Because this work served as the basis for her doctoral dissertation, the project had a well-defined research component, with a stronger theoretical foundation than is usually encountered in community programs. The theories used illustrate how health education draws from and integrates theories from many disciplines. Here we see interactionist, communications, gerontological, linguistic, social networking, and adult learning theories, all synthesized for the development of this course.

The needs assessment process occupies a central role in this case. It is reasonable to assume that the research interests made possible the comprehensive assessment. This five-month, five-phase assessment might not have been possible in a project whose prime focus was provision of services. Apart from the comprehensive nature of the assessment, the methods used are important to note.

Data were collected from a variety of sources through a number of different methods. The sources of data can be divided into the target group, that is, people with arthritis, and professional experts such as rheumatologists and other providers who work with arthritis. The multiple sources of data and methods of data collection allowed for triangulation and cross checking of data, which strengthened the conclusions derived from the assessment (Patton 1980). Another example of a multistep assessment is found in the Falck case (p. 362).

The course was conducted by leaders who were specifically solicited and trained for the program. Generally, the leaders were lay volunteers. This choice of leadership raised a number of issues. The ability of lay leaders was questioned by professionals. The question of lay leader quality is usually explicitly asked. But implicit to this discussion is the question of whether volunteers take jobs away from professionals.

Any agency that utilizes volunteers on an ongoing basis needs to develop a personnel policy for volunteers that includes screening, selection, training, and supervision. Written agreements that spell out the role and responsibilities of both the agency and the volunteer are highly desirable (Gaby and Gaby 1979). In this case, three volunteer leaders were terminated for different reasons. Many agencies often have difficulty in terminating a volunteer, but hard decisions need to be made when the goals of the program are in jeopardy. For this program, it would be interesting to know whether different project outcomes resulted from the use of different volunteers.

One professional operating procedure that is important to consider when dealing with clinical issues is consultation with physicians. This consultation occurred throughout the course of the project and was necessary for its success. By including physicians in the planning, the project gained their support. Without this support the course might never have gotten off the ground, for the physicians were the central gatekeepers of potential participants, even though they did not refer their patients to the course. The authors' statement that physicians are not the enemy is interesting. It is true that many physicians (as well as other medical care providers) are wary of, or at best don't understand, health educators and health education. But health educators can ill afford to ignore or treat as the enemy the power center of the health professions. The more prudent and more profitable course is to gain influence with the medical sector through cooperation and demonstration of competence in terms that physicians understand. This does not mean that health educators should assume the medical model for their own use.

Finally, chocolate chip cookies are a practice management tool not commonly encountered in health education practice. Their use is not fully understood and perhaps kindles a certain amount of guilt. Although some would justifiably question their nutritional and dental implications, their value in group process is beyond question when they are judiciously used by a facilitator.

References/Select Resources

Gaby, P. V., and Gaby, D. M. 1979. *Nonprofit Organization Handbook.* Englewood Cliffs, N.J.: Prentice-Hall.

This handbook is highly recommended for those who administer nonprofit community organizations. A variety of useful information is presented, such as training and utilizing volunteers, developing personnel policies, raising funds, getting publicity, and developing a board of directors.

Levin, L. S.; Katz, A. H.; and Holst, E. 1976. *Self-Care: Lay Initiatives in Health.* New York: Prodist.

This book was one of the first works to promote the concept of self-care and provide a framework for self-care research. The case by Lorig and Laurin is a good example of what Levin and his colleagues recommended be accomplished under Clinical and Educational Studies in Self-care, which is the second section of a four-part typology that delineates research issues in self-care.

Milio, N. 1982. "Self Care in Urban Settings." In *SOPHE Heritage Collection of Health Education Monographs*, vol 2: *The Practice of Health Education*, edited by B. Mathews. Oakland, Calif.: Third Party Publishing.

In discussing the potentials of self-care for urban groups, the author states that if self-care systems are to prosper, they must be based on community action rather than just on individual or family activities. Such systems should include an information base, methods of dissemination to the community, support structures to enable people to utilize the information, and methods for evaluating the self-care program.

Patton, M. Q. 1980. *Qualitative Evaluation Methods.* Beverly Hills: Sage Publications.

This is the necessary book for anyone interested in qualitative methods in program evaluation. The author offers a checklist that indicates when qualitative methods should be used. The methods themselves are thoroughly described and include qualitative interviewing, observation, and nonreactive research, as well as methods for analyzing the gathered information.

Discussion Questions

1. How would you apply grounded theory in the Lorig/Laurin case if it were your responsibility to assess needs for this project?

2. This program did not fare very well in a minority community. What information would you want from a needs assessment to increase the likelihood of success in a minority community?

3. How would you use adoption-diffusion theory in disseminating this project?

4. How could learning/social change principles be substituted for the wide range of theories that were used in this case?

5. What other chronic illnesses would be appropriate for a similar self-management program? What barriers could you anticipate in developing and implementing the course that would be specific to the disease?

East Side Health District's Cervical Cytology Demonstration Project

Stanley G. Rosenberg, M.A., M.P.H.

BACKGROUND AND PURPOSE OF THE PROJECT

In 1960, the county cancer society in East St. Louis, Illinois, had a cervical cancer detection program at one of the county hospitals. State funding was obtained when the clinic was "opened" to persons on welfare. At the same time, the clinic moved from the hospital to the East Side Health District. A subsequent review by the state revealed that a small group of physicians in the county were sending patients whom they considered medically indigent to the clinic, but few of the welfare recipients were benefiting from the program.

Representatives from the state and district health departments and the cancer society met to determine ways of making the cancer detection test available to more welfare recipients. The plan to test the best way of bringing women on welfare in for Papanicolaou smears called for sociologists, available at the local university, to seek information about the recipient population. This information was to be used by a health educator to determine the best methods of encouraging these women to seek early cervical cancer detection.

The teaming of two university sociologists with a practicing health educator was an innovative approach in 1960. The sociologists were to describe the knowledge and attitudes of the target group,

---

Stanley G. Rosenberg is the President of Rosenberg and Associates in Bozeman, Montana. He was formerly a Health Education Consultant with the Cancer Control Program for the U.S. Public Health Service.

and the health educator was to plan and carry out an educational effort utilizing this information.

It is important to make clear that the purpose of the project was *not* to have all women in the target group examined for cervical cancer. It was to determine and test the most effective method(s) of persuading the women to accept the screening technique.

Funding for the project was provided by the Public Health Service (PHS) and the Cancer Control Program as well as the state and local health departments. Approval for the project was secured from the county medical society and the county cancer society. At the request of the state and the East Side Health District, a PHS health educator was assigned to coordinate the project.

GATHERING THE DATA: THE FIRST MAILING

Before I (the PHS health educator) arrived, the two sociologists carried out a long, elaborate demographic study of the target population. They utilized the services of several of their students to record data from case files in the general assistance offices and the offices of the Public Aid Commission. They collected information on marital status, age, number of children, recency of last delivery, religion, education, length of residence in the county, the number of places they lived over a period of time, and so on. The purpose of the data collection was to draw a comprehensive picture of the universe of women on welfare. The sociologists also developed an interview schedule that they presented to me shortly after my arrival. Much of the information sought related to their thesis that the women saw themselves as "baby dolls," and as such did not perceive themselves as ill or subject to illness. This interview schedule had over 300 questions. Most of these related more to the need of one of the sociologists to collect data for his doctoral dissertation than to the needs of the health departments. After much discussion and restatement of the purposes of the project, the interview schedule included questions that elicited relative information on gatekeepers, opinion leaders, communication patterns, health knowledge, attitudes, practices, and support systems. The instrument was pretested, revised, and finally accepted. There were 15 pretests and 35 interviews conducted.

While I was working with the sociologists and doing preliminary planning for the project, the cancer society felt that the Cervical Cancer Detection Clinic should not cease operation and that the public should be informed about the new location of the clinic. The sociologists objected to any activity that might tend to contaminate their study. They finally agreed to a simple notice mailed to the study group. This was printed on a three-by-five sheet of paper. It stated that the Cervical Cancer Detection Clinic formerly held at the hospital was now at the health district and that no appointment was necessary. The women were informed not to douche 24 hours prior to the examination. No information concerning the type of examination to be given was on the notice. The address of the health district was noted.

The original universe, that is, women on welfare, as specified by the sociologists totaled 7,500. The names were obtained from lists in the general assistance offices and the offices of the Public Aid Commission. Excluded were 1,679 Old Age Assistance recipients. After further checking, the population was reduced by another 1,185 because of duplications and males.

The presentation of the sociologists' report in March 1961 concluded their contract with the project. Although the information was valid and some of it useful, the generalizations drawn from the data were too broad for practical use.

The consultants from the state (an M.D. and a health educator) and I agreed a new approach was in order. We decided to mail a pamphlet to the target population and to interview a sample of those who did not respond, that is, did not have a Pap smear, to learn their reasons for not responding. We knew from previous experience that the response to the pamphlet would be negligible (Griffiths and Knutson 1960).

The pamphlet was based on work carried out earlier by Hochbaum and Rosentock, providing information on susceptibility, seriousness, and curability of cervical cancer (Hochbaum 1958). It was pretested among groups of women attending Well Child Conferences at the health district. Two and one-half percent of the women receiving the pamphlet had a Pap smear.

A sociologist was hired to interview a sample of those who did not come in for the examination. This approach had to be dropped when she had to resign because of ill health. A third approach was then developed.

PHYSICIAN REFERRAL SYSTEM

After reviewing data available from clinic attendance records, interviews with referring physicians, clinic patients, public assistance files, and the sociologists' report, I decided physician referral would be a logical means for getting women to accept cervical cancer detection.

In the review of the data I found the following:

1. Slightly better than 26 percent of all Pap smears given at the health district from May 1960 to February 1961 had been the result of physician referrals, according to the patients (see Table 1, page 218).
2. The physicians who most frequently referred patients to the clinic wanted permission to refer all their welfare patients for Pap smears.
3. According to the sociologists' report, recipients looked to the physicians to provide information about their illness or health (see Table 2, page 218). The only other persons named more frequently, and then only when taken as a group, were family members.
4. Physicians who received the largest amount of money from the Public Aid Commission and the Township General Assistance Offices were most frequently named as their private doctors by patients coming to the clinic for a Pap smear through self-referral. In other words, the doctors who were treating the re-

Table 1
Source of Referral for First Pap Smear, Indigent and Recipient Persons, May 1960–February 1961

	Number	Percentage
Physician referral	253	26.7
Caseworker referral	18	2.0
Relative and friend referral	23	2.4
Public health nurse referral	4	.4
Total referral	298	
Response to announcement (Self-referral)	608	64.3
No information noted on card	40	4.2
Total	946	100.0

Table 2
Frequency and Percentage Distribution of Persons with Whom Respondents Most Frequently Discussed Illness, February 1961

Person	Number	Percentage
All	296	100.0
Physician	99	33.6
Husband	50	16.9
Mother	32	10.8
Neighbors	29	9.8
No one	27	9.1
Female relatives	25	8.5
Female children	20	6.8
Other	6	2.0
Male relatives	4	1.3
Social worker	1	.3
Clergyman	1	.3
Precinct committeeman	1	.3
Druggist	1	.3
Father	0	.0
Male children	0	.0

cipients coming to the clinic through self-referral were, by and large, the same physicians who treated most of the patients receiving assistance in the health district. Table 3 summarizes this information.

5. Data obtained from the interview schedule showed that 90 percent of the women receiving assistance had visited their physicians at least once in the previous year, and 60 percent had visited their physicians at least once in the previous three months (Table 4).

Since the recipients visited their physicians fairly often, it seemed that using the physician as the referring agency should prove feasible (Weeks 1961). I reasoned, therefore, that the community to be organized should not be the community of recipients, but rather the molders of opinion among them, their physicians.

The interviews I had with nine physicians suggested organizing them might not be too difficult. We made it clear that the public health role was detection. The physician's role was patient care. We assured physicians that the case-finding technique was acceptable to the medical society and that patients with questionable findings would be referred to them for care. The majority of the physicians we spoke with were comfortable with this arrangement.

I identified a physician sympathetic to the cause to assist in planning and checking the mechanics of a physician referral system. After we worked out the mechanics, I asked him to suggest others who he thought might cooperate. We contacted these nine physicians and invited them to the home of the physician who had helped work out the mechanics. Seven were unable to come. This was a social gathering during which we asked them to refer their patients to the clinic on a routine basis.

The greatest problem with the referral system was maintaining a sustained level of interest among the physicians. After I made a visit to their offices, they would refer patients in greater numbers for two or three weeks. Then the referrals would begin to decline, sometimes dramatically. The reasons given were always valid and logical. They just had too much morbidity to take care of. A discussion of the advisability of having a Pap smear for early cancer detection had a low priority on the day's agenda.

The solution, as I saw it, was to set up some sort of office routine so the physician could not forget to refer. This routine took the form of the receptionist's attaching a referral slip and pamphlet to the patient's chart. The nurse could ascertain from the chart whether the patient had had a recent

Table 3

Relative Position of 16 Physicians in the Health District Concerning Specific Relationships with Recipient Groups in Three Selected Areas, February 1961

Physician by Code Number	General Assistance Monies Received	Illinois Public Aid Commission Monies	Number of Times Named by Patients Not Referred by Physicians
34	1	1	2
22	2	2	3
63	3	3	5
30	4	4	1
64	5	5	8
61	6	8	12
35	7	6	4
19–20	8	11	None
28	9	NIA*	10
32	10	NIA	None
38	11	12	6
46	12	9	None
41	13	10	None
49	14	13	11
21	NIA	7	7
50	NIA	NIA	9

*No information available.

Table 4

Frequency and Percentage Distributions Showing the Last Time Respondents Visited a Physician, February 1961

Recency of visit	Number	Percentage
All	295	100.0
Never	9	3.1
Within past month	126	42.7
Within past three months	52	17.6
Within past six months	51	17.3
Within past year	37	12.6
Within past three years	13	4.4
Within past five years	1	.3
Over five years	6	2.0

smear. If so, she would remove the referral slip. The referral to the clinic was to be made by the physician who could not forget to refer *because the slip acted as a reminder.* This reminder also allowed the physician to refer *before the patient described her current illness,* so the patient would not feel she was being referred because of a suspected carcinoma.

Each physician made minor changes in the routine. Those who followed the routine maintained a sustained high referral rate. The dynamics of clinic attendance as a result of physician referral can be seen in Figure 1 on page 220.

CASEWORKER REFERRAL

Two additional methods were tried in an effort to determine the most effective means of persuading women to have a Pap smear.

The first method was caseworker referral. Even though our data did not indicate caseworkers would be a viable referral source, reports from a Florida program indicated a great deal of success from caseworker referral. A request was made to the casework supervisor of the Public Aid Commission to secure the assistance of caseworkers to refer their clientele for Pap smears. A test program was worked out whereby a group of six caseworkers referred individuals to a viewing of the film "Time

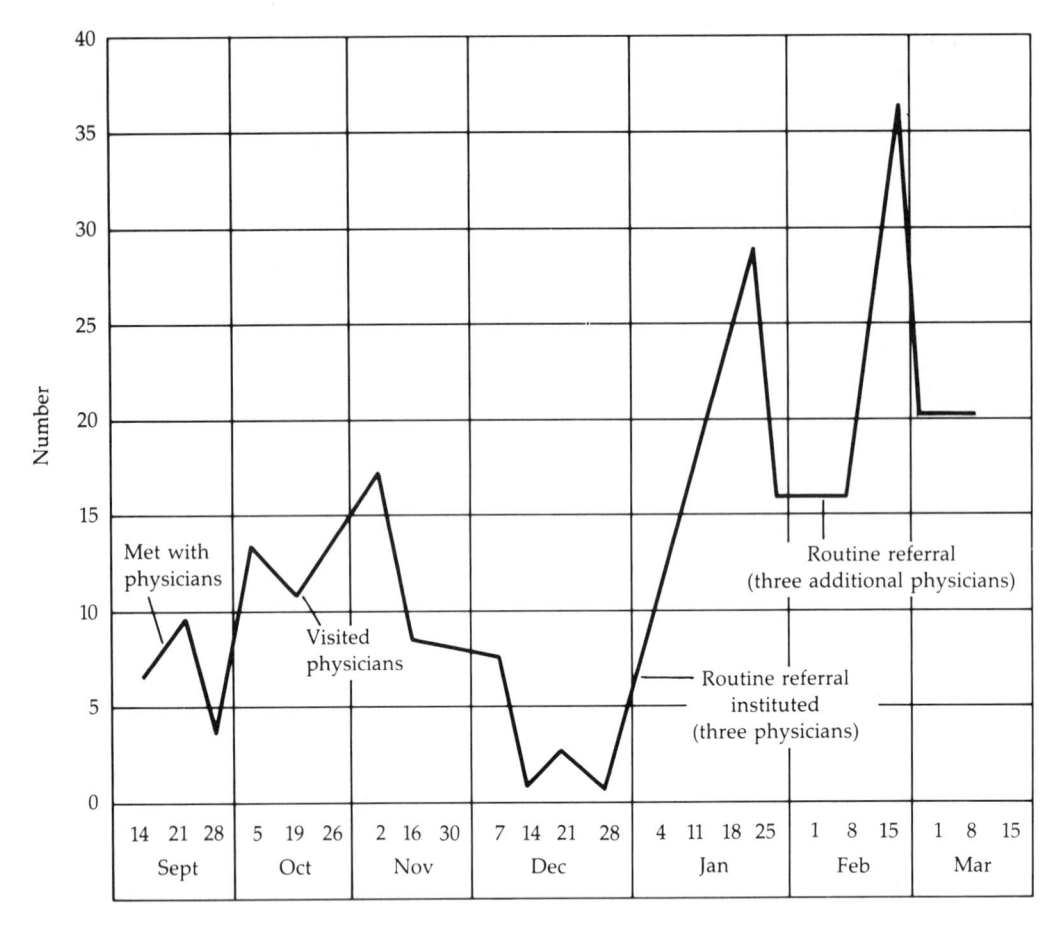

Figure 1
Clinic Attendance as a Result of Referral by 14 Selected Physicians for Initial Pap Smear, September 14, 1961, to March 15, 1962

and Two Women." After the film and a discussion, the women were asked to sign appointment slips to have a Pap smear. A total of 95 women were invited to a series of six film showings that were held in different housing projects in East St. Louis. Of the 95 women invited, 27 came to the movies and 12 came in for Pap smears. The percentage response was about equal to that from the first mailing.

As a second method, an authoritarian letter by the "man who sends the checks" was tried. A response of 18–23 percent was recorded. We did not know whether that response was due to the cumulative effect of several efforts, to the fact that over 1,000 of the women had already had the test, or to the perception that refusal to have the test might jeopardize their income. None of the staff was willing to use this approach.

PATIENT EDUCATION

An analysis of experiences in the clinic during the early part of the project revealed that 10 of the first 30 women with suspect cytology refused prompt follow-up recommended by their physicians. Interviews with patients revealed a high anxiety level regarding the results of the examination. To help deal with this problem, I designed a pamphlet that provided a complete explanation of the examination and the need for appropriate follow-up. The nursing staff used this together with counseling their patients to help relieve anxiety. After use of this technique there were fewer refusals for follow-up care.

We also discovered a sizable portion of the women had refused necessary repeat smears. To help overcome this problem, a routine was worked out whereby on examination day between the time of registration and the appearance of the examining physicians, two films were shown ("Time and Two Women" and "Breast Self-Examination"). I led a discussion on breast self-examination and also emphasized the possible need for a repeat smear, pointing out the possibility of a broken slide or our failure to obtain sufficient material during the examination because they perhaps douched before the examination. A good deal of humor was engendered in this portion of the session. After the patient education sessions were instituted, there were no refusals for repeat smears.

STAFF EDUCATION

Staff education was given on an as-needed basis. I initiated this approach in conversation with the director of nursing. We had four formal sessions dealing with the purpose of the project, attitudes and knowledge of the client population regarding cancer of the cervix, and interviewing skills. A good deal of informal education occurred with the nurses at clinics and in our day-to-day encounters.

CONCLUSION

The Public Health Service contract with the East St. Louis Health District for my services was for two years. The two years were up, and I was assigned to a new post. We left the district with a plan for interesting the women on welfare in having a Pap smear at the East Side Health District Clinic. The plan called for the physician referral system and periodic contact with the target population through mailings and the media. We also left them with an understanding that getting the women in for the Pap smear was only part of the job that needed to be done. Once they came in, the system had to be set up so each test was adequate and so those with suspected cytology got to an appropriate referral source. The administration was also made aware of two essentials: the need for renewing and constantly updating the technical and human service knowledge and skills of the clinic staff, and the need for a trained health educator to carry out the function of planning, coordinating, and evaluating the components of a program such as the one we had just completed.

REFERENCES

Griffiths, W., and Knutson, A. L. 1960. "The Role of Mass Media in Public Health." *American Journal of Public Health* 50:515–523.

Hochbaum, G. M. 1958. *Public Participation in Medical Screening Programs: A Socio-psychological Study.* PHS Publication no. 572. Washington, D.C.: Government Printing Office.

Weeks, H. A. 1961. *Family Spending Pattern and Health Care.* Cambridge: Harvard University Press.

Analysis

This case focuses on the health educator as a planner, coordinator, and evaluator. The central task was to determine the most effective means of persuading women on welfare to accept a Pap smear. Determination of the most effective method required two steps: (1) determining what would motivate women on welfare to have a Pap smear, and (2) trying out the method to see whether or not it worked.

In carrying out this task, the health educator encountered the traditional research/practice dichotomy. It is often difficult for the researcher and the practitioner to work together and achieve the purposes of both, because their goals are often in conflict.

The case illustrates two points critical to the practice of health education: (1) Incorrect assumptions can result in failure to reach program goals; and (2) available data must be sought and examined before collecting additional data. The assumption that the women on welfare were the target population seemed quite reasonable, but proved invalid when available data were carefully examined. The target population was in reality the physicians who served the women on welfare.

Although a number of theories and models could apply to this case, such as PRECEDE (Green et al. 1980) and a systems model (Argyris 1973), we believe the best theoretical fit is provided by Rogers's concept (1983) of the influence of the opinion maker on the adoption of a new practice.

Rogers states (p. 27):

> Opinion leadership is the degree to which an individual is able to informally influence other individuals' attitudes or overt behavior in a desired way with relative frequency. . . . Opinion leadership is earned and maintained by the individual's technical competence, social accessibility and conformity to the system's norms.

As Rogers points out, this definition implies a "leadership-followership relation." For leadership to occur, there must be a change in the behavior of the follower as a result of contact with the leader. In the East Side Health District the physicians appear to be the opinion makers for the welfare women in matters of health behavior.

Two concepts of learning/social change apply to this case. First, there is the concept of credibility: People learn from what they perceive to be a credible source. For example, a local physician who had credibility with his peers was enlisted to help the health educator develop a mechanism for getting physicians to refer welfare patients for Pap smears.

The second concept is that of reinforcement: People learn over time as the result of a number of different learning experiences. For example, the health educator made repeated visits to the physicians' offices to remind them to refer patients. This was not sufficient reinforcement—the referral slip, a constant reminder, was necessary. The behavior, referral of women for a Pap smear, was not sufficiently meaningful to the physicians for them to integrate it into their daily routine, that is, to learn and apply it.

Three strategies were used for identifying effective ways to motivate women to have a Pap smear:

1. Surveys
2. Interviews
3. Analysis of available data

The following strategies were used to try out the method:

1. Identification of a credible physician to help develop a referral mechanism
2. Training of clinic staff to carry out the screening of patients
3. Follow-up of patients as appropriate

The key to the successful use of the first set of strategies was to focus on program goals, keeping the end product in mind. That sounds fairly simple to do. On the contrary, as you will note from the case, it was not easy to keep those involved with the project focused. Sometimes a person's interests that may be related to, but not really the same as, the project goals can divert a project from its goals. Note the sociologists' questionnaire. To keep the end goal in mind, it is continually important to ask, "Where are we heading?" Too often the methodology takes over and becomes the goal rather than the method to reach the goal.

The strategies for trying out the method are directly related to the opinion leadership theory. The use of this theory was suggested by the data analysis.

The educational programs for those who needed a return visit for a second smear probably would not have been attended if they hadn't been planned for presentation at the time the women were coming to the clinic. By working the programs in at that time, the staff assured the patients' attendance. To have planned the programs for a different time would have required a second visit, which would have been impractical. This is a valuable operating procedure to keep in mind.

The physician who helped the health educator devise a means of interesting other doctors in referring women on welfare for Pap smears invited these doctors to his home for a social gathering at which they could learn more and ask questions about the referral system. Social events, if appropriate and sponsored by someone with credibility, can often turn the tide. They add a note of pleasure and fun to a project; they are informal and often enjoyable so that the professional can relax. Perhaps most important, whoever sponsors the event doesn't have to do so. So this voluntary support gives the project a kind of credibility that a formal or professional endorsement does not have.

Prevention as a priority in medical care surfaces as an issue in this case. Rosenberg points out that the number of referrals from physicians increased after he made a visit to their offices to remind them to refer. But, as he could not continue to make these visits, he devised a simple tool, a referral slip attached to the medical record, to help ensure ongoing referrals. Had this tool not been used, physicians might not have continued to refer patients for a Pap smear even though they claimed to believe in it. As they pointed out, prevention was secondary to morbidity on their agenda for any given day. The Bartlett case (p. 134), set 20 years later, illustrates the same issue.

Although the events described in this case study occurred 23 years ago, the processes and theory applied are relevant today. Had the case occurred in 1984 rather than 1960, the health educator's task of data gathering and analysis would have been easier because of the advances in computer technology. The public health problem, that of motivating low-income women to have a Pap smear, is still with us (see the Windsor case, p. 273).

References/Select Resources

Argyris, C. 1973. *Intervention Theory and Method: A Behavioral Science View.* Reading, Mass.: Addison-Wesley.

In this book, Argyris, a leading behavioral scientist, applies a systems model to effecting change in organizations. This model can also be applied when community change is the focus. Argyris points out that in approaching any system, an accurate diagnosis is required to explain present conditions. The changes needed and their sequence, as well as the resisting forces, must be stated. Theories of change and intervention should be utilized and, finally, evaluation is necessary to measure the effectiveness of change.

Blalock, H. M. 1979. *Social Statistics*. 3d ed. New York: McGraw-Hill.

As in the Rosenberg case, very often the health education specialist will have either partial or complete responsibility for data analysis. For those who fear statistics, this readable book noticeably reduces anxiety. An excellent introductory text, it emphasizes a conceptual understanding and application of statistical procedures. Less emphasis is placed on calculation and derivation.

Green, L. W.; Kreuter, M. W.; Deeds, S. G.; and Partridge, K. B. 1980. *Health Education Planning: A Diagnostic Approach*. Palo Alto, Calif.: Mayfield.

This seminal work in health education describes a health education planning model known as PRECEDE, which is an acronym for "predisposing, reinforcing, and enabling causes in educational diagnosis and evaluation." The model consists of six phases: an epidemiological and social diagnosis (phases 1–2), a behavioral diagnosis (phase 3), an educational diagnosis (phases 4–5), and an administrative diagnosis (phase 6). These phases are present in the Rosenberg case. For example, the initial data gathering can be seen as phases 1–2, while the development of a physician referral system falls under phases 4–5 as a reinforcing factor.

Rogers, E. M. 1983. *Diffusion of Innovations*. 3d ed. New York: Free Press.

A tremendous increase in diffusion research has occurred since Rogers's first publication on diffusion in 1962, when he reported on 405 studies; for this third edition, he reviewed 3,085 studies. In now extending diffusion theory to include factors that antecede and follow the adoption process, Rogers poses some new questions. For example, where do innovations come from, and how do their origins and development affect diffusion? What problems are encountered, and how are they solved as innovations are implemented? Readers of the Rosenberg case will find chapter 8 very informative on the effect of opinion leadership.

Discussion Questions

1. Suggest methodologies for reaching the physicians other than that used in this case. Compare the effectiveness of these with that of the one used.

2. Describe a data collection and analysis project that you feel you, as a health educator, could handle, and then describe one for which you'd need expert assistance (e.g., sociologists specializing in survey techniques).

3. Develop a plan for orienting the nurses working in the clinic to the cervical cancer detection project and their role in the project.

4. Which staff training skill would a health educator need in a case like this?

5. Compare the methods that were employed in this case with those used in the Windsor case (p. 273).

Cooperative Problem Solving: The Neighborhood Self-Help Project

Rosalind P. Thomas, M.P.H., Barbara A. Israel, Dr.P.H., and Guy W. Steuart, Ph.D.

This case will describe challenging aspects of a Neighborhood Self-Help Project in North Carolina that was a collaborative effort of the Health Education Department at the University of North Carolina at Chapel Hill (UNC), the Alamance/Caswell Area Mental Health and Mental Retardation Center (which we will refer to simply as the mental health center), and residents of two small neighborhoods in the Burlington area. The project was initiated by a request from the mental health center to UNC's School of Public Health for assistance in involving hard-to-reach groups in the center's preventive service programs.

This 14-month (July 1980–August 1981) project was partially funded by Title I-A, Higher Education Act of 1965. Under a technical assistance agreement, the project was considered a demonstration activity of the mental health center's Consultation, Education and Prevention Program. Mental health center staff served as counterparts to the UNC team throughout the planning and implementation process.

The project focused on promoting mental health by strengthening community identity and community problem-solving capacities in blue-collar neighborhoods. We shall present first the conceptual framework for the project, then a brief description of how the project was carried out, and finally a detailed analysis of the difficulties and challenges encountered in trying to adhere to project principles in three different phases of the project: (1) neighborhood entree, (2) neighborhood adoption of full program responsibility; and 3) the balancing of evaluation and delivery goals. A more detailed description of the project is available elsewhere (Thomas et al. 1981).

CONCEPTUAL FRAMEWORK

Many programs in health education target change at the individual level, where the desired outcome is for individuals to make particular changes in behavior. However, social environmental conditions have been identified as predisposing or as protective factors in the illness process, and these must be addressed more directly by systems-level interventions. Although policy has been one arena in which systems-level solutions have increasingly been targeted, another important action arena is that of enhancing the functioning of local community systems.

This project was based on a conceptual framework that ties the development and maintenance

---

Rosalind P. Thomas is Community Service Program Director and Clinical Assistant Professor in the Department of Health Education at the University of North Carolina School of Public Health in Chapel Hill. Barbara A. Israel is an Assistant Professor in the Department of Health Behavior and Health Education in the School of Public Health at the University of Michigan in Ann Arbor. Guy W. Steuart is a Professor in the Department of Health Education at the University of North Carolina School of Public Health.

The authors would like to acknowledge the important contributions to the Neighborhood Self-Help Project made by Nancy Lamson and Maria Ricardo (Department of Health Education, University of North Carolina) and by Ruth Wright, Judy Little, and Yvette Bogan (Alamance/Caswell Area Mental Health and Mental Retardation Program), and especially highlight those made by the residents of Amity and Blanton.

of the mental health of community members to the relative capacity of their community system to provide certain functions. According to Klein (1968), three factors that have a direct impact on positive mental health as a reflection of community functioning are security and physical safety, support at times of stress, and a context for obtaining self-esteem and significance.

How people perceive and experience their community is one of many sociocultural and psychological factors that may serve as a mediator in stressor situations by influencing both perceived resources and the extent to which any situation is experienced as stressful and hence potentially detrimental to health. Therefore membership in a competent community may be seen as an important but, of course, not a sufficient condition for good mental health.

Several authors have developed constructs of "community competence" (Bloom 1977; Iscoe 1974). We modeled many of this project's goals on Cottrell's (1976) profile of the competent community. He describes (pp. 196–197) a competent community as one where the various component parts have the following abilities:

1. They "are able to collaborate effectively in identifying the problems and needs of the community."
2. They "can achieve a working consensus on goals and priorities."
3. They are able to "agree on ways and means to implement the agreed upon goals."
4. They "can collaborate effectively in the required actions."

For the purposes of this project the community development approach was selected as an action strategy for enhancing community competence and thereby the mental health of the communities involved.

INTERVENTION STRATEGY

As a backdrop for the discussion of the three practice issues, the following brief summary of the sequence of project contacts and activities will provide a general overview of the process involved.

The first three months of the project were spent in planning tasks and in developing a working relationship with mental health center staff. Respective roles for the UNC team and mental health center staff were negotiated, and general strategy sessions were held to discuss and agree upon practice principles and details of the intervention plan. Given staffing and time constraints, we focused the intervention and evaluation primarily on the neighborhood/community level. Other components we had projected working with—for example, social networks, families, individuals, and agencies—received minimal direct attention.

GOALS AND OBJECTIVES OF THE NEIGHBORHOOD/COMMUNITY COMPONENT

Following is a list of the goals and objectives of the neighborhood/community component:

1. Increase the proportion of community members who believe that they can positively influence decisions that affect them and their neighborhood (i.e., influence either directly or by influencing powerful others).
2. Develop or strengthen the problem-solving capacity of neighborhood members involved in the project.
   a. Facilitate the identification and assessment/analysis of problems and strengths of the neighborhood as a whole and of subunits of the neighborhood, including individuals, families, and organizations.
   b. Facilitate the development or strengthening of a problem-solving structure in the neighborhood (e.g., a group or organization).
   c. Serve as a catalyst in helping neighborhood members reach a consensus on goals and priorities.
   d. Increase the knowledge level of neighborhood members regarding the range of possibilities and alternatives available for dealing with identified problem situations.
   e. Increase the knowledge level of neighborhood members regarding where and how to acquire resources.
   f. Serve as a resource in helping neighborhood members select, implement, and evaluate appropriate action strategies for reaching identified goals.

g. Reduce the negative effects of at least one neighborhood-identified problem (stressor) previously thought by neighborhood members to be intractable.
3. Increase the proportion of neighborhood residents active in the neighborhood problem-solving structure.
4. Increase the proportion of neighborhood residents who take an active versus passive role in the project (e.g., take responsibility, make concrete suggestions, carry out project activities).
5. Promote cooperative working relationships among neighborhood groups with similar interests and goals, especially where linkages are weak or nonexistent.
6. Increase the proportion of project activities being planned and carried out by community members rather than by project staff until such activities can be initiated and sustained without staff input.

CHOICE OF NEIGHBORHOODS

A major activity was familiarizing ourselves with the town and then mapping the boundaries of neighborhoods in the Burlington area. This was done after collecting information on neighborhoods from numerous sources, including agency staff and long-term residents. *Neighborhood* was defined as a residential area within specific geographic boundaries, where residents felt a sense of shared identity. This was the most practical operational definition, given the methods available for community identification in a short period.

We chose two neighborhoods to approach as potential project participants. Criteria for selection included the mental health center staff's perceptions that these neighborhoods were underserved by the center's prevention programs and were at high risk for family stress, plus the apparent existence of a degree of neighborliness and neighborhood identity among residents.

Following is a brief description of each of the neighborhoods, which will be called Amity and Blanton.

Amity is comprised of approximately 200 households, located within the city of Burlington, North Carolina (population 37,266). Historically, the area was a mill community, the houses built and owned by a large textile mill bordering the neighborhood. Over the last several decades, however, these houses were purchased by individual owners. The community is primarily white, working class, with many persons employed in nearby mills, others in factories and service operations. There are two somewhat distinct sections within the neighborhood. One of these consists mainly of families who own their own homes and have resided there for years. Many of the adults grew up in the area and have extended family members living in the same house or close by. The other section has become mostly rental houses in recent years, with the residents being younger, with younger children; these families are the most transient. Throughout both sections are a significant number of widows, living alone, who have been there for many years. Many community members attend one large church in the neighborhood, which also draws its membership from the entire Burlington area. Other residents go to churches outside the neighborhood.

Blanton is comprised of approximately 250 households, located outside the city limits of a small town (population 2,403) at the outskirts of Burlington. This is a semirural area, where even though houses are close together, most available open space is used for gardening/farming purposes. The community is primarily black, working class, with many persons employed in local mills, factories, and public agencies. One part of the neighborhood has predominantly older, wood-frame houses, some of which have recently been rehabilitated through a federal HUD Community Development grant. Water and sewer services and paved streets were also installed in conjunction with this grant. Another section of the neighborhood is mostly newer, brick homes. Many of the persons living in this newer section grew up in the older area and still have family and close ties there. Numerous churches within the neighborhood draw their membership mainly from residents of the community.

KEY NEIGHBORHOOD ACTIVITIES AND EVENTS

The second phase of the project, that of initial neighborhood entree, began in the third month and extended through the fifth month. Community leaders in each neighborhood were identified, contacted, and interviewed. Most expressed interest in the project and agreed to meet with others from the neighborhood to explore shared interests.

At the initial meeting in each neighborhood, held in the sixth month of the project, the project's purpose was reviewed. Those attending were asked to share and discuss first their perceptions of neighborhood strengths and then their concerns. Both groups expressed interest in becoming involved in the project and in meeting again.

Following is a summary of subsequent activities, events, and key meetings of each neighborhood group:

Blanton (largest meeting attendance, 60+; average attendance, 15–20)

Quickly focused on problems of teenagers in the area. Teens, parents, and other concerned residents were involved.

Decided to try to establish a local community center, a centralized place for social and educational activities.

Formalized their group by forming an advisory committee and electing officers, agreeing on a name (Citizens United for Neighborhood Achievement), and writing bylaws.

Initiated a process to lease the closed neighborhood school building from country officials, arranging for a local church with nonprofit status to act as the official sponsor.

Applied for a grant from a private foundation to get funding for renovation and program initiation activities for the community center.

Organized and conducted with high community participation, two clean-up days at the school in anticipation of the lease.

Negotiated with the mental health center for funds available for fun fairs. Planned to hold a fun fair as the kickoff activity for the center.

Four-month postproject period

Tried, through community action, to regain a lease option after the county put the school building up for sale.

Held fun fairs at local churches as fund-raisers. Received a $13,000 grant from a foundation.

Moved to incorporate. Attempted to secure the school or some other site for the community center. (Note: the school building was subsequently sold.)

Amity (Largest meeting attendance, 24; average attendance, 6–8)

Kept trying for wider participation. The small group of residents interested in the project finally decided to focus on improving the neighborhood climate for unsupervised youngsters, who had been causing problems in the neighborhood.

Decided to hold a neighborhood field day, with emphasis on involving kids from the neighborhood and their parents in the activities.

Held a field day at a neighborhood park; group was encouraged by the turnout.

Decided to have a second field day in the fall. Interest expressed in starting a community watch.

Contacted the police department, scheduled a community watch meeting. Drew the largest attendance of any meeting.

Negotiated with the mental health center to use fun fair funds for the second field day; submitted proposal describing activity and needs.

Four-month postproject period

Held the second field day. On processing the activity, planned to have another one the following spring.

Stated interest in following through on a community watch. No organized group was expected to continue.

FACILITATIVE AND CONSULTATIVE ROLE OF STAFF

Our general strategy in working with each neighborhood was to play a facilitative and consultative role by asking relevant probing and guiding questions and by helping the group work sequentially through the following problem-solving steps:

1. Identify priority needs and issues.
2. Select an issue to work on by consensus.
3. Consider various action alternatives.
4. Select and develop an action plan.
5. Implement the designated action plan.
6. Evaluate their work.
7. Begin again, recycling the process, as appropriate.

Our emphasis was on helping each group consider things that they could do on a neighborhood basis to address their concerns and perceived problems. In addition to facilitating neighborhood meetings, staff members made informal visits and follow-up phone calls to foster relationship building as well as to facilitate the planning process.

What we perceived as the phase-out period began in the twelfth month of the project. Although the project officially continued for three more months, we used the approaching deadline to focus on getting neighborhood residents to consider becoming even more active in carrying out key roles and activities. In addition, project staff, who had negotiated an informal consultative role for the transition period, kept in close touch with the groups for four months after the official completion date of the project, participating in the special events scheduled by each group.

Against this backdrop, we will present and analyze challenges that arose in carrying out the project on a day-to-day basis and that reflect important practice issues in health education.

PRACTICE ISSUES

Although there are numerous experiences we would like to share and analyze, the areas of neighborhood entree, neighborhood adoption of full program responsibility, and the balancing of evaluation with delivery goals seem particularly central when using community development as a health education strategy.

ISSUE 1: NEIGHBORHOOD ENTREE

A form of reputational leadership analysis was used as a means of entree in each neighborhood. People who were respected and seen by residents as important to getting something done in the neighborhood were identified and approached for interviews.

As would be expected, we were perceived as outsiders and had to allay suspicions about our motives to gain even cautious acceptance. Increasingly, however, we were able to use referrals from other residents in introducing ourselves. Project staff had good interpersonal skills and were successful at building relationships and establishing rapport. Nonetheless, there was a major difficulty in getting across the self-help nature of the project and in convincing people that we were offering to help neighborhood residents find ways to achieve their own goals rather than having our own specific outcomes in mind.

This problem was particularly challenging in initial telephone contacts. In a short call, we had not only to explain what the project was about but also to arrange to meet. Although we got some refusals, most people who were contacted in the neighborhood did agree to meet with us.

We developed and used detailed interview guidelines that outlined numerous questions about neighborhood identity and boundaries, resources and strengths, concerns, ways people usually dealt with the problems they had, helping roles, interest in the project, and so on. We tried to cover the following points about the project as an introduction:

1. We were working with several local agencies on an outreach project.
2. These agencies realized there was a lot of helping going on in neighborhoods they would like to learn more about.
3. This neighborhood had been identified as one that seemed to have a sense of identity and where people helped one another out.
4. Project staff had received a small grant (covering 14 months) and in that period was trying to identify two neighborhoods that might be interested in a self-help project.
5. The focus of the project was on strengthening support for families at the neighborhood level and on helping with day-to-day pressures before these grew into serious problems.
6. At this point we were trying to meet people in the neighborhood to find out what it was like to live there, whether they felt the project was something others in the neighborhood might be interested in getting involved in, whether they could suggest other people we should talk with, and so on.

Although people were very willing to talk about themselves and about the neighborhood in these interviews, it became clear to us that they had more difficulty grasping the self-help focus of the project than we had anticipated. This was especially noticeable in Amity, but it also occurred to a lesser extent in Blanton. The following statement, made by an Amity resident in an interview at the end of the project, captured this confusion:

Well, I asked you the day you came and you explained to me what you were doing, but I still didn't quite understand. . . . Even after I talked with you all, I didn't understand exactly what it was except that you wanted to get something going in the community, but I didn't really know how we were going to go about it until we had the meetings and all of us got together and we finally got something planned. . . . I didn't really understand what we were trying to do.

Some of the factors contributing to this difficulty in communication were preconceptions of traditional roles of agencies in "delivering" services, the emphasis on process rather than on a specific issue or content area, and variations on prior experience of neighborhood residents with community efforts of this kind.

Not surprisingly, people perceived human service agencies as resources of last resort—resources people go to for help with the expectation of tangible service to be provided when they have serious problems that they cannot solve themselves. At the same time, we were told about negative experiences with agencies, and many people expressed pride in not having to use their services. Such attitudes, expectations, and experiences sharply contrasted with the approach of our team, which, on entering the neighborhood affiliated with an agency, wanted to learn about the neighborhood and to work alongside its residents on issues they identified.

A second challenge was to communicate that it was the *process* of the neighborhood coming together that we were interested in, and that the project did not focus on any predetermined problem. Because professionals were seen as having expert knowledge in special problem areas (e.g., child abuse, food stamps, housing), our description of our focal interest and expertise as facilitating the process of cooperative problem solving with neighborhood residents represented an unfamiliar notion that was accepted only over time.

Finally, a key dimension that seemed to affect the relative understanding and acceptance of the self-help focus of the project was the prior organizing experience of each neighborhood. Amity residents had no recent experience in collective neighborhood efforts to address a shared problem, and reciprocal helping roles were confined largely to individual initiatives in helping neighbors who were in need or distress. By comparison, some of the Blanton residents we talked with had been involved in a number of informal organizing actions (e.g., attending zoning hearings, organizing a food cooperative) and recently had worked with the local community action program to obtain a HUD Housing Rehabilitation grant. In general, they had a greater understanding of the potential benefits of neighborhood self-help.

At the very first group meeting in Blanton, a prominent resident introduced us by explaining that this project was "a self-help affair, not agencies giving you something; no money, only some people trying to help you come together to do something to make the neighborhood a better place to live in." Those present seemed to understand and accept this, and the group's action took off from there. By contrast, it was not until the fourth group meeting in Amity that people seemed to understand that we were not going to do anything unless *they* wanted to, nor would we suggest what should be done. The head start by the Blanton group was reflected in all stages of the project, with resident participation higher than in Amity.

We believe that some initial confusion should be expected with this type of intervention, and that one has to strive to counteract community members' expectations and perceptions that the consumer is simply the recipient of predetermined services. We were able to elicit an initial willingness by neighborhood residents to work along with us for a while, and hoped that a successful experience would be the ultimate "teacher" of self-help and community development principles for those participating.

ISSUE 2: NEIGHBORHOOD ADOPTION OF FULL PROGRAM RESPONSIBILITY

At the heart of the cooperative problem-solving strategy is the pervasive issue of the complementary roles of staff and neighborhood residents. At almost every staff meeting, held weekly throughout the project, questions arose concerning how fast and to what extent neighborhood residents should assume responsibility for project planning and development. Attempting to strike the optimal balance of staff and community contributions was a continual challenge.

There was a consistent effort in all individual

and group contacts to stimulate the initiation of action by neighborhood residents and to hold to the principle of "never do for people what they can do for themselves," in order to increase the likelihood that the neighborhoods could take viable problem-solving action in future situations, beyond the life of the project. But it proved difficult to translate what appeared to be a rather simplistic maxim into an appropriate, consistent, and effective intervention strategy.

Our role was prominent and clear-cut at the early neighborhood intervention meetings, where we set the agenda and facilitated. In these initial stages we tried to involve community members in limited but active roles: for example, introducing us and the project at the first meeting; bringing refreshments; calling other residents to remind them of meetings or to talk about the project; summarizing decisions made at the last meeting; and actively participating in the meetings. We focused more intently on strengthening the initiative and roles of residents at the point that each neighborhood identified a problem it wanted to address and work to resolve.

At various stages of project development it proved difficult to decide which roles and tasks were *most* important to transfer. In addition, it was harder than we thought to identify and recognize signs of community members' preparedness to take on specific roles or tasks. People often seemed to have the ability but lacked the confidence to try. Finally, both time constraints and community members' expectations of us led us to carry out some roles and assume some tasks.

It was the seemingly endless small details about practical day-to-day arrangements that were particularly difficult to make decisions about. It was obvious that we should refrain from imposing our own agenda and from expressing our opinions about what we felt the problems or priorities to be. But so far as more routine matters were concerned, we had constantly to grapple with judgments about which actions should not be compromised on and which actions community members really needed to carry out. Is arranging for a meeting place a small thing, or is it symbolic of who is in control and therefore extremely important for a neighborhood resident to handle? What about reminder phone calls, publicity for meetings, and informal visiting? What, if anything, should we do besides asking facilitating questions and engaging in limited follow-ups between meetings? More than once, after facilitating the division of tasks among group members, we were directly asked what *we* were going to do. Although it was our goal to play the role of facilitating consultants to a neighborhood effort, it often seemed that people viewed us as equal members of the group, and therefore as responsible for carrying out a share of the work. This perception was incompatible with our general strategy and goals.

In addition, questions of appropriate techniques to use in facilitating people's adoption of roles and ownership dominated many staff planning meetings. When will expending significant effort to persuade residents to do something themselves increase commitment and participation rather than result in their feeling burdened by our expectations? How does one know how much, if any, guidance is needed by a person to successfully complete a task and thus feel good about it? When will doing the task oneself serve as a modeling or coaching strategy that community members can learn from instead of creating the assumption that it takes special "expert" skills? How does one help a group consider and recognize its often latent resources and therefore achieve the best match of tasks with talents and skills. When one feels a resident is making a mistake in project planning, to what extent does one intervene or rely on other residents to intervene?

A prime example of this last issue is a situation that arose at the end of the project, when we had officially phased out the project but were still in frequent contact with the action group in Blanton. At that time it became known that the lease option of the neighborhood for the empty local school was sidetracked, because someone was interested in buying the building. There were numerous important questions, some deeply involved in local politics, that needed to be explored. After much discussion, the team chose to limit its role to asking directed questions and sharing our ideas about options with several residents who were in leadership positions in the group. But they did not pick up on most of those suggestions (to have a community meeting, get answers to additional questions, use their own contacts, etc.) Should we have stepped in and "modeled" more assertive actions, such as helping neighborhood residents pressure administrators for straight answers? Or were we right to remain fairly inactive and refrain from influencing the neighborhood's action and decisions?

It is a common assumption that what happens in successful community development is the community members' total adoption of the roles and skills of the external change agent. A more realistic outcome may be a continuing interdependence, a service role that Lenrow and Burch (1981) have identified as an underdeveloped aspect of professional helping.

This project was clearly not long enough to test the appropriateness of continuous interdependent relationships with these two neighborhoods. We had been very explicit with the agency and the neighborhoods that there was a 14-month time limit to UNC's involvement in the project. This short time frame was an artificial limitation imposed on the community development process and on the transference of skills to community and agency personnel. At the project's inception we expected continuation funds to be available for extending the period to at least three years, but Title I funds were rescinded by Congress.

Incorporated into the project design was the stipulation that our local agency counterparts were to integrate our model into the center's programs and to continue working with the two project neighborhoods as well as expanding to work with others. But halfway through the project it became clear that, owing to budget cuts and an accompanying move by the mental health center administration to a fee-for-service model for prevention services, this would not be possible. Although center staff were very interested in continuing the program, there was no one to "pay" for the staff's time spent on neighborhood self-help, so they could not justify this activity to the administration.

Each neighborhood group did ultimately move through at least one problem-solving cycle and successfully completed several projects that they had set out as goals for themselves. In reviewing progress with the group in Amity at a special neighborhood meeting at the end of the project, we found that they had decided to continue working on two activities, a field day and a "community watch" antiburglary program sponsored by the police. However, no concrete plans were made, and it seemed clear that the organized group originally established would not continue, at least in the form it had assumed during the program. In light of both an incomplete assumption of roles and skills by residents and the goal of promoting long-term problem-solving capacity, it was obviously premature to phase out the project. If we had remained to work with them on additional activities over a longer period (perhaps several years), their profile as a "competent community" would have been much more complete.

By the time the project phased out, Blanton had formed a standing community group that was moving toward incorporation and had applied for and received a grant from a North Carolina foundation. Even with this strong evidence of internal organization, it seemed to us that much would be gained by their having a continuing partnership in problem solving with official agencies. Outside facilitators would have continued to be helpful in averting potential problems on the horizon: stemming the alienation from the group by some residents angry over the loss of the school building, developing leadership skills of neighborhood youth, creating and maintaining a financial base to operate the community center after the grant ran out, and addressing other needs that had surfaced.

The community development process in the longer term is often a cyclical process with periods of heightened and of reduced activity. Monitoring and involvement by outside change agents serving as catalysts may be important in maintaining momentum, although their involvement may also be cyclical. We feel a need for further exploration of whether the ultimate success of cooperative problem solving is a total assumption of all roles and skills by community members or rather a continuing interdependent relationship.

ISSUE 3: BALANCING EVALUATION AND DELIVERY GOALS

Trying to integrate our evaluation and intervention strategies posed a difficult challenge, and hindsight revealed a number of misjudgments and missed opportunities during the course of the program. One error in judgment we made in the early stages of the project was not to give community members full partnership in the evaluator role. A great deal of professional time was spent discussing techniques for transferring different roles and responsibilities to neighborhood residents without considering the residents' potential role in project evaluation. Evaluation instruments that were developed were used almost exclusively by staff. As usual, hindsight was clearer than foresight, and halfway into the project we realized we had labeled evaluation expertise as "professional expertise," and were thus keeping our questions, our instruments, and our "official" measures to ourselves. We had translated being unobtrusive (which was one of our criteria for selecting evaluation methods) into evaluation methods invisible to community members.

For example, one evaluation tool was a map and coding system to document the level and type of participation in the project on a house-by-house basis. We anticipated obtaining the necessary information on participation from our detailed process notes, matching participants and addresses by using the telephone book. This method was unsuccessful because many people in Amity had unlisted phone numbers, and in Blanton a number of people had rural route numbers, not addresses listed in the phone book. The better alternative would have been to have elicited community help in the mapping from the beginning. Neighborhood members could have been asked to mark their own houses and those of family members and to identify meeting places in the neighborhood. Had the map been prominent at group meetings, it might have served to focus many of the discussions about increasing participation by providing a bird's-eye view of who was not involved and who had dropped off in participation.

It strikes us that most health educators are not well versed in effective ways of explaining the importance and purpose of evaluation to community members. We usually learn about evaluation and about community development as distinctive skill areas, and are left to integrate the two on the job. Consumer participation in evaluation will not replace the evaluation responsibilities of professionals. But consumers do know what they want to accomplish and can often assist not only in developing techniques and data collection methods that are culturally and linguistically appropriate, but also in legitimizing evaluation efforts. Furthermore, citizen involvement in evaluation is important as a means of enhancing the skills of community members in this important phase of the problem-solving process.

Another problem area in evaluation was in trying to evaluate the community development process itself. We had hoped to adopt or adapt an already tested instrument, but found very few useful evaluation studies in the community development literature. When we tried to specify intermediate outcomes and respective indicators of the various stages of the development process, we were struck with how difficult it was to specifically define, let alone measure, outcomes in community development. We considered the options of measuring changes in the individual capabilities of the participants, of measuring improved effectiveness of the neighborhood groups in problem solving, and of documenting the functioning of the neighborhood as a system. But none of these options seemed particularly adequate indicators of community development.

Attempts to measure the enhanced problem-solving capacity of the neighborhood groups as an indicator both of "community competence" and of effective interaction and decision making proved insufficient. We had developed a framework outlining certain necessary conditions for, and essential processes of, community development, but we found it unwieldy to code information from process notes indicating successful establishment of certain conditions or completion of certain processes. We were not even sure that the framework was a valid index of the community development process.

Given the relatively short duration of the project, we began implementing the intervention and designing the evaluation almost simultaneously. In the first few months of the project, evaluation decisions usually got pushed behind planning and making day-to-day neighborhood and agency contacts. By the time we caught our breath on the intervention component and began to spend substantial time on the evaluation component, it was evident that we simply would not be able to achieve the quality of evaluation we wanted.

What is particularly frustrating about all this is that we were unable to determine, describe, and document everything that seemed to have been accomplished by this project. We have a substantial amount of data, in many forms, that suggest the real potential of the strategy we adopted. Blanton did form a citizen-based organization that sought, and was awarded, a $14,000 grant to develop a community center. In closure interviews, residents of both neighborhoods expressed feelings that something different and important had happened in their neighborhood and that they had learned something about themselves and their abilities to solve problems. A minister in Blanton had the following comment:

> Receiving the grant has given everyone a lot of encouragement. If nothing else, and there will be a lot else, people have seen that if they sit down, put their heads together, and plan things out, they can accomplish something. This type of experience is something that people in the community for the most part have been able to see, to enjoy, or to participate in.

In reading through the field note volumes, subtle and developmental changes in participation, commitment, and problem-solving capacity can be seen. The mental health center staff expressed excitement about having reached people who had never before used their services and others they had seldom been able to reach and work with previously. In spite of evaluation shortcomings, we hope that many of the evaluation experiences, mechanisms, and tools from this project can be built upon and refined as a useful starting point in designing the evaluation component of future projects of this type.

POSTSCRIPT

The Neighborhood Self-Help Project emphasized mental health promotion goals because our local counterpart agency was a community mental health center. Although there are increasing roles for health educators in consultation, education, and prevention programs in mental health settings, a community development strategy such as we attempted here is of course relevant to both physical and mental health issues. Community development, with its focus on competency development, may have mental health implications intrinsic to the process itself, but it is directed toward achieving increased community capacity of a sufficiently generalized nature to be relevant to the solution of a wide range of health and welfare problems.

Health educators employed in local agencies have the opportunity to include a community development component in the health education program alongside many others that may focus on other units of practice or on specific health problems. Over time, in living and working in an area, it is possible to identify various communities, analyze their leadership and natural helping patterns, and consider the possibility of a step-by-step neighborhood application of the strategy.

Of more immediate interest, in this era of scarce resources, is the potential for tapping resources in the form of consumer and community expertise that can significantly supplement the resources available from the agency base to address important health problems. We grant that only certain types of problems can be addressed or prevented at the small neighborhood level. But many linkages can be made among communities skilled at problem solving to address problems of broader social origin; and as byproducts of neighborhood action, certainly many linkages can be forged among individuals who may be able to help one another with problems at a much more personal level.

REFERENCES

Bloom, B. 1977. *Community Mental Health: A General Introduction.* Monterey, Calif.: Brooks/Cole.

Cottrell, L. 1976. "The Competent Community." In *Further Exploration in Social Psychiatry,* edited by B. Kaplan and R. Wilson. New York: Basic Books.

Iscoe, I. 1974. "Community Psychology and the Competent Community." *American Psychologist* 29:607–613.

Klein, D. 1968. *Community Dynamics and Mental Health.* New York: Wiley.

Lenrow, P., and Burch, R. 1981. "Mutual Aid and Professional Services: Opposing or Complementary?" In *Social Networks and Social Support,* edited by B. H. Gottlieb. Beverly Hills: Sage Publications.

Thomas, R., ed., with Israel, B.; Lamson, N.; Ricardo, M; and Steuart, G. *Problem Solving at the Neighborhood Level: A Project Handbook.* Chapel Hill: University of North Carolina, School of Public Health, Department of Health Education.

RECOMMENDED RESOURCES

Bloom, B. L. 1979. "Prevention of Mental Disorders: Recent Advances in Theory and Practice." *Community Mental Health Journal* 15(3):179–191.

Cassel, J. 1976. "The Contribution of the Social Environment to Host Resistance." *American Journal of Epidemiology* 104(2):107–123.

Cox, F. 1976. "Alternative Conceptions of Community: Implications for Community Organization Practice." In *Strategies of Community Organization*, 3d ed., edited by F. Cox, J. Erlich, J. Rothman, and J. Tropman. Itasca, Ill.: F. E. Peacock.

Froland, C.; Pancoast, D.; Chapman, N.; and Kimboko, P. 1981. "Linking Formal and Informal Systems." In *Social Networks and Social Support*, edited by B. H. Gottlieb. Beverly Hills: Sage Publications.

Hamburg, B., and Killilea, M. 1979. "Relation of Social Support, Stress, Illness and Use of Health Services." In *Healthy People: Background Papers*, The Surgeon General's Report on Health Promotion and Disease Prevention, DHEW Publication no. (HHS) 79-5507IA. Washington, D.C.: Government Printing Office.

Leighton, D. 1979. "Community Integration and Mental Health: Documenting Social Change through Longitudinal Research." In *Psychological Research in Community Settings*, edited by R. Munoz, L. Snowden, and J. Kelly. San Francisco: Jossey-Bass, 1979.

Leighton, D., and Stone, I. 1974. "Community Development as a Therapeutic Force: A Case Study with Measurements." In *Sociological Perspectives on Community Mental Health*, edited by P. Roman and H. Trice. Philadelphia: F. A. Davis.

Steuart, G. 1975. "The People: Motivation, Education and Action." *Bulletin of the New York Academy of Medicine*, 2d ser., 51(1):114–185.

Warren, D. 1980. "Support Systems in Different Types of Neighborhoods." In *Protecting Children from Abuse and Neglect: Developing and Maintaining Effective Support Systems for Families*, edited by J. Garbarino and S. Stocking. San Francisco: Jossey-Bass.

Warren, R., and Warren, D. 1977. *The Neighborhood Organizer's Handbook.* Notre Dame: University of Notre Dame Press.

Wellman, B., and Leighton, B. 1979. "Networks, Neighborhoods, and Communities: Approaches to the Study of the Community Question." *Urban Affairs Quarterly* 14(3):363–390.

Analysis

This case focuses on the health educator as a facilitator of the community development process. The role could also be described as a facilitator of the learning process (a teacher) helping individuals and groups in the community identify and solve their own problems.

This case illustrates the difficulties of carrying out this type of project when it is limited in time by funding restrictions. Had the project been funded by an established organization, as in the Robinson and Campbell/Williams cases (pp. 68 and 288), staff would have been much likelier to reach their goal of helping the community identify and solve their own problems. Initially, it was assumed funds would be available for three years. When the project began, it was learned funds were available for only 14 months. As the authors point out, this was too short a time to enable a community for the first time to identify and work out its own problems. In addition, the local counterpart agency was not able to take over the staffing role at the end of the grant period as had been anticipated.

Several theoretical perspectives are helpful in understanding the issues in this case. Adoption-diffusion provides a good fit (Rogers 1983). Amity had no experience with community development projects and therefore began at the basic level of the adoption process. The community of Blanton, on the other hand, had experience with several grants for community projects. The members of the community began farther up the scale, perhaps at the persuasion stage.

Adoption-diffusion theory explains why Amity did not get on the bandwagon immediately and why, when the project was terminated after 14 months, the community was apparently not going to continue on its own. The residents had not moved far enough up the adoption scale to value the behaviors associated with community development sufficiently so that they were ready to adopt them or substitute them for existing behaviors.

We could examine this project from the perspective of learning or social change (Pine and Horne 1969; Zaltman and Duncan 1977). Fundamental to both these theories is that the individual must feel a need to change or a need to learn. We do not know why the residents of Amity who were involved in the 14-month project got involved. They could have had many reasons besides an interest in or a need for learning or changing. Perhaps they wanted something to do. Perhaps they wanted to associate with people who were involved. Perhaps they thought the project was something it was not. In 14 months there was barely time for individuals to understand the project and to sort out their own motivations and their own interest in participating. A similar issue is raised in the Hamrell/Raiser case (p. 181) about the motivation of trainees.

The common expression "give a man a fish and he'll eat for a day; teach him to fish and he'll eat for the rest of his life" expresses the basic philosophy of community development, the strategy employed in this case. It is a philosophy with which few will disagree. The problems occur, as the authors indicate, in executing the philosophy.

A common problem is the difficulty a population has in understanding the concept of skill development for the sake of skill development. The strategy of incorporating this concept has been used much more in developing countries than in the United States. It fits well in these countries because the communities usually have multiple fundamental problems such as sanitary disposal of waste (as in the Morehead case, p. 199) or economic development. These problems are usually obvious and give the community a substantive issue of concern to sink their teeth into. It is more difficult to use this technique in communities where problems or their solution are not quite so obvious.

Nonetheless, the concept of helping people learn to solve their own problems can be integrated into just about any health education project whether it is long- or short-term. If it is short-term, the health educators will not see their long-term goal attained, but they can get individuals and groups started on the road. That's what happened in this case. Despite the authors' frustrations, they did get the neighborhood residents together and did get them moving on issues they had identified. Just the process of identification of issues is a valuable learning experience. It would have been more satisfying to have stayed with the community long enough to have seen individuals take great steps in skill development, but that luxury is not always possible. Sometimes we have to be satisfied with small gains.

The case raises the issue of readiness to learn. The staff's dilemma in trying to determine when to offer help to a community and when to let the community go it alone is a dilemma common to parents and teachers. That is, when is the child ready to fly on his or her own?

Bruner (1971:29) states that "the idea of 'readiness' is a mischievous half truth. It is a half truth largely because it turns out that one teaches readiness or provides opportunities for its nurture. One does not simply wait for it." In other words, a teacher builds a curriculum in such a way that the student is ready. In community development, events shape the curriculum; the experience is the curriculum, and usually a very effective one. Even if one could develop a structured curriculum in Bruner's sense, there would still be the issue of time.

The authors identify the basic problem with evaluation, that is, "implementing the intervention and designing the evaluation almost simultaneously." This is a trap into which many health educators fall. Evaluation too often takes a back seat in order to get the job done. By designing the evaluation together with the implementation, the authors would have identified the evaluation issues they encountered as they tried to evaluate the project.

This case offers another example of a funding agency that seems unaware that people learn over time as the result of a number of different learning experiences (see the Hamrell/Raiser case, p. 181). What does staff do when they are faced with carrying out a project that is funded for much less time than they know it will take to reach the desired goal? Give the money back? Most people do the best they can in the time they have.

What is really needed is not short-term funding but stable, staffed, funded community agencies that can help the community deal with community issues over time (Campbell/Williams case, p. 288).

This case illustrates both the challenges of getting neighborhoods involved in self-help activities and the frustrations encountered in trying to help a community learn/change in a short time. It suggests the need for staff available in funded, local community agencies to work with communites over time so that individuals and communities can be allowed time to learn/change and offered a chance to have a number of different learning experiences. Both time and variety of experiences are usually necessary if meaningful learning/change is to take place.

References/Select Resources

Bivins, E. C. 1979. "Community Organization—An Old but Reliable Health Education Technique." In *Handbook of Health Education*, edited by P. M. Lazes. Germantown, Md.: Aspen Systems Corp.

This paper describes a number of successful community organization projects carried out in rural and urban areas in North Carolina and elsewhere. Bivins provides a list of elements necessary in community organization for health as well as a list of characteristics that the community organizer should possess.

Bruner, J. S. 1971. *Toward a Theory of Instruction*. Cambridge: Harvard University Press, Belknap Press.

Bruner describes the eight essays in this volume as "efforts of a student of the cognitive process trying to come to grips with the problems of education." Although he writes about the education of children, his thoughts are also applicable to adults. All the essays provide the health educator with thought-provoking ideas about teaching and learning. Bruner's concept of the need to provide opportunities to encourage *readiness* is particularly applicable to this case. Community organizers like teachers cannot simply wait for things to happen. Bruner's concept as applied to teachers is discussed in Chapter 2, "Education as Social Intervention."

Mico, P. R., and Ross, H. S. 1975. *Health Education and Behavioral Science*. Oakland, Calif.: Third Party Associates.

This is the first book-length discussion to link health education with behavioral science. The authors identify three basic technologies for change: personal growth (PG), for change that affects people as individuals; organizational development (OD), concerned with effecting change in organizations; and problem-oriented applied behavioral science (PO-ABS), with the goal of bringing about change in social systems such as communities. Chapters 8 and 13 describe and apply the third technology, PO-ABS, which can be used in any community organization effort.

Pine, G., and Horne, P. 1969. "Principles and Conditions for Learning in Adult Education." *Adult Leadership* 18(4):108–134.

The principles and conditions outlined in this article are useful to health educators who practice in a variety of settings. These are as well closely akin to the principles of social change outlined by Zaltman and Duncan (see below) that were applied in this case.

Rogers, E. M. 1983. *Diffusion of Innovations*. 3d ed. New York: Free Press.

In this edition of his work on the diffusion of innovations, for which he reviewed 3,085 studies, Rogers notes the tremendous increase in diffusion research since his first publication in 1962, when he reported on 405 studies. In contrast to the second edition, this new edition extends diffusion theory to include factors that antecede and follow the adoption process, so that such questions as the following arise: Where did the innovation come from? Which comes first, the need or the innovation? What kinds of problems are encountered, and how are they solved as the innovation is implemented? The basic diffusion model (p. 165) is useful in explaining the communities' behavior in the Thomas/Israel/Steuart case.

Zaltman, G., and Duncan, R. 1977. *Strategies for Planned Change*. New York: Wiley.

In this book, which is basic reading for the health educator as change agent, the authors define and describe the steps in the process of change. Part 2 is relevant to the Thomas Israel case. It offers great detail on the various strategies for change. Each strategy (e.g., reeducative, persuasive) is illustrated with case studies that are discussed in terms of the appropriateness of the strategy for a given goal.

Zander, A. 1982. "Influencing People in the Face to Face Setting: Research Findings and Their Application." In *SOPHE Heritage Collection of Health Education Monographs*, vol. 1: *The Philosophical, Behavioral, and Professional Bases for Health Education*, edited by S. K. Simonds. Oakland, Calif.: Third Party Publishing.

This article points out the need for health educators to be familiar with and skilled in applying concepts of social psychology that relate to influencing others. Although Zander is concerned primarily with influence at the group level, his model for change, developed in this article, can be applied to broad community organization efforts such as those described in the case study by Thomas and her colleagues. Zander's model includes the following five concepts: creating a favorable cognitive structure; arousing motives; putting motives in control of behavior; developing supportive group standards; and establishing the change.

Discussion Questions

1. Assume you are the executive of the Alamance/Caswell Area Mental Health and Mental Retardation Center. Your monthly report on the use of the center's services shows little use of preventive services by Amity and Blanton. The demography of those communities suggests to you that they should be making more use of these services. Identify three ways in which you would try to increase the use of preventive services by those communities; exclude the methodology used in this case. Specify the advantages and disadvantages of each of the three methods.

2. Would you have gone to the authorities with the residents of Blanton or would you have left matters as the staff in the case did?

3. Write a letter to the funding agency explaining why 14 months' funding is not adequate to reach a desirable goal in Blanton and Amity.

4. Given the goals of this project and the time constraint—14 months—specify (short-term) evaluation criteria and a methodology different from those considered in the project.

5. Given the reason for the grant, would you have introduced the project to the community the same way as it was in this case? If not, how would you have introduced it? Explain.

Planning for Effective Health Education

Zora Travis Salisbury, Ed.D., M.P.H.

AN EXPLANATORY NOTE

As you review the following sequence of events, your awareness of setting and context is essential to understanding the control and decision-making issues touched on in the case study.

The South Carolina Department of Health and Environmental Control serves citizens by providing traditional public health services through its central office and 15 public health districts. In the central office the health education unit has been placed with various programs over the years. It was phased out in 1973 and reestablished in late 1975 as part of the Office of Educational Resources. In 1980, it was designated the Office of Health Education, one of five discipline offices (nutrition, nursing, dentistry, social work, and health education) in the agency, all of which constitute the Office of Professional Services. The responsibilities of the discipline offices center on (1) setting and maintaining standards of practice, (2) providing consultation and technical assistance, and (3) providing resource support. Over the last five years, health education staffing has remained fairly stable. As of June 1981, there were 35 health educators in the agency, 10 in the central office, and 25 in the districts.

On paper, the discipline director, that is, the state director of public health education, has responsibility for the professional supervision of the health education staff in the central office and districts; the administrative supervision is the responsibility of the program director (in almost all cases this would mean the family planning program director). In practice, the supervisory lines blur. To accomplish practice objectives, the discipline director depends on persuasion and a reasoned approach far more than on administrative mandate.

Unlike most state health departments, in South Carolina there is a direct administrative link between the districts and the central office. The districts do, however, retain a great degree of autonomy. The district medical director (DMD) has the designated responsibility for the district public health programs. The district nursing director has administrative and professional supervisory responsibility for the nursing staff. She or a nurse under her professional supervision may also have supervisory responsibility for other discipline staff (nutritionists, health educators, social workers, physical therapists) assigned to specific program areas. There are approximately 900 nurses in the system. In those districts where a health educator is designated as district director of public health education, that person reports directly to the DMD as do the district directors of nursing, social work, environmental sanitation, and so on.

Zora Travis Salisbury is a Post-Doctoral Fellow in the Division of Health Education at Johns Hopkins University. Formerly, she was the Director of the Office of Health Education for the South Carolina Department of Health and Environmental Control.

The author warmly acknowledges the many contributions of the health educators who have been a part of this effort over the past few years and the valuable support of other agency staff. A special thanks to Fran Owen, Ruth Martin, and Peter Lee for their work in developing and maintaining the effort, and to Lawrence Green for providing us with a framework to build on.

At the district level, the field health educators, even those designated as district director of public health education, feel that they have little direct influence or power in shaping decisions that affect health education. The reasons for this are that (1) the funding has historically been categorically based, with control of resource allocation residing with program directors and district administrators; (2) health educators are frequently recruited to meet already established program requirements for patient or community education; and (3) inexperienced staff and/or staff with no formal training in health education are frequently recruited even when there is no direct professional supervision available in a district. This situation has changed somewhat over the last few years, especially in regard to the third factor.

Most of the health education staff working in the health departments were trained in schools in the state. A school of public health opened in 1974, so courses in epidemiology, biostatistics, and public health administration became available. By 1979, four of the central office's health education staff working on the planning and evaluation effort had graduated from the M.P.H. programs in health education or administration. One health educator had an M.A. in teaching (health education). Taken together, these young professionals had had courses in program evaluation, curriculum development, sex and drug education, nutrition, public health planning, and public policy, in addition to the epidemiology, biostatistics, and environmental health courses that were required. The missing element in the health education training program was the linking of public health education practice to its epidemiological, educational, and behavioral science foundations, either in theory or in application. Increasing frustration with the inability to make those connections and recognition of their importance served as stimuli for identifying planning and evaluation of public health education as the top priority for the Division of Health Education in 1978.

Thus a major long-term effort was undertaken to increase the planning and evaluation skills of the health educators. Primary to these efforts were recruitment and training of central office consultants, development of planning and evaluation workshops, acquisition of supportive resources, and continuing follow-up consultation with and assistance from health educators, program staff, and other agency personnel.

THE BEGINNING

At first public health educators were exposed to concepts of program planning and evaluation through the family planning program. A statewide workshop for health education staff was held on family planning as early as 1975. Some progress in understanding the need for specific measurable objectives was made, but a critical piece was missing: On what basis did one determine the best health education method(s), the percentage of increase or decrease to strive toward, or even which particular aspect of the problem to tackle? There simply had to be some way to make some systematic, rational decisions about the detail and focus of health education practice.

The training brochure from Johns Hopkins University outlining the Educational Diagnosis and Evaluation Workshop, July 1978, was like manna from heaven. From the description it sounded as though we all needed it. We couldn't afford to send everyone to the workshop, so plans were immediately made to have three central office staff attend. Follow-up efforts would then be directed to holding a similar workshop in South Carolina for health educators and other appropriate staff.

The information was new and exciting, and the planning sessions provided a theoretical framework for health education that was essentially new to the South Carolina contingent.

So we returned to South Carolina with heads and notebooks full of ideas directed toward changing the practice of health education in South Carolina. A vacant staff position in the Division of Health Education was designated for "planning" and was filled by one of the persons attending the Johns Hopkins workshop. The health education consultant from the Bureau of Maternal and Child Care/Family Planning, who also attended the workshop, wholeheartedly endorsed the new approach to the practice of health education and joined in efforts to support a skills development program. The director of the Division of Health Education (now Office of Health Education) was the third person who attended the workshop. Together these three central office health educators charted a course and shared a vision.

THE ENTHUSIASM OF THE NEWLY CONVERTED

Our enthusiasm was practically boundless. And it was with a real sense of excitement and growth that plans were made, remade, refined, and changed some more.

Realizing the inherent problems of implementing any significant change if it was planned in a vacuum, and building on the expressed interest and commitment of other programs in the agency, we undertook to coordinate our efforts with agency health education staff representing the Bureau of Maternal and Child Care (MCC) and Early Disease Detection (EDD) programs. In addition, both the MCC bureau chief and the EDD program director had expressed their interest in working with the Division of Health Education on this new effort. In fact, both programs contributed substantial funding support.

A BACKWARD GLANCE

Armed with lots of enthusiasm and a fledgling understanding of the new concepts, we didn't factor in soon enough how hard it would be to "convince" other health education practitioners that something was really missing in our current approach to the practice of health education. Add to that a combination of organizational apathy, resistance to change, and lines of responsibility, and we had a sleeping tiger by the tail.

SPREADING THE WORD

Whenever two or more health educators were gathered together, there was someone to press our case. Never mind that it sounded like Greek, meant "more work," and was something those central office people were pushing. The workshop planning went forward. To build a broader base of support, cooperation, and understanding, plans were made to invite representatives of various descriptions and programs to an April 1979 planning workshop that was to be conducted by Lawrence Green. Green had developed and conducted the training program at Johns Hopkins. We reserved slots for students and faculty from the School of Public Health, representatives of the Health Services Administration, and health educators, nurses, and other health education providers from our own agency. Representatives from the powers that be—district medical directors and district nursing directors—were specifically invited. Total costs of the workshop were assumed by the three offices, thus removing an economic barrier to participation.

PREPARATION

Our preparations went on. Making full use of an already available closed circuit TV system, we developed a four-part preworkshop training series. To increase their readiness and understanding, potential participants were strongly encouraged to watch the programs, which sought to explain what was involved in a planned approach to public health education and the importance of a data base and evaluation to the process. Resources and worksheets were provided, and viewers were encouraged to contact the office for additional information.

Presentations and individual conversations about this new approach and the upcoming workshop were made at meetings of the central office's family planning staff, the district medical directors, the Improved Pregnancy Outcome Project staff, and the discipline directors. Both central office and district health educators were exposed to existing health data to identify problem areas. The commissioner and the director of the Office of Educational Resources (to whom the health education director reported) were fully informed of the content and purpose of the workshop and the new emphasis on planning. The memos going out to the rest of the agency went through them, as appropriate and consistent with communication policy. Generally speaking, representatives of all groups were contacted, with *all* health educators being specifically contacted.

The million details of the workshop were worked out, materials ordered, state and local data on health problems pulled together. Discipline efforts were centered on this project, and it was clear that all senior health education staff would participate. And with skepticism and something less than unrestrained enthusiasm, they planned to endure a workshop that simply did not seem relevant to the day-to-day demands of their jobs. It's probably a testament to their sense of responsibility or identity as health educators that they didn't openly revolt.

A last step here was a change inserted into the health education section of the policy manual: "Health education plans will be submitted as requested." That is, health educators would submit plans as requested/required by their professional supervisor (the state director of public health education), or designee (program health educator), or professional supervisor of a unit (director of the Division of Health Education). It should be noted that policy manual changes were submitted and approved by the agency administrator as required by agency policy.

A BACKWARD GLANCE

In retrospect the video training sessions were far too intense and complicated. The load of new information was just too much to absorb, and though we offered to work with people on an individual basis, our services were not in demand. And that's not surprising, because it sounded as though everything everyone had been doing was now somehow wrong.

LOBBYING THE DECISION MAKERS

We certainly gave attention to the decision makers. Lobbying was done through the team role of the EDD and MCC health educators who were involved in the planning and through the advocacy of the Division of Health Education with the administration in the central office. Memoranda on record indicate that the commissioner, program directors, and district medical directors were fully informed of the rationale, objectives, and expectations of the planning and evaluation efforts. Support was evidenced by the authorization of agency funds for staff development, by policy changes, by lack of verbal opposition, and by permission for staff to participate in a training program.

THE WORKSHOP

The workshop went off on schedule. Predictably it turned out to be a beginning for some, created complete confusion for others, and engendered the active resistance of a few. For the workshop planners, it provided a combination of delight and dismay. The delight came with the reconfirmation that there were some guidelines for how one went about deciding what health education services to provide; the dismay surfaced when it later became resoundingly clear that, on the whole, the participants really didn't see the information and approach as being especially relevant. "I don't have time to plan—I have to do" was their cry. What we didn't hear clearly was another equally important message: "I don't make the decisions. I'm not the decision maker you have to deal with."

THE MIRAGE OF A PLANNED APPROACH

Our planned approach turned out to be only a mirage. Like all mirages, it shimmered for an instant, but when we went to touch it, it wasn't really there. Family planning health educators were used to completing "plans," and so, given the new direction and emphasis, health educators were expected to apply the principles to their 1979–1980 plans. It simply didn't happen. Some cheerfully ignored the new and held on to the old way of doing things; others expressed more open resistance. When submitted, the family planning plans looked remarkably as they had in years past. We were severely disappointed.

TAKING STOCK

We looked around to see where we were. Within a brief span of time, major staffing changes had been made. The commissioner and the director of the Office of Educational Resources had left the agency, and one of the core health education staff had signed on with another agency program. All this required adjustment. And we were forced to confront the question, What now? The options were somewhat limited in that health education staff (both central office and field) were a long way from having a full complement of planning skills and, for the most part, discipline leadership/influence rested on the power of persuasion and advocacy rather than on administrative mandate. One of our problems was that we hadn't developed a well-defined "after the workshop" plan of action.

REGROUPING

We decided to work with those who were interested and to remain constant in our advocacy. And there were some bright spots, some beginning efforts to think through certain practice decisions by using the framework. Colleagues in the School of Public Health were also placing increasing emphasis on health education planning and evaluation. A support network was developing. It was slow going and especially frustrating for the newly hired planning and evaluation consultant. Add to that mixed messages and conflicting opinions on what to do and how to do it, and it was not an easy time.

One thing became clear. We had to invest more heavily in providing a data base for practitioners. Resource materials were purchased and a limited literature file (affectionately known as the "Black File") was reestablished and made available to anyone requesting or requiring data relevant to health problems or state-of-the-art health education information.

A MAJOR DECISION

Looming on the horizon was a major decision. The first workshop had only mentioned evaluation. Originally, plans had been made to have an evaluation workshop within six months. Given the response to the first workshop and the notable lack of substantial gain in planning skills, we had decided to delay. Now the question resurfaced: Do we or don't we proceed with the evaluation workshop when we know full well people don't fully understand the planning side? Some staff said yes, some said no. The decision was yes, the rationale being that some progress had been made and that it would be helpful if the whole process (planning and evaluation) was described, even if imperfectly understood.

TRYING AGAIN

We planned an evaluation workshop for April 1980. We shaped the content around South Carolina problems, used a local university professor as workshop leader, and once again tried for representation from all disciplines and personal health programs. Again memos outlining objectives and intent were sent to and through the commissioner, the DMDs, and the program directors.

And once again it was a resounding success. Only this time, the participants thought so too. The whole process was beginning to make sense to most; and a few saw evidence of great strides. There was a fledging cause for optimism and a belief that, though progress would continue to be slow, the concept of public health education practice had, indeed, undergone change. Now we were really ready to prepare health education plans, effective July 1980. We had had more than a year to get ready; now it was time to put talk into practice. A memo approved by the commissioner went out to all professional health educators requesting that they submit to the Office of Health Education a plan for the health education services provided through their unit.

A FIRESTORM

Then a firestorm erupted, ignited by the DMDs. Never mind that the policy manual had earlier been changed, through all the proper channels, saying plans would be submitted as required. It would not happen. The agency management, at both the central office and district level, expressed the view that health education was a support service and therefore did not require a plan. And though it might be nice from an academic point of view to do all that planning, health educators were too few and far between to waste precious time in planning. They were to "do."

Both the commissioner and assistant commissioner expressed support, but they obviously were not willing to go to the mat on the issue of plans for health education.

In all the uproar over territory, responsiblity, and authority of the Office of Health Education and the DMDs, the intent of the plans was largely ignored. In an unforgettable meeting with the DMDs, it also became clear as never before, that there was one set of rules for nurses and another for health educators. Because, after all was said and done, the fact that district nursing directors submitted yearly plans to the Office of Nursing was not questioned. And though those plans were less comprehensive than those desired by the Office of Health Education, the basic intention and administrative links were the same. We lost the round . . . and we lost ground. Again, we took the means available to us and pressed forward. We worked with those health educators who *were* interested *and* had the support of the DMDs (there were some), and together we made progress.

A BACKWARD GLANCE

Our intentions were not or should not have been a surprise to anyone. Certainly the memos, the plans, and the funding approval all attest to the fact that this was not a clandestine operation. One can speculate, then, that the disruption occurred for the following reasons:

1. The decision makers did not really understand what we envisioned as an expected outcome.
2. The decision makers never paid much attention as long as nothing was immediately required from district staff.
3. The DMDs were fed up with central office people "telling them what to do," and health education was the fall guy.
4. We hadn't done a good enough job in communicating with the decision makers.
5. We confused the issue of "requiring a plan" with using the planning process.
6. We didn't have the health educators' support from the ground up.

Looking back, I think probably all of these factors and then some contributed to the events of the summer of 1980.

NOTABLE PROGRESS

Despite all the setbacks, notable progress was made during the last two years covered in this account (1980–1982). Some significant outcomes:

1. The district and central office staff have shown progressive improvement in the development of plans or plan components.
2. The Office of Health Education has put its money where its mouth is. A mini-grant program has been initiated to encourage and give tangible support to planned health education efforts.
3. There has been increasing Office of Health Education involvement with central office programs to stimulate and support change at the program level.
4. An emphasis on a planned approach to health education has been incorporated in the School of Public Health's health education curriculum.
5. In some cases district health educators have been recruited, with planning and evaluation skills being a primary consideration.
6. Professional health education meetings in South Carolina have taken on a different shape and focus by incorporating issues and concerns related to a "planned approach."
7. Library facilities (now part of the Office of Health Education) now include computer search capabilities and a comprehensive selection of professional journals. Use has increased significantly and the library is now regarded as a most valuable support service.
8. The South Carolina *Manual of Practice for Public Health Education* has a section on planning and evaluation.
9. A Health Education Rapid Access File (an expanded version of our "Black File") has been established in cooperation with the School of Public Health in the Department of Health Education at the University of South Carolina.
10. Continuing education programs have focused on increasing the skills of health education providers. Recent examples are workshops on "A Systematic Approach to Problem Solving," "Group Facilitation," and "Consultation," all funded by the Office of Health Education.
11. The contribution of district health education staff to the identification of local problems and appropriate health education intervention has been noted by program directors at state and local levels.

All these advances give testimony to a new set of expectations for health educators. It is now more clearly understood that health educators can contribute to the planning process, and they are therefore increasingly involved in district/program planning efforts.

The breakthroughs with both administration and the health educators came slowly. The major factors in changing the attitudes to the extent they have been changed were probably two: (1) increasing calls from the outside for accountability, and (2) a slow, steady, consistent advocacy that allowed for something less than a textbook approach when dealing with real-life situations.

OPTIMISM PREVAILS

Even if slightly dampened in these times of continued scarce resources, our continued optimism appears well-founded. We've been making our case and now slowly but surely we've gained support for a planned approach. The concepts and jargon are increasingly well understood by people both inside and outside the agency.

The Health Education/Risk Reduction grants funded through the Center for Disease Control have supported our concept and provided training resources for others in our state. Additionally, the Child Safety Seat Grant awarded to the Office of Health Education has provided an opportunity to demonstrate the use of data to plan and support a community-based intervention.

The agency is increasingly supportive of services and plans based on community needs assessments. Using the data base has proven helpful in shaping program plans.

We aren't alone anymore.

A BACKWARD GLANCE

We've learned to be better consultants over the years—becoming more sensitive to the different roles, responsibilities, and perspectives of central office and field staffs.

We didn't involve field practitioners during the initial problem identification and planning stages, and we paid for it. Learning from the experience we took care to include others when we developed the quality assurance standards of practice.

We expected too much, too soon. The changes being sought—whether from an administrative or discipline standpoint—were substantial, and change takes time.

It was sometimes a case of the blind leading the blind. We've gained expertise and so have our colleagues.

WHERE TO NOW?

The question now, of course, is: Where do we go from here? As cuts in program funds require staffing reductions, it is increasingly important to connect with all health education providers to ensure to the extent possible that health education efforts contribute to the desired program outcomes. An increased role in staff development is projected, as is an increased involvement of both central office and district health educators in the development, implementation, and evaluation of the health education components of state and local programs. Considering the growth we have experienced over the last several years, I am convinced that by strengthening our skills in planning and evaluation, we have indeed strengthened the practice of public health education in South Carolina.

Analysis

In this case study, Salisbury describes the process undertaken to increase the planning and evaluation skills of health educators employed by a state health department. Although this case centers on the training of working health educators, it has important implications for the health educator as trainer of other health professionals. Salisbury was one of three health educators of the state's central office who planned and implemented the training program.

Although the trainers managing the program did not identify a theoretical base for their activity, one can assume they, like other practitioners, utilized what Argyris terms "theories in use" (Argyris 1976). These theories in use may not be the theories that the individual says he or she operates under, but they actually are the basis for behavior. The health educator's theories in use appeared to evolve over time in this case. Initially, the trainers assumed that new knowledge that would benefit the target population would readily be diffused, assimilated, and utilized after presentation. Once this theory in use proved not to work in practice, the health educators modified it as they regrouped. They apparently recognized that more development work needed to take place within the health department. Their theory in use now appeared to be a form of organizational change theory: Zaltman's theory of innovations in organizations (Zaltman and Duncan 1977).

The most prominent strategy reported in the case was a series of workshops, some of which made use of closed-circuit television. After the initial failures, the trainers continued to work with those staff members who expressed the most interest. Greater emphasis was now placed on developing support services for the health educators—for example a health education rapid-access file and computer search capabilities.

Lynton and Pareek (1978) in their seminal work, *Training for Development*, provide a very useful framework for developing training programs. They state that training is the responsibility of three partners: the participant's organization, the participant, and the training organization. If one or more of these actors abdicates responsibility, the results of training will be less than desirable. Lynton and Pareek divide the training process into three phases. The first phase, *pretraining*, begins with understanding the situation that calls for more effective behavior by the prospective trainees. This circumstance demands an operational description of the job as it is actually carried out. The second element of this phase that needs to be understood is how receptive the organization will be to the trainee's new behavior. Further, who feels the need for the new behavior? Is it the trainee, an immediate supervisor, or a distant central office?

In the second phase, *training*, once the participant reaches the training program a five-stage sequence should occur:

1. Selection of some items for learning
2. Initial trial or experience
3. Feedback from the initial trial or experience
4. Reinforcement and continued practice
5. Internalization of what has been learned

The third phase, *posttraining*, is probably the phase of the training process that receives the least attention, with the resulting failure of the whole process. When the trainee goes back to his/her organization, will there be encouragement to utilize new knowledge and skills, or does something else happen, such as a lack of support from colleagues or even outright resentment? The latter are obviously conditions that are unfavorable to utilizing the new skills and will lead to withdrawal of support from supervisory personnel.

Within this case we see several issues that are identified in the Lynton and Pareek model. In the pretraining phase it was acknowledged that the field practitioners were not involved enough in planning and that the roles and responsibilities of the central office in the training process were not clearly understood. Salisbury also notes that change takes time—that is, the training phase consists of a number of steps that need to be followed before adequate training can be assumed. Finally, changing conditions during the posttraining phase (e.g., budgetary cuts) made it more difficult to utilize the new skills gained from training.

Apart from training, this case illustrates a number of other issues important to the practice of health education. It is particularly interesting and disturbing to note that agency management at the central office and at the district level viewed health education as a support service and thus not in need of an annual plan. What we see here is a basic lack of understanding of the purpose of health education by those who hire and supervise a health education staff. This flaw is rather surprising in a state that maintains a staff of 35 health educators.

Salisbury also notes that inexperienced staff or staff with no formal training in health education were recruited even when there was no direct professional supervision. This by no means is an unusual circumstance, and the reasons for it can be complex. But the reason that stands out is the tenuous position that health education occupies as a profession. Although health educators may as a group see themselves as having achieved professional status, they have been slow to gain recognition by other health professionals. It is safe to say that, outside of the disciplines of health and education, health education is unknown as a separate professional entity. Considerable effort is now being made to professionalize the field, as witnessed by the Role Delineation Project and heightened interest in certification (U.S. Department of Commerce 1982). However, it is uncertain whether these efforts will be enough. It is interesting to speculate how much one article in the *Reader's Digest*, perhaps entitled "Health Educators that I Have Known," could do for professionalizing health education in the minds of others.

References/Select Resources

Argyris, C. 1976. *Increasing Leadership Effectiveness.* New York: Wiley.

Argyris, C., and Schon, D. A. 1980. *Theory in Practice: Increasing Professional Effectiveness.* San Francisco: Jossey-Bass.

Chris Argyris is someone health educators from all settings should become familiar with. He has much to say to the health educator who is either in or aspires to a leadership role or has responsibility for working with other professionals within an institutional context. He has also written elsewhere on training methods such as role playing.

Boissioneau, R. 1980. *Continuing Education in the Health Professions.* Rockville, Md.: Aspen Systems Corp.

Although this book is not specific to health education, the information on the organization and implementation of continuing education is of value to anyone who has responsibilities in this area.

Lynton, R. P., and Pareek, U. 1978. *Training for Development.* West Hartford, Conn.: Kumarian Press.

This book should be part of every health educator's professional library. Although it is primarily directed at those who have responsibility for developing training programs, the material presented is applicable to anyone who is faced with developing a program for the public, special groups, or other professionals.

U.S. Department of Commerce. National Technical Information Service. 1982. *Role Refinement and Verification for Health Education; Final Report.* Access no. (HRP) 09–04273. Springfield, Va.

This document represents the work of many health education specialists who have been actively working to strengthen the profession through an empirical determination of the health educator's role. This work has now led to the development of a list of basic competencies for health educators.

Zaltman, G., and Duncan, R. 1977. *Strategies for Planned Change.* New York: Wiley.

In this basic text for the health educator as change agent, the authors define and describe the steps in the process of change. Chapter 11, which presents the authors' ideas on innovations in organizations, should be of particular interest in regard to the Salisbury case.

Discussion Questions

1. Besides training courses, what methods could be used to diffuse new knowledge to staff?
2. What arguments could district medical directors make for health education being just a support service?
3. What distinguishes a profession from job categories that are nonprofessional?
4. How would you reorganize the health department on the basis of the information provided in the case?
5. Describe the content that would be appropriate for workshops on a "A Systematic Approach to Problem Solving," "Group Facilitation," and "Consultation," which are mentioned in the case.
6. How might the adoption-diffusion theory or organizational change theory apply to this case?

Consumer-Planned Health Education in Comprehensive Health Planning

Marcia Pinkett-Heller, M.P.H., and Noreen M. Clark, Ph.D.

This case will describe the development and the implementation of consumer education courses in the early 1970s. The purpose of these courses was to help consumers "learn to articulate health needs of their community and develop both planning and administrative skills." These courses took place in central Harlem in New York City; they were developed by the Harlem Health Alliance, Inc., in cooperation with the Program of Continuing Education at Columbia University's School of Public Health.

This case occurred from 1970 to 1974, and the data presented reflect the circumstances of that time. During this time, federally sponsored health planning efforts, Comprehensive Health Planning, provided greater opportunities for consumer involvement in health care provision than ever before.

Two health educators, staff members of the Program of Continuing Education at Columbia, "staffed" this project, the first doing so for six months during the planning phase, and the second for the two years the project was implemented.

We will describe first the setting in which the project occurred and the political background, and then the development and implementation of the courses and the influence they had on the behavior of the participants. Finally, we'll discuss the role we health educators played in the project.

Marcia Pinkett-Heller is a Visiting Assistant Professor at Hunter College, School of Health Sciences. When this case was written, she was Assistant Director of the Program of Continuing Education at Columbia University. Noreen M. Clark is Associate Professor of Health Behavior/Health Education at the University of Michigan School of Public Health.

THE SETTING

Central Harlem is an area of 3½ square miles in the middle of Manhattan Island, New York. In 1970 there were 182,730 people living in 70,140 housing units; 94.1 percent of the population were Black (U.S. Bureau of the Census, 1970), compared to 21.1 percent of the New York City population (New York City Planning Commission 1973). The average family income in central Harlem was $6,137 per year (U.S. Bureau of the Census 1972).

It is a predominately Protestant, residential community with small businesses along the major north-south avenues and scattered side streets. The majority of these businesses are in the personal service category (e.g. beauty parlors, dry cleaners, and barber shops). There are also many restaurants and taverns in the community. The major shopping and entertainment area is concentrated on one wide, east-west thoroughfare.

At the time of this case there was one municipal and two voluntary hospitals in the central Harlem Health Center District and only 116 private physicians practicing in the area. The shortage of private health practitioners had not helped central Harlem lower its shockingly high infant and maternal mortality rates (Table 1). It is not surprising that in 21.7 percent of the total births in central Harlem, the mother had little or no prenatal care (U.S. DHEW 1973).

The high incidence of diseases such as tuberculosis, diabetes, and lead poisoning; the high crime rate and higher narcotic use rate; the deteriorating housing, congestion, and poverty—all have combined to make central Harlem appear to be the prototype of urban ghettos. The factor that sets it apart, however, is its people.

Table 1
Comparison of Infant and Maternal Mortality Rates in Central Harlem and Manhattan, 1971

	Central Harlem	Manhattan
Live births	16.2 (rate per 1,000 population)	12.9
Maternal deaths	10.1 (rate per 10,000 live births)	4–5
Infant deaths	29.3 (rate per 1,000 live births)	21.4

Sources: U.S. DHEW, Health Services Administration, Bureau of Health Statistics and Analysis (1973); New York City, Department of Health (1971).

There are a large number of people living in Harlem who care about their community. This case will explore how some have attempted to translate their concern into positive action. Providing the background will be a chronicle of events leading up to the writing of a request for specific funds to provide education for health consumers.

POLITICAL BACKGROUND

A center for teaching Comprehensive Health Planning at Columbia University was established in 1967, focusing on training health planners at the master's and doctoral levels. From the outset, the Program of Continuing Education at Columbia, staffed by health educators, had great interest in the role of consumers in Comprehensive Health Planning and sought to include them as often as possible in Continuing Education courses and learning activities.

After long discussions between faculty of the academic program in Comprehensive Health Planning and Continuing Education faculty, it was agreed that a project in consumer education be included in the Harlem Health Center's continuation request for support to the Community Health Service of the Department of Health, Education, and Welfare (DHEW).

Staff of Continuing Education began to explore the interest and relevance of consumer education to community groups in the metropolitan area. At the same time, Mayor John Lindsay named an Organizational Task Force to prepare for establishment of an areawide "B" agency for health planning in New York City. The task force, in turn, designated eight local demonstration units in planning, which were to be forerunners of community health planning advisory boards. Several of the local demonstration units expressed interest in Continuing Education's plan to seek support under Section 314c of the Public Health Service Act, for consumer education.

Continuing Education staff met with representatives of these community groups over the three-month period prior to preparation of the grant application; many community groups and organizations had a good grasp of the issues and problems facing Comprehensive Health Planning on the local level. Their insights were necessary in preparing the application.

A major factor concerning the proposed consumer education was the role Columbia University would play. Many people viewed the School of Public Health as generally unresponsive to needs of local communities and wanted to be sure that consumer education would address problems and issues from the consumer's perspective. Continuing Education, as a program of the School of Public Health, had done much to ameliorate the general suspicion of community groups outside the university. For several years, it had worked in a variety of New York City neighborhoods through a series of "Voice of the Community" courses. In these courses, community providers and consumers studied specific health problems and developed alternatives for solution. Even though some of the persons represented in local demonstration units had been involved in these activities, many who had not were cautious about becoming involved with the school. There was, in the main, concern about who would have the say in curriculum development and implementation. Long, and often heated, periods of deliberation occurred in which community representatives weighed the advantages and disadvantages of collaboration with Columbia. These deliberations finally led to formation of a core of representatives from the local demonstration units who were to work with Continuing Education staff in drafting a grant proposal to ensure relevance and effectiveness from the community point of view.

During this period, the gap between the local demonstration planning units and the mayor's Organizational Task Force widened over the issue of community control and power of local boards. Plans for consumer education moved along, but were influenced by the emerging conflict. As the application deadline neared, the core committee of community representatives and Continuing Education staff developed a comprehensive and, in their view, potentially effective design for broadening the awareness of Comprehensive Health Planning in communities and preparing individuals for active involvement in the process.

The central issue that then emerged was whether the training must come under the aegis of the mayor's Organizational Task Force, the community, or some combination of both, or whether training would be removed from the political interests of each, a condition that seemed as unlikely as it was unrealistic. When it became clear that any proposal to foster the concepts of Comprehensive Health Planning would logically and administratively need to be submitted for review to the mayor's Organizational Task Force, several local demonstration units felt their best interests would not be served in the joint venture with Continuing Education, because they believed review by the task force might weaken their stance on other issues.

Of the original seven local units involved in developing the proposal, only one, the Harlem Health Alliance, decided to take its chances with the project. The Alliance had long been the strongest and best organized of the community planning groups growing out of the demonstration units and, in addition, had had previous contacts with Continuing Education. It is an umbrella organization comprised of 43 groups working to improve the quality of health of the people of Harlem. This history, along with the belief of the Alliance members that education is necessary for effective consumer participation, resulted in the members agreeing to cooperate with Continuing Education should the collaboratively developed proposal receive federal support.

The consumer education proposal was subsequently reviewed at a regular meeting of the mayor's Organizational Task Force, where Continuing Education representatives reiterated their intention to work with the Harlem Health Alliance, though not to the exclusion of other community groups and organizations interested in Comprehensive Health Planning. The Advisory Board of the task force found the proposal acceptable, and it was submitted through the regular channels for funding. Over one year later, Continuing Education received notice of the grant award and, on paper, the project became a reality.

It would be worthwhile at this point to examine the motives of the agencies involved in this novel venture: the Harlem Health Alliance, the Program of Continuing Education, and the Department of Health, Education, and Welfare.

The objectives of the Harlem Health Alliance, as stated in its bylaws (1967) are as follows:

1. To draw and effect the implementation of a comprehensive health plan for the Harlem community.
2. To focus on certain high-priority health problems in order to coordinate fragmented facilities and programs, to better utilize existing facilities, and [to] establish innovative methods for resolving these problems.
3. To coordinate and evaluate data on health facilities, their deficiencies, and their absences in order to determine the true health needs of the community.
4. To serve as a health-advocacy force to maximize the impact of Harlem providers and consumers in resolving the key health issues affecting the community.
5. To establish and maintain an up-to-date consumer education and public information system for central Harlem residents, with mechanisms for effective feedback on health needs and priorities from the community. These mechanisms will include newsletters to consumers, planned conferences, the mass media, etc., with special emphasis on coordinating the fragmented consumer-education projects designated for Harlem residents.

6. To serve as a forum for discussion on the merits of all health proposals which will directly or indirectly affect the Harlem community. The Alliance may then choose to adopt a public position reflecting the views of its membership majority.
7. To form working relationships with outside groups or facilities to offer input into development of specific health programs or proposals deemed to further Alliance goals.

The Program of Continuing Education stated its objectives in the original grant application: "To help citizens recognize their health rights, gain confidence in the importance of their role as consumer representatives, learn to articulate the health needs of their community and develop both planning and administrative skills."

It would seem from the Comprehensive Health Planning legislation that the objectives of the federal government (DHEW) were as follows (National Association of Counties Research Foundation 1968:32):

To encourage both providers and consumers of health services to reach agreement on . . . a) Health needs of a community; b) Goals and priorities of a health delivery program; c) Resources and measures appropriate to achievement of goals; [and] d) Recommendations of actions by the public and private sectors which might enhance the effectiveness of the existing resources and activities and which could develop those needed for the future."

CURRICULUM DEVELOPMENT AND IMPLEMENTATION

In the interim between submission of the grant and the notice of funding, Noreen (the second author) worked with the members of the Harlem Planning Committee to outline the first 16-session course on communication. When the project was funded, the first course was ready to go. However, shortly after the notice of the grant award, Continuing Education staff met with the Harlem Health Alliance Executive Board to officially reconfirm their interest in the project. A Consumer Education Committee of the Alliance (for the most part the Planning Committee for the project) was formed to work with Continuing Education staff in developing courses and workshops in central Harlem.

The committee members determined that a public meeting should precede any further curriculum development. They did, however, identify three "areas of knowledge" they believed necessary for consumers involved in the planning process:

1. *Communication* (already developed)—emphasis on how community organizations and health agencies get health information to consumers
2. *Administration*—emphasis on understanding administration in light of the increasing administrative functions of consumers in their roles as community leaders, advisory board and committee members, and so on
3. *Economics and politics of health*—the financing of health care, funding of programs, and organization of health care services to meet consumer needs

A general meeting of community residents was called two weeks later in central Harlem. About 70 people attended, including several members of the Harlem Junior Health Workers Association, a group of young people whose active involvement is encouraged by the Harlem Health Alliance. At the open meeting, there was agreement on the need for consumer education and support was voiced for the joint effort to develop courses. Suggestions for three topic areas were made, and it was agreed that the subjects of greatest importance could be fitted within the general headings "communication," "administration," and "economics and politics." The group broke into three brainstorming workshops, each focusing on one of the three topic areas. Each group developed a list of specific subjects under the topic heading it wanted to learn about during the consumer education courses.

Three committees were then formed of people who volunteered to work on developing the courses. Utilizing the data from the large group as a starting point, the planning committees held ongoing meetings to further develop each subject area into a 16-session, 32-hour course. It was agreed that the faculty for the courses should be drawn as much as possible from resources available in central Harlem, but several other criteria were also involved in the faculty selection. The consumer committees agreed they wanted to have the "best that's available" to discuss specific subject matter, they wanted faculty with empathy and understanding of the community, and they wanted an opportunity for consumers to conduct a dialogue on health with important figures in government. The process of identifying and verifying possible faculty was carried on by the committee members during this period. An attempt was made to minimize misunderstanding between student and faculty participants by encouraging each to verbalize their expectations of themselves, one another, and the courses.

Each planning group decided on the hours and scheduling of class sessions. In every instance, the decision was made to hold evening sessions to allow working people to attend. It was also decided that the Harlem Hospital Center was both a central and safe place to hold the sessions. Arrangements were made to utilize classroom space in the Martin Luther King, Jr., Pavillion.

The courses utilized a variety of methodologies. There was much use of group dynamics. Class sessions were problem-oriented and dealt with specific questions. Lectures/discussions were used frequently, as were workshops and panel discussions. Class size was limited to 35 people in each course to ensure maximum participation of all. A coordinator was chosen from the original planning committee for each course. This person was responsible for introducing the faculty and leading discussions at each session. Also selected from the planning committee was a person to take notes of the sessions and record attendance of the participants. These community people each received an honorarium for those tasks.

Announcements of the classes were widely distributed to organizations and individuals in central Harlem. The word-of-mouth process undoubtedly alerted a sizable number of people as well. Each planning committee became the admissions committee to check applications. The major criterion for acceptance was that the person applying had demonstrated in some way interest in the health of the community. It was felt that any further criteria might block those who could be potential contributors to the Comprehensive Health Planning process.

Participants were recruited in many ways. One member of the Harlem Health Alliance, hostess of her own program on a local radio station, invited course planners to discuss the issues of consumer education for health planning during the course recruitment period and provided enrollment information to interested participants. The Harlem Junior Health Workers distributed course announcements around the community, and news of the courses was given out at regular meetings of the community organizations in the Alliance. In addition, the director of each Alliance member organization was contacted personally and encouraged to assist in consumer recruitment.

Participants were selected on a first-come, first-served basis and a stipend of three dollars per session was made available to needy consumers to pay for such out-of-pocket expenses as carfare and babysitting.

Typically, participants were employed in health-related jobs, almost exclusively at the paraprofessional, clerical, or technical level. Half a dozen described themselves as community health workers or aides; several were technicians, clerks, and licensed practical nurses. One directed a family planning clinic, another a nursing home. A handful were registered nurses. There were no physicians, hospital administrators, or public health officials among the "provider" participants. The "consumer" participants seemed fairly representative of low-income community residents. Several described themselves as community organizers; others were school aides, bookkeepers, students, blue-collar workers, and housewives.

The three different courses extended over a period of six months, with two weekly sessions each. Provision was made for an introductory session and a wrap-up evaluative session in each of the three courses. This plan gave students an opportunity for discussion and evaluation of each course. Discussions usually included students' reactions to speakers, session content, and the degree of usefulness they believed each topic had for their own needs.

Briefly described, the three courses were as follows:

Course 1—Communication. The objective of this course was to help the participants improve their interpersonal relationships at home, in the community, and in business, especially in the health field. Inter- and intra-agency communication was discussed. A presentation was made to develop speaking, listening, and observing skills as beneficial tools, basic to strengthening self-confidence and communication in all areas of endeavor.

Course 2—Administration. The course was developed to serve as a vehicle for maximizing the consumer's participation in the decision making that affects the health of the community. The course began with a definition of the subject as it relates to health. Among the topics covered were planning for services, general responsibilities of the administrator, the decision-making process, community board involvement in decision making, and municipal and statewide planning for health services to the community.

Course 3—Economics and Politics of Health. The purpose of the course was to aid the participants in their development of insight into the political aspects of health, from the financing to the organization of services. An identification of health issues was followed by a review of health planning in the past. Subsequent sessions covered funding for health care, revenue sharing, current health provision systems, federal and state responses to health needs, and an overview of the health planning effort in New York City. Near the end of the course, there was a concentrated period for the development of skills in proposal writing.

A consumer mini-library was established in the Harlem Hospital Center Library to provide materials and books that might be useful to persons attending the courses who might wish to supplement their classroom activities and learning.

At the end of the six months, the students gave their evaluation of the three courses. Sessions were rated by each student in a scale with four headings: poor, fair, good, excellent. They were also asked to rate the sessions as to their usefulness, from very little use to extremely useful. Ninety-five percent of the participants stated that overall the courses were either good or excellent. They made requests for additional classes and workshops and asked for further elaboration on particular topics. The community participants wanted more advanced courses in health and the health care system, building on the first three courses.

In response to the request of the consumers, a two-day, weekend session was held with participants from all three courses. Again, the planning of the curricula and selection of faculty were done by Harlem residents. This session required the participants to work together, utilizing the knowledge and skills gained from the previous class sessions to determine how others might become more aware of health and planning for its improvement. The workshops resulted in the decision of the group to write a pamphlet describing the process and content of courses that had been developed. The Harlem Health Alliance members felt such a brochure would help motivate other community groups interested in developing training programs. This pamphlet is now being written by a committee of volunteers from the weekend workshop.

The participants in that first weekend retreat also selected 30 of their peers, who demonstrated leadership potential in the consumer education courses, to receive further training in leadership skills. The group selected developed their own curricula for three consecutive weekend leadership workshops.

EVALUATION

One immediate effect of the Harlem consumer education courses was felt in the spring of 1973. The Comprehensive Health Planning steering committee, for the central Harlem area, was selected, and of the 13 providers and consumers on that committee, 10 of the consumers had attended one or more of the consumer education courses. Many other participants are now serving more effectively on patient councils or advisory boards for local hospital and other health providers in the area.

A second effect of the Harlem consumer education program has been the interest aroused in community groups in other areas of the city for similar courses. Word-of-mouth description of the program and the process for community planning and involvement has caused interested consumers from other communities to contact the Program of Continuing Education and request assistance in developing consumer education. Some subsequent requests have come from the other original demonstration units, which had elected not to participate in the granting process.

The Institute for Adult Development, Larchmont, New York, evaluated several aspects of this consumer education program in 1974. Of those participating in the course, 115 responded to a questionnaire.

We were particularly interested in the respondents' perception of the educational outcome of the courses. Participants were asked: "How much did you learn about community health problems as a result of your participation in the Consumer Education Program?" Only 8.7% indicated they learned a little they didn't know before; 32.2% said they learned some things they didn't know before; and 59.1% said they learned many things they didn't know before.

A related question asked: "How much did you learn about the organization and workings of the health care delivery system in your community as a result of the Consumer Education Program?" Ten percent indicated "little," 35% "some," and 55% "a great deal." Not surprisingly, only 40% of those employed in the health field said they learned a great deal, compared with 62.5% of the consumer group. Also not surprisingly, a larger proportion of those who took two or more courses reported learning a great deal (62.5% compared to 44.4%).

Respondents were also asked: "To what degree, if any, did the Consumer Education Program improve your ability to participate effectively in community health care decision making?" About 13% reported that the program helped little; 40% reported it helped some; and 45% reported it helped a great deal. There was a substantial difference on this item between those who took only one course and those who took two or more courses. Only 25.5% of the former group reported that the course "helped a great deal to improve my ability to participate effectively," compared with 61.5% of the latter group.

After the evaluation, the Harlem Health Alliance continued to be interested and involved in consumer education and cosponsored courses in health with the Program of Continuing Education.

THE ROLE OF THE HEALTH EDUCATORS

We—the health educators involved in the project, Noreen Clark (for the first six months) and Marcia Pinkett-Heller (for two years)—have evolved a similar style in working with groups: relatively low-key and nondirective. We both tend to function as facilitators and/or clarifiers.

In the beginning our role was that of convenor.

After the Harlem Health Alliance agreed to participate in the project and the grant proposal was written, there was a hiatus of three or four months. Noreen worked with the Harlem planning committee to outline the first 16-session course on communication. This work included identifying topics that should be covered and possible speakers for each topic. The technique most frequently used in these meetings was brainstorming. The health educator was just one member of the group, albeit one with many external resources. All members had equal chances to speak, and all were identified as "experts" by virtue of their many years of community involvement and interest in health matters. Both Noreen and I were careful not to present ourselves as all-knowing. Indeed, given the Harlem community's suspicion and resentment of Columbia University, we played an even lower-key role than was probably necessary to avoid being considered "colonialists."

At a typical planning meeting, the health educator usually took notes of issues raised, suggestions made, topics to be covered, and so on. These notes became the minutes of the planning meetings. The health educator was responsible for getting the minutes typed and distributed to everyone, writing the letters of invitation to the speakers (based on what the committee wanted said), mimeographing and mailing the course announcement (contents based on committee input), answering telephone queries—in short, we carried out staff functions for the group.

An important point to reiterate here is that the community people were volunteers and as such often had full-time jobs. We had our own office, secretarial staff, and access to university resources such as telephone, postage, and letterhead stationery, plus credibility in the larger community. Access to these resources was important to the Harlem group.

The planning committees for all the courses met maybe four to six times, for one to two hours each time.

When the grant funds finally came through, the first Harlem course was ready to begin. Noreen bowed out and I took over the project. Over 50 people applied for the course. Thirty-five were selected and not one of them missed a session.

At the time the first Harlem course got under way, another community group made overtures to

Table 2
Community Group Involvement in Consumer Education Project

Community	Number of Courses Offered		
	1972	1973	1974
Harlem	{ X X X	X X X X X	X X
Williamsburg, Greenpoint, Brooklyn	X	X X	X
Lower East Side, New York City		X X	X
Bedford-Stuyvesant, Brooklyn			X

Continuing Education to take part in the project. The people in the Williamsburg section of Brooklyn had organized themselves into a planning committee after hearing what was going on in Harlem.

In all, four community groups got involved with the project and stayed with it over a two-year period. The Harlem group was involved the longest. Table 2 identifies the communities involved and the number of courses offered in each. Each X represents a 16-session course (two hours each session). Many of the people who attended the first course continued on through subsequent courses. All told, over 325 community people participated in the project.

The major problems encountered in carrying out this project had to do with trust—first too little and then too much. When the planning committees first started meeting, every detail had to be agreed on by the committee. If a committee member missed a meeting, actions taken and decisions made had to be explained and justified later to the absent member, and sometimes decisions and courses of action were scrapped or turned around at subsequent meetings because the person who had been absent didn't want anything to be "put over." This was particularly true in the planning of the Lower East Side group, the one in which the individuals had the least amount of previous interaction. A leadership power struggle developed among some members of the committee, and if one leader was absent, everything had to be done from scratch at the subsequent meeting. This complication occurred in three or four meetings until I called the group's attention to the fact that time was passing and other groups in the city wanted to develop courses. The group agreed that decisions made would be binding, and planning went forward.

By the middle of the second year, things were going so well and enough trust had been developed between the community groups and Columbia University staff that the planning committees didn't want to meet. Rather, they entrusted yours truly to "take care of things," because, as they pointed out, "you know how the community wants it done." I balked at this, reminding the Harlem Health Alliance members at one of their meetings that they were cosponsors of the project and had some responsibility. I also claimed inability to be three places at one time, because by that time there were courses going on in Harlem, Brooklyn, and the Lower East Side on Tuesday and Thursday evenings. My nonavailability forced the community planning groups back into action. I deliberately missed meetings, and all of the groups rolled along without me. Even though physically absent, however, I was always available by telephone, and the groups knew this.

Problems? There weren't too many, amazingly enough. Two come immediately to mind. First, speaker "no shows." This situation happened twice when elected officials were invited to attend, and in both instances the community groups wrote and phoned the official's office to voice their anger. At subsequent meetings someone from that official's office was there! The second problem was administrative or bookkeeping problems on our end. Participants were paid a stipend for attending (three dollars per session), and the checks were issued from the Columbia bursar's office. Once or twice there was a considerable delay in sending out the checks, and boy, was I pounced on!

Part of what seemed to make the project function so smoothly was totally serendipitous—the personalities of the people involved. Another contributing factor to success was the personal and professional philosophy of the health educators. Noreen Clark, the original project coordinator, obtained her master's degree in adult education and was (and is) a strong advocate of the philosophies of education proffered by Paulo Friere, Ivan Illich, and Carl Rogers. I (Marcia Pinkett-Heller) had obtained an M.P.H. from the University of Michigan's School of Public Health at a time when that program focused on community development, and I had been steeped in the community organization approach of Saul Alinsky as part of Peace Corps training.

REFERENCES

National Association of Counties Research Foundation. 1968. *Comprehensive Health Planning: A Manual for Local Officials*. Washington, D.C.

New York City Department of Health. 1973. "Summary of Vital Statistics, 1971, the City of New York." New York.

New York City Planning Commission. 1973. "Health Area Profiles, Part 1: Population and Housing." New York.

U.S. Bureau of the Census. 1970. First Count Tapes, 1970 Census.

U.S. Bureau of the Census. 1972. *1970 Census of Population and Housing: Census Tracts, New York, N.Y.* PHC (1)–145. Washington, D.C.: Government Printing Office.

U.S. Department of Health, Education, and Welfare. Health Services Administration. Bureau of Health Statistics and Analysis. 1972. "Services and Vital Statistics by Health Center Districts, New York City, 1970." Washington, D.C.

U.S. Department of Health, Education, and Welfare. Health Services Administration. Bureau of Health Statistics and Analysis. 1973. "Services and Vital Statistics by Health Center Districts. New York City, 1971." Washington, D.C.

Analysis

This case describes how a large institution developed a consumer education course with the goal of increasing consumer involvement in the planning and provision of health services. Two health educators of the institution's continuing education unit had prime responsibility for planning and implementing the course. It is important to note that the health educators saw themselves primarily as facilitators and clarifiers. Unfortunately for health educators, these functions are often not highly valued by others, although they are necessary for the successful implementation of any project. Generally, the health educator as facilitator needs assurance from administration or management that the functions required are understood, have value, and directly relate to the project's outcome.

Although the theory the health educators based their activities on is not directly stated, the consumer education courses appear to have a firm basis in adult learning theory. Following are some of the principles of adult learning theory that are employed in successful adult education programs (Pine and Horne 1969:109):

- Learning is an experience which occurs inside the learner and is activated by the learner.
- Learning (behavioral change) is a consequence of experience.
- Learning is a cooperative and collaborative process.
- One of the richest resources for learning is the learner himself.

It is also worth considering some of the conditions under which learning best takes place. According to Pine and Horne (1969:110, 126), an atmosphere that facilitates learning has the following characteristics:

- It "encourages people to be active."
- It "promotes and facilitates the individual's discovery of the personal meaning of ideas."
- It "tolerates ambiguity."
- It encourages people "to trust in themselves as well as in external sources."

The health educators employed a variety of strategies in carrying out this project. They included organizational development within the institution to ensure commitment. Community organization was another major strategy, because diverse groups needed to be brought together for planning and implementation. As the authors state, the whole process was politically sensitive, especially since there was considerable distrust among community groups. Group process was also extensively used within committee meetings and the courses themselves.

As facilitators, the health educators were responsible for staffing the planning committee in which much of the work on the project took place. Committee work demands many functions that are very important, though they often masquerade as being trivial. One such function is note taking. An accurate record of what takes place in a meeting is essential not only to meet one's own needs but to ensure the continued functioning of the committee. Moreover, minutes may under certain circumstances be legal documents.

The need and utility of consumer participation have long been an established principle in health education practice (Nyswander 1980). As involvement increases, commitment to achieving the objectives of the program increases, and very often active participants have much to contribute to the program by way of knowledge and experiences that they alone possess apart from the skills of the expert. It was understandable that with the passage of the Comprehensive Health Planning Act in 1966 (PL 89-749), which mandated consumer involvement, health educators would find employment in health planning agencies. The framers of the health planning legislation wisely recognized that the consumer who is the supposed beneficiary of the health care system has a vested interest in planning for the system. The legislation stated that policy decisions of planning agencies were to be made by volunteer councils composed of a majority of consumers "broadly representing the geographic and socio-economic distribution of the area's population" and of "providers of personal, environmental and preventive health services." The Comprehensive Health Planning Act was replaced in 1974 by the National Health Planning and Resources Development Act of 1974 (PL 93-641), which in 1979 was amended and strengthened and which, at least on paper, heightened consumer involvement in health planning. Both laws resulted in the establishment of statewide and regional health planning agencies with the goal of making health and medical organizations more efficient and responsive to human needs.

Consumer involvement, then, was to be an important factor in health planning. But its full potential would not be realized unless consumers could effectively function in the council and committee arena to promote their interests, which were very often contrary to those of the providers. It thus became the responsibility of health planning agencies to provide orientation and education for consumers as well as to reach out into the community to ensure diverse consumer representation. Some health planning agencies took this role very seriously. Other agencies at best assumed only a passive role, which resulted in provider dominance that negated the intent of the legislation in regard to consumer participation.

What we see in this case study is a successful example of how consumer involvement can be increased through education. As the authors note, consumers who attended the course were later well represented on the Comprehensive Health Planning committee for their area and in other health planning bodies. An external evaluation indicated that the course met its objectives of increasing participants' understanding of the health care system and provided them with the tools to function effectively on committees.

References/Select Resources

Knowles, M. 1973. *The Adult Learner: A Neglected Species.* Houston: Gulf Publishing.

We recommend that anyone who has responsibility for an adult education program consult this book. The process of adult education, andragogy, is distinguished from the process of childhood education, pedagogy.

Metsch, J. M.; Berson, A.; and Weitzner, M. 1975. "The Impact of Training on Consumer Participation in the Delivery of Health Services." *Health Education Monographs* 3(3):251–261.

This paper documents the evaluation of training for consumer advisory groups, including content analysis of minutes of meetings as one interesting approach to the impact of training.

Nyswander, D. 1980. "Public Health Education: Sources, Growth and Operational Philosophy." *International Quarterly of Community Health Education* 1(1):15.

In this paper, first delivered at the University of Massachusetts, Dorothy Nyswander reviews some of the principles underlying the practice of health education. Her discussion is based on her experience as one of the leaders in health education during its formative years.

Pine, G. J., and Horne, P. J. 1969. "Principles and Conditions for Learning in Adult Education." *Adult Leadership* 18(4):108–134.

The principles and conditions outlined in this article are useful to health educators who practice in a variety of settings. The discussion clearly illustrates the close affiliation that health educators have with other educators.

U.S. Department of Health, Education, and Welfare. 1976. *Educating the Public about Health: A Planning Guide.* DHEW Publication no. (HRA) 78–14004. Washington, D.C.: Government Printing Office.

This planning guide, which was originally developed for staffs in health planning organizations, is of value to health educators who are responsible for developing and implementing community programs.

Discussion Questions

1. What are some of the arguments for and against consumer participation in health planning?

2. What kinds of experimental exercises would you include in the three courses described in this case?

3. The consumer education program was supported by federal money. How could the project have been otherwise supported?

4. What are some of the problems that could occur during the group meetings like those in this case, and how would you as the health educator deal with them?

5. This case occurred in an urban environment. How would you proceed if it were a rural environment, and what barriers would you anticipate?

Changing Tuberculosis Treatment from Inpatient to Outpatient Care and from Sanatorium to General Hospital Care

Frances R. Ogasawara, M.S.

BACKGROUND

Prior to the discovery in 1945 that antibiotics were effective against the tubercle bacilli, care of the tuberculosis patient consisted of bed rest, often for many years, or of surgical procedures designed to collapse and rest the lungs. The patient was kept in isolation in a sanatorium or tuberculosis hospital usually located in rural areas or the mountains.

In the late 1940s physicians used antobiotics for critically ill patients. Then they utilized the drugs as an adjunct to rest cure but continued the isolation, the bed rest, and other measures (e.g. clean air, good food).

In the early 1960s there was enough experience to show drugs to be effective in rendering patients noninfectious, in abating symptoms, and in restoring health. Many physicians recognized that patients could be treated in their communities or could be discharged from inpatient care after a relatively short stay. They also recognized many could resume work and other usual activities without harm to themselves or others while continuing to take medication.

The American Lung Association (ALA) board committee charged with the tuberculosis program, the Committee for the Guidance of the Tuberculosis Program, decided in 1966 that the time had come to promote the "modern methods of tuberculosis care." The major components of "modern methods" were chemotherapy as the treatment of choice; outpatient, clinic-based care; and general hospitals instead of specialized tuberculosis hospitals for those who needed hospitalization.

The ALA and its medical section, the American Thoracic Society (ATS), provided leadership and guidance in encouraging these changes throughout the country. The Tuberculosis Control Division of the U.S. Public Health Service's Center for Disease Control was a partner in this effort. State and local branches of the ALA carried out the program to bring about the desired changes in their areas. All members of the ALA and ATS did not immediately accept the "modern methods." Activities to convince ALA members of the efficacy of these methods were going on simultaneously with activities to convince other institutions and organizations to make changes.

The development of the program to effect change is described in terms of the activities of committees. This is because in lung associations, all policy issues are developed by committees appointed by the president of the board of directors. Often committee work is augmented by ad hoc subcommittee(s) appointed by the ALA president to carry out a specific and time-limited task.

These committees make recommendations to the board, which in turn makes decisions on the association's policy and direction. The association's staff carries out the decisions made by the board, determining the details of implementation on the basis of their professional knowledge and expertise. In actual practice, volunteers and staff work as a team. An ALA staff member is assigned to work with all committees.

This case study describes the role of a health educator in her function as staff to the committees

---

Frances R. Ogasawara is the Director of Constituent Relations for the American Lung Association. She was formerly a Special Consultant for the Tuberculosis Program.

that promoted a change in the preferred method of care for tuberculosis patients. The case chronicles ten years of activity at the national level. At the state and local level, activities were conducted to implement the policies and positions promoted by the national association. During these years, the organization changed its name twice, from the National Tuberculosis Association (NTA) to the National Tuberculosis and Respiratory Disease Association (NTRDA) in 1968 and then to the American Lung Association (ALA) in 1973. All three are used in this story.

STAFF FUNCTION

The health educator assigned to the Committee for the Guidance of the Tuberculosis Program worked closely with the chairman, bringing to her attention problems, issues, proposals, suggestions, recommendations, or decisions for which there was need for discussion. Together they decided what the salient points were about each issue, what background materials were needed, whether guests should be invited as resource people, and what action was needed by the committee. The health educator developed a tentative agenda for committee meetings and reviewed it with the chairman. (This procedure is critical for a productive meeting. The chairman and staff should know before a meeting what they expect from the committee's discussion, what they hope the outcome will be.)

They also planned housekeeping details in scheduling a meeting: selecting a site (city and hotel), date, and times for the meeting. If there were meal functions, menus were selected. (Arrangements have much to do with attendance at a meeting. Convenience for the majority of the committee members, smoothly running arrangements, and good food affect the ability of the committee to work as a productive group.)

Two weeks before a meeting date, the health educator sent the committee all the background materials needed. These included the charge to the committee, the names and addresses of members, the tentative agenda, information on each agenda item, background reading, and an indication of the questions or issues for each agenda item.

The health educator worked in the same way with the chairman of the ad hoc committees appointed to deal with specific aspects of introducing the "new methods."

Committees concerned with program issues usually met two or three times a year for one or two days. Ad hoc committees met as often as necessary to complete the assigned tasks. Committees dealt by mail or phone to the extent possible. These procedures are still followed.

APRIL 1966—IDENTIFYING THE PROBLEM

In promoting "modern methods" for the treatment of tuberculosis, the Committee for the Guidance of the Tuberculosis Program recognized the use of general hospitals as the most controversial of these methods. To begin the promotion of the new concepts, the committee decided on two strategies. They invited a proponent of general hospital treatment to meet with them and discuss the issues, and they requested that an ad hoc committee be appointed to explore the problems associated with the treatment of tuberculosis in general hospitals and make recommendations to them.

The proponent, Carl Muschenheim, M.D., of New York Hospital and Cornell University Medical School, a highly respected pulmonary physician, told the committee he had been trying to change the attitude of hospitals and the pattern of hospitalization for tuberculosis for 10–15 years!

The ad hoc committee was chosen with great care. The members included physicians, a hospital administrator, a nurse, a representative from the Public Health Service, and Richard L. Riley, M.D., an expert on airborne infections. The chairman and the committee members were proponents of treating patients with tuberculosis in general hospitals.

DECEMBER 1967—THE FIRST RECOMMENDATIONS AND A PLAN FOR ACTION

The Report of the NTA Ad Hoc Committee on Treatment of Tuberculosis Patients in General Hospitals was completed. It described the problems associated with the admission of tuberculosis patients to general hospitals and the infectiousness of tuberculosis. Recommendations were made for six specific steps to be taken:

1. Get wide publicity for a statement, "Infectiousness of Tuberculosis," by Dr. Richard Riley.
2. Conduct a broadly based educational campaign to inform relevant groups, professional and lay, about the true nature of the infectiousness of tuberculosis so as to make admission of tuberculosis patients to general hospitals acceptable and routine.
3. Repeal legal barriers.
4. Assure that insurance benefits cover tuberculosis.
5. Produce educational materials for hopitals.
6. Approach the Public Health Service for approval of the statement "Infectiousness of Tuberculosis."

The report was accepted by the Committee for the Guidance of the Tuberculosis Program. It was recommended that a new ad hoc committee be appointed to prepare specific recommendations for working with general hospitals on treatment of patients with tuberculosis. The new committee was appointed in April 1968.

NOVEMBER 1968—"GUIDELINES FOR GENERAL HOSPITALS"

The committee for the Guidance of the Tuberculosis Program accepted the report "Guidelines for the General Hospital in the Admission and Care of Tuberculosis Patients," submitted by the new ad hoc committee.

This statement said:

> The general hospital is the logical place for treatment of those tuberculosis patients who need hospitalization—a development in patient care made possible by the proper use of antituberculosis drugs and modern methods of controlling infection. The following procedures and policies are offered by the NTRDA as a guide to facilitate the orderly transfer of this responsibility to the general hospital.

In the introduction, Julia M. Jones, M.D., who was chairman of the Committee for the Guidance of the Tuberculosis Program, explained that the committee noted the trend to treat tuberculosis patients in general hospitals and that such hospitals have the same responsibility to tuberculosis patients as to any sick person. She also stated that the guidelines are directed to individuals and agencies that have decided to plan for the treatment of tuberculosis patients in the general hospitals within their communities; they do not attempt to identify the many factors that may influence this decision.

When the statement was prepared, the ALA prepared an educational kit, "Tuberculosis in the General Hospital," including reprints of articles and statements on the various aspects of providing care, primarily the treatment and control of infectiousness.

The statement was published in April 1969 in the *American Review of Respiratory Disease,* the scientific journal of the ATS. It was also published in May 1969 in the NTRDA *Bulletin,* a monthly 16-page publication for lay volunteers, although read widely by health professionals too.

Publication of the guidelines provided lung associations, tuberculosis controllers (each health department has one such official who is responsible for the control of tuberculosis in the area of the department's jurisdiction), and pulmonary physicians with an authoritative statement that they could use in their communities to gain acceptance of the concept by the general hospitals. It should be noted that for years private patients had received care for tuberculosis in general hospitals. If hospitalization insurance did not cover tuberculosis, the patient was hospitalized under the diagnosis "bacterial pneumonia."

At the state and local levels, the nonmedical aspects of continuing tuberculosis hospitals had to be addressed. Many involved in the operation of these hosptials were reluctant to make changes. Many of these institutions were large and isolated. Often they were the major employer in a small community. The economic and social implications of closing these hospitals were far-reaching. What would happen to the employees? How many jobs would be lost? What about the contracts for providing supplies and services to the hospital? What about the responsibilities of the boards of trustees of the hospitals? Because the situation differed from place to place, these problems had to be solved locally.

The largest organized effort to fight the concepts outlined in the "Guidelines" of 1968 came from a group of southern states with large state hospital systems. This group presented a resolution to the national board of directors objecting to the policy on where tuberculosis patients should be treated.

In response, Dr. Jones pointed out that the "Guidelines" did not recommend *where* patients should be treated. The "Guidelines" were for people who wanted to know how general hospitals could prepare for accepting tuberculosis patients. Words in the statement were selected with great care so that their literal meaning could not be misconstrued. However, in issuing such a statement, the committee members implied that treatment in a general hospital was a good idea. Indeed, they intended to convey this.

A different type of barrier to acceptance of the "new methods" came from another source. Some young pulmonary physicians who were not in practice in the pre-chemotherapy era tended to view with disdain the older physician who chose to continue long-term bed rest in a tuberculosis hospital while prescribing chemotherapy. They made their feelings in this regard very clear by ignoring the older physicians, not listening when they spoke, and in some instances ridiculing their opinions. This treatment tended to harden the stance of those physicians who continued to follow the outdated regimen.

The leadership ability, prestige, and credibility of Dr. Jones, the chairman of the Committee for the Guidance of the Tuberculosis Program, was helpful in dealing with this barrier. She was professor of medicine and chief of the pulmonary service at a leading medical school, a recognized and highly respected clinician and teacher. She worked well with people at all levels of professional and social status. Her ability to encourage others to do their best and her sensitivity to the feelings of those who did not immediately accept the "modern methods" saved the day on more than one occasion. She was careful to allow everyone to express an opinion and to protect the self-respect and dignity of the individuals regardless of their opinions.

While the committee was trying to strike a balance between suggesting a good idea and telling people where and how to treat patients, and also trying to deal with conflict between the younger pulmonary physicians and some of the older physicians who chose not to accept the new ideas, it received a request from a respected pulmonary physician to develop criteria for the quality of care. He called attention to the fact that patients were still being treated by old-fashioned methods more appropriate to the pre-chemotherapy era. To deal with this referral, Dr. Jones appointed the Ad Hoc Committee on Quality Care.

The committee approached the quality issue from the perspective of total care. The site of treatment, the proper use of chemotherapy, and the length of inpatient care are interrelated. For example, it appeared that patients were often not discharged to outpatient care when they should have been because of the need to keep beds in the tuberculosis hospital filled.

MAY 1970—"STANDARDS FOR TREATMENT"

The result of the work of the Ad Hoc Committee on Quality Care was the statement "Standards for Tuberculosis Treatment in the 1970's," approved on May 27, 1970.

The first paragraph states:

> Although highly effective methods for the treatment of tuberculosis patients are known, they are not available to all patients. The quality of care provided tuberculosis patients varies to a considerable degree in many places in the United States. There are differences in quality both in the treatment of tuberculosis and [in that] of other diseases a patient might also have.

In this statement, for the first time, it was recommended that "the tuberculosis patient should receive most and sometimes all of his treatment as an outpatient, either in a clinic, health center, or physician's office," and that "when hospitalization is required, selected general hospitals should be available and utilized."

The preparation of this statement was a turning point in the transition from the old to the new. The appointment and work of this ad hoc committee were handled with great prudence, quality of care being a very controversial issue. The health educator worked closely with the chairman of the parent committee, Dr. Jones, in appointing the committee. Experience with other committees on controversial matters taught us that if all sides are equally represented, a consensus or a meaningful statement that presents a cohesive point of view is not possible. In appointing a committee, the chairman and staff must know the objective of the task to be carried out. If the purpose is to foster change, it is necessary that committee members have experience with the change and can provide constructive suggestions on how to implement the change.

The experience of the chairman, Dr. Roger S. Mitchell, in tuberculosis care spanned many years. He had been a patient at Trudeau Sanatorium, Saranac Lake, and worked there. Other members included a public health nurse and pulmonary physicians who were in private practice, conducted big city clinics, conducted rural clinics, or were associated with county tuberculosis hospitals and with general hospitals. Dr. Mitchell guided the committee through many stormy meetings as committee members struggled with the content of the statement, getting consensus or agreement, and working over the exact wording.

Individuals on the committee threatened to resign if their strongly felt points of view were not included or if someone else's strongly held point of view was included. In the end, one member who strongly supported tuberculosis hospitals felt he could not sign the statement and resigned from the committee.

Despite the fact that almost everyone on the ad hoc committee believed in the major points on treatment (outpatient care and general hospital use), the statement went through 24 drafts. For all the rewriting, the health educator collated the comments and revisions, worked with the ad hoc committee's chairman in preparing a revised draft, and sent it to the committee for further comments. This process was continued until the final draft was agreed upon.

APRIL 1971—THE AMERICAN HOSPITAL ASSOCIATION

We approached the American Hospital Association (AHA), asking its help in implementing the transition in tuberculosis care. The AHA is the member organization for hospitals; it is looked to by members for advice and counsel on issues that arise in the operation of a hospital. Therefore AHA support was critical.

The AHA leadership assigned the task of preparing a statement on "Care of Patients with Pulmonary Tuberculosis in General Hospitals" to their Committee on Infections within Hospitals. The resulting statement was the product of three meetings between representatives of the ALA/ATS and the AHA committee. It too went through many drafts. The final version was a compromise between the beliefs of the committee members of the two agencies. The staffs of AHA and ALA articulated these beliefs and worked out the compromises. Much of the "working out" was the selection of words.

The ALA health educator played an interesting role during these negotiations. Dr. Jones attended the first AHA committee meeting and presented the problems and our request of the AHA. In subsequent meetings, Dr. Jones asked the ALA staff to attend. A physician from our staff was assigned by the executive director to be the official representative. He was accompanied to meetings by the health educator.

All members of the AHA committee were physicians, infectious disease specialists. We sat at a large table; there were fewer than ten of us. During these discussions, the health educator sat next to the ALA physician, giving him answers to questions asked and feeding him questions to be asked of the committee. Since the health educator worked with the ad hoc committees, she was thoroughly familiar with all the details of the committee's work on infection control, whereas the physician was totally unfamiliar with the committee's work. It became ludicrous to continue the discussion through the physician. The committee members finally talked directly to the health educator, and she joined in the discussion.

However, ALA would not have approached the AHA committee with a nonphysician as spokesperson. The physician was perceived by AHA to have the proper credentials and the appropriate knowledge to be credible, that is, the medical degree. Backing up the physician with the person who had detailed knowledge of the subject got the job done.

The AHA statement was approved by the AHA Board of Trustees in November 1971, published as a joint statement of the AHA and ALA in the AHA Journal, *Hospitals*, January 16, 1972, and reprinted as a leaflet available for wide distribution. This statement gave the lung associations the endorsement needed to continue the educational efforts at the community level.

In April 1972, the ATS's Scientific Assembly on Tuberculosis appointed an ad hoc committee to work with ALA staff in developing a consultation service to assist the health departments of general hospitals and the lung associations in educational programs with hospital staff members on treating tuberculosis.

During this period many task forces were organized and seminars held throughout the country by the local association staff and volunteers in cooperation with health departments. These activities focused on in-service education and on examining the tuberculosis care system and bringing about change gradually. The health educator was invited to be a participant as speaker or resource person at some of these activities. Some states asked her for assistance in planning, for suggestions of names of speakers or resource people, or for information about what other states were doing.

The experiences of states that had successfully made the changes were described in national publications and at national annual meeting sessions.

From 1966 to 1972, the aforementioned activity at the national level and the activity in states that picked up the innovation early on and implemented changes resulted in interest among most local associations in promoting the use of the "modern method" for the care of tuberculosis patients. The corner had been turned in the acceptance of the innovation by the majority of those who had to adopt it if change was to occur.

However, the job was not done. There were other issues to be considered.

OCTOBER 1972—HOSPITAL INSURANCE

The Committee for the Guidance of the Tuberculosis Program addressed one of the deterrents to achieving the transition of care to general hospitals—the question of hospitalization insurance. Because tuberculosis care was established at public (tax) expense, many insurance policies excluded coverage for it. Further, when the preferred method of treatment was long-term bed rest, the length of hospitalization was a real barrier to including tuberculosis care in a health insurance plan. When the length of hospital stay was considerably shortened, discussions about inclusion in insurance plans were feasible. In 1972, the Blue Cross Association notified member associations that they could include coverage for tuberculosis care when it was requested. Many private carriers followed suit. Local association staff and volunteers met with local Blue Cross plans to encourage changes in coverage.

APRIL 1973—"MINI-SANS"

The Committee for the Guidance of the Tuberculosis Program was asked about special units for tuberculosis patients in general hospitals. Its response was: "It is neither necessary nor desirable to set aside specific beds, rooms or floors." The committee was concerned that hospitals would create "mini-sans," thereby isolating patients in a manner that would compromise the quality of care.

MARCH 1973—HOSPITAL INFECTION CONTROL

The concern of nurses for infection control in general hospitals was brought to the attention of the ALA and the Public Health Service's Center for Disease Control (CDC). These two organizations sponsored a meeting of four nurses, specialists in infection control, with the health educator. A booklet, "Guidelines on Prevention of Transmission of Tuberculosis in Hospitals," coauthored by a nurse from the Tuberculosis Control Division of the CDC and the ALA health educator, was the result of this meeting. It was published in 1974 and described in an article in the ALA *Bulletin*, September 1974.

During the next few years the health educator participated in several continuing education seminars for infection control nurses. The other faculty were physicians and nurses. The physician described how tuberculosis is treated; the nurses described infection control procedures and public health aspects of nursing care; and the health educator reviewed the change in concepts and the reasons for the change. These seminars helped to alleviate fear and to correct misconceptions about tuberculosis patients in the 1970s.

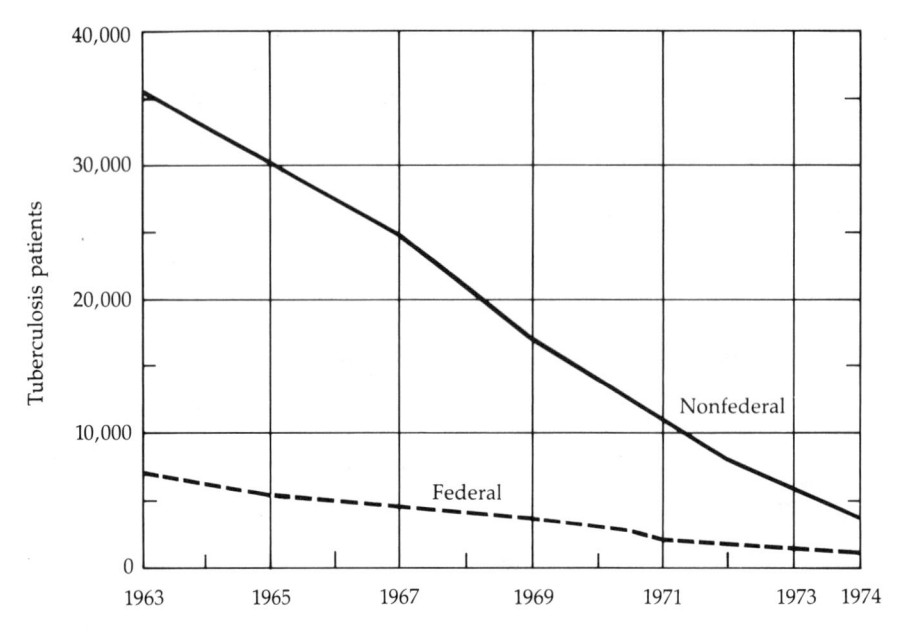

Figure 1
Tuberculosis Patients in Hospitals, United States, 1963–1974 (Beds Occupied on June 30)

Source: U.S. Department of Health, Education, and Welfare, Public Health Service, Center for Disease Control, *Reported Tuberculosis Data, 1973* (Washington, D.C.: Government Printing Office, December 1974), 22.

MAY 1978—STANDARDS UPDATED

The ATS Council adopted as an official statement, in May 1978, "Toward Eradication—A Contemporary Tuberculosis Control Strategy," an update of the 1970 "Standards."

In time the 1978 statement will be revised. The provision of quality care requires constant review and revision of standards.

POSTSCRIPT—1982

The information in "Toward Eradication" was accepted without controversy. It was recognized as a summary of the status of tuberculosis treatment and control in 1978.

By that time the specialized tuberculosis hospitals had been converted to other uses—mental hospitals, developmental centers for the mentally retarded, long-term care facilities for the elderly, or nonmedical uses such as prisons. Figures 1 and 2 illustrate this change dramatically.

Since then there have been further improvements in tuberculosis care, especially in the development of shorter courses of chemotherapy. Over the years, numerous other statements were issued to deal with various aspects of tuberculosis care: screening, laboratory aspects, return to work, and so on. All of these, including "Toward Eradication," are now being updated and consolidated into two statements to describe the present state of the art: one on therapy and one on public health control.

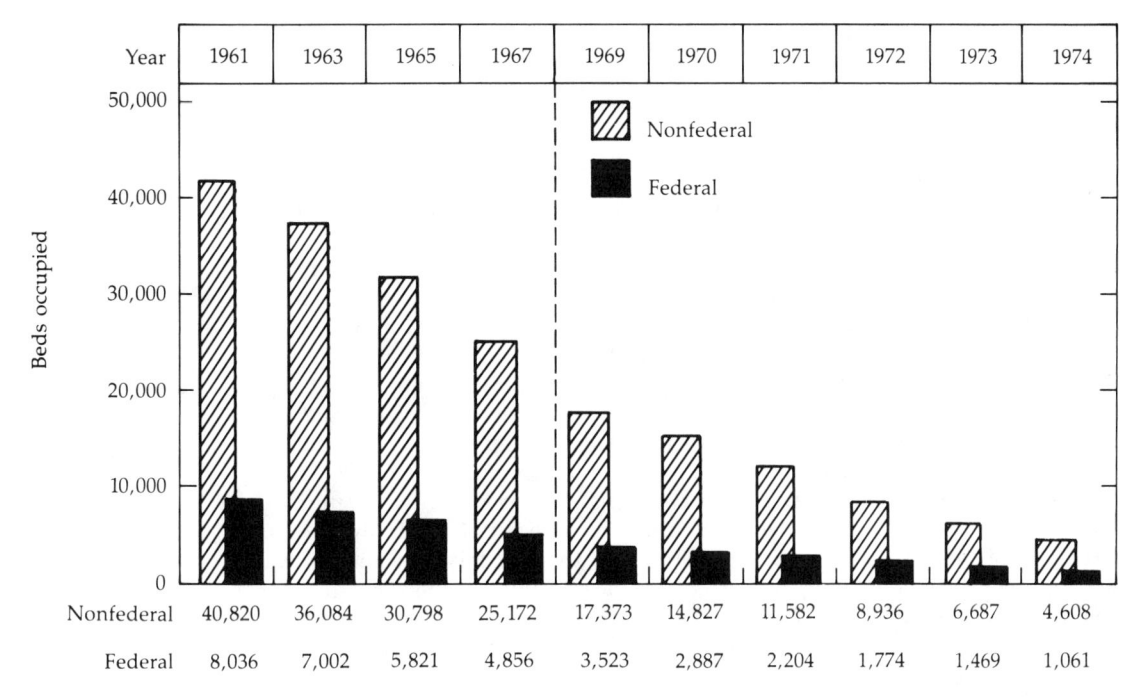

Year	1961	1963	1965	1967	1969	1970	1971	1972	1973	1974
Nonfederal	40,820	36,084	30,798	25,172	17,373	14,827	11,582	8,936	6,687	4,608
Federal	8,036	7,002	5,821	4,856	3,523	2,887	2,204	1,774	1,469	1,061

Figure 2
Tuberculosis Hospitals, United States, 1961–1974 (Beds Occupied on June 30)

Source: U.S. Department of Health, Education, and Welfare, Public Health Service, Center for Disease Control, *Tuberculosis Programs, 1973* (Washington, D.C.: Government Printing Office, December 1974), 31.

Analysis

This case describes the ten-year effort of the American Lung Association to promote modern methods of tuberculosis care based on chemotherapy, outpatient care, and the use of general hospitals. The health educator served as a staff member to the committees that were promoting the new method. Adoption-diffusion of innovation provides the best theoretical fit for this case. Rogers (1973:76) defines as "an idea, practice, or object, perceived as new by an individual" and diffusion as "the process by which innovations spread to members of a social system."

This example of planned change was designed to influence the power centers within, or tangential to, tuberculosis care. Top-down change was the intended basic strategy. As Rogers (1973) notes, top-down change is more likely to succeed than is bottom-up change. Medical practice is clearly one sector where this is difficult to dispute. Bottom-up change generally results in more conflict than does the top-down variety. The general assumption has been that if conflict is minimized, change is more likely to occur. However, under certain circumstances, conflict is necessary if change is to be brought about. The targeted power centers in this case included hospitals, medical schools, medical specialty societies, health departments, and the state lung associations.

The American Lung Association wisely recognized that only physicians would be able to directly influence the practice of other physicians. This is the principle of homophily, which states that the transfer of ideas (an innovation) occurs more frequently and in a shorter time span between a source and a receiver who are alike than between those who are unalike (Lazarsfeld and Merton 1964; Rogers 1983). Although this is true, and was true in this case, it is important to note that the health educator was an important link in this communication. We saw this directly in her assistance to the proponent physician during committee meetings and indirectly through the nonglamorous but necessary work of seeing that the committee functioned properly. This work included site preparation, agenda building, and the provision of background information to committee members.

Policy statements and national reports were prime vehicles in disseminating the innovation, but we also see an effective use of in-service training in the face-to-face transmission of the new concepts. To a great extent this transmission was made possible by the existing network of lung associations at the state and local levels. The change agents, therefore, did not have to develop new networks of communication or learn how to use existing networks, as is often necessary in planned change.

Although the prime focus of the change effort was to promote a new method of care, the change agents had to consider a number of issues apart from the therapeutic value of the new and old methods of care. They needed to analyze what structures supported or were supported by the old method and what structures would be needed to support the new method. For example, as was mentioned, many chronic care hospitals that had been developed to specifically serve the tuberculosis patient had an economic interest in the old method of long-term in-hospital care. Conversely, there was a need for new systems such as third-party payment if in-patient tuberculosis care was to be assumed by general hospitals. Under the old system, tuberculosis care was tax-supported. The method of care could not be viewed apart from the larger system. In any change effort, the practitioner must step back during the planning phase to analyze just what change means, what it will involve, and how it will affect the larger system.

If we apply force-field analysis, we must consider the strength of the restraining forces, for example, the vested interests versus those interested in change. It is naive to believe that those who have an economic interest in an old method of care will acquiesce quietly even in the face of overwhelming evidence for the new method. Consider for a moment how a relatively simple cure for cancer would disrupt the cancer research and cancer care industry.

Another important issue in planned change is the degree to which it is proper for the change agent to manipulate the situation to achieve the goals of planned change. To thoroughly explore this issue, the question of what constitutes manipulation would have to be answered. Is *manipulation* an ideal term, in the philosophical sense, that can be understood external to any circumstance, or is it understandable only within the context in which it might occur? Although this issue cannot be satisfactorily determined here, it behooves you to consider how the Ad Hoc committee on Quality Care was appointed. As Ogasawara states, quality of care was a pivotal concern in shifting from the old to the new method. The goal was to develop a meaningful policy statement based on committee consensus. This goal would not be achieved, it is asserted, if all views were equally represented on the committee. The implication, then, is that the change agents should, at least under certain circumstances, exclude dissenting opinions when the task is to develop policy statements. To do this may call for a degree of manipulation that the change agent must either accept or reject. It is important to note here that the ALA felt the evidence for the modern method of care was beyond question; hence there was no need to debate the issues again.

References/Select Resources

Bennis, W. G.; Benne, K. D.; Chin, R.; and Corey, K. E. 1976. *The Planning of Change*. 3d ed. New York: Holt, Rinehart & Winston.

This book of readings has been one of the standard sources on planned change since it first appeared in 1961. Among the many notable contributors are Chris Argyris, Ronald Lippitt, Edgar Schein, and Jay W. Lorsch.

Lazarsfeld, P. F., and Merton, R. K. 1969. "Friendship as Social Process: A Substantive and Methodological Analysis." In *Freedom and Control in Modern Society*, edited by M. Berger, New York: Octagon.

In this article two prominent sociologists provide an early statement of the principle of homophily. Although the emphasis is on friendship, the findings and the methodology employed can be of use to health educators who are involved in group work as facilitators, participants, or leaders.

Rogers, E. M. 1973. "Social Structure and Social Change." In *Processes and Phenomena of Social Change*, edited by G. Zaltman. New York: Wiley.

This article offers a concise statement of many of Rogers's ideas that are presented at greater length in *Diffusion of Innovations*. The collection in which it appears is an excellent source book on social change up to the early 1970s.

Rogers, E. M. 1983. *Diffusion of Innovation*. 3d ed. New York: Free Press.

Rogers reviewed 3,085 studies on diffusion for this edition, whereas in his first publication in 1962 he reported on 405. He now extends diffusion theory to include factors that antecede and follow the adoption process, so that new questions arise. Where did the innovation come from? Which comes first, the need or the innovation? What kinds of problems are encountered, and how are they solved as the innovation is implemented?.

The Ogasawarea case offers an excellent example of the persuasion stage of the diffusion process. Several different activities were carried out over time to persuade physicians to decide to adopt the new method of treatment. These included policy statements, national reports, and in-service education.

In his discussion of homophily, Rogers accepts the general principle that homophily promotes diffusion, but he states that it can at times serve as a barrier to diffusion throughout a system. "New ideas usually enter a system through higher status and more innovative members. A high degree of homophily means that these elite individuals interact mainly with each other, and the innovation does not 'trickle down' to non-elites" (p. 275), so ideas spread horizontally rather than vertically.

Discussion Questions

1. Can you identify examples of bottom-up or grass-root changes that are now taking place in medical practice? If yes, why are your examples of change following a bottom-up rather than a top-down course?

2. Why does better communication take place when the source and receiver are homophilous?

3. How might a committee that has equal or near representation of opposing views be more effective in promoting change than one less balanced? How would the facilitator/health educator function differently with this heterogeneous committee than with the more homogeneous Ad Hoc Committee on Quality Care described in the case?

4. Although this case is an example of top-down change, why did the young physicians who were perhaps lower on the hierarchy tend to be early adopters?

5. In your judgment, under what circumstances does manipulation by the health educator become unacceptable or unethical?

Planning and Evaluation of Public Health Education Programs in Rural Settings: Theory into Practice

Richard A. Windsor, M.S., Ph.D., M.P.H.

The application of health education principles, methods, and procedures in a practice setting often seems difficult and at times impossible. This difficulty in the application of theory is, in part, a function of the diversity of settings that a health education specialist may encounter. It also reflects two common problems and constraints, limited resources and lack of staff expertise, either in the program planning or in its implementation. The purpose of this paper is to discuss how a consortium of public health professionals dealt with a variety of issues common to many health education programs serving rural residents. The group consisted of personnel employed by the Alabama Department of Public Health (SAPH), the Alabama Cooperative Extension Service (ACES), and the University of Alabama in Birmingham (UAB). The case study discussed should be of particular interest to the practitioner because it was conceived, implemented, and completed without grant or contract support. Case material from this recently completed rural health education project confirms that much more can be done in a rigorous and analytical fashion than meets the eye: Ongoing public health programs can examine the behavioral impact of their health education efforts. The discussion is divided into two sections: (1) planning issues and (2) evaluation issues.

BACKGROUND

The ADPH's Cancer Screening Program (CSP) was established in rural communities, initially with National Cancer Institute support, to remove or reduce existing barriers to service use: availability, access, acceptability, and cost. At the end of 1981, this project was available in 50 of 67 counties and had screened approximately 110,000 women. Ninety percent of the screenees were members of families below federally established levels of poverty. Of those screened, 57 percent reported they never had had a Pap smear, had not had one within the last two years, or did not remember ever having one. This project represents one of a number of ongoing public health projects in rural areas of Alabama in which public health education expertise and competency are reflected. The objective of the project was to increase CSP use by high-risk target groups, women over 35 who had never been screened for cervical cancer (ADPH 1981).

In 1978, a series of discussions with representatives of the ADPH, the ACES, and the UAB's School of Public Health was held. Since the development of motivational strategies to increase service use was an ongoing interest of the CSP, it

---

Richard A. Windsor is the Director of the Division of Health Education–Health Behavior and Professor of Public Health in the School of Public Health at the University of Alabama in Birmingham.

The author would like to express his thanks to the following persons for their assistance with the implementation and evaluation of this project and in the preparation of several published reports on which this case study is based: Jennie J. Kronenfeld, Ph.D., Department of Health Administration, University of South Carolina School of Public Health; Gary R. Cutter, Ph.D., Department of Epidemiology, School of Public Health, University of Alabama in Birmingham; Linda A. Goodson, Project HELP, University of Alabama in Birmingham; Max G. Cain, Division of Cancer Detection, Bureau of Clinical Services, Alabama Department of Public Health, Montgomery; Evelyn Edwards, County Agent—Home Economics, Hale County Cooperative Extension Service, Greensboro, Alabama.

became apparent that an opportunity and need existed to apply principles of health education planning and evaluation. In approaching this project, a number of important issues were apparent, one of the first of which was the epidemiologic issue of the appropriateness of the Pap smear as a method of cervical cancer detection.

THE EPIDEMIOLOGIC ISSUE

The problem faced in this program presented a classic epidemiologic example that health education specialists have to deal with in collaborating with others to develop disease prevention programs. The periodicity of cervical cancer screening, a secondary prevention method, has been considerably debated in recent years. Because of the existing controversy about the Pap test, I felt it particularly important to perform an extensive examination of the literature on its efficacy. In this case, as in other situations faced by health education specialists, the controversy necessitated a careful examination of the available evidence in support of the association between a given health behavior (e.g., having a Pap smear) and improved health status (e.g., decreased delay and increased cervical cancer survival rate). The level of consensus among oncology and health services research specialists with respect to the efficacy of Pap smear was sought and assessed.

A review indicated that though there was evidence of a significant decline over the last 25 years in the incidence of invasive cancer of the cervix, cervical cancer still accounted for approximately 16,000 new cases and 7,400 cancer deaths in the United States in 1980. The observed decline was felt to be due in part to the broad acceptability of the Pap smear by the medical profession and many women. But most of the observed mortality attributable to cervical cancer was preventable, because the majority of invasive cancer occurs in women who have never been screened. Although much of the argument relating to cervical cancer screening focused on the interval between Pap smears for women, most critics agreed that periodic screening at an interval appropriate to a woman's risk should be conducted (Anonymous 1980; Clarke and Anderson 1979; Foltz and Kelsey 1978; Fruchter, Boyce, and Hunt 1980; Guzick 1978; Kleinman and Kopstein 1981, Rutstein et al. 1976; Silverberg 1980). The NIH Consensus Development Conference on Cervical Cancer Screening: The Pap Smear, held in 1981, included such a recommendation to the medical community and public (Anonymous 1981).

An ongoing concern to cancer control programs in the United States is the large proportion of high-risk people who have remained unscreened either because of limited availability and accessibility of health services or because of missed opportunities by health services and hospital personnel when caring for these high-risk individuals. Past public health education efforts have been successful in motivating more educated and wealthy women to get screening and reduce delay. A continuing problem, however, exists in reaching women with high-risk profiles, often demographically characterized as Black, lower-income, and rural female residents (Fruchter, Boyce, and Hunt 1980).

It is this kind of inquiry and evidence that public health education specialists must examine as they begin to conceptualize and plan disease prevention programs. Health education specialists must examine existing epidemiologic, clinical, and behavioral evidence that establishes a clear association between health actions and health status indicators. In this case, though a debate existed about the effectiveness of the Pap smear, the evidence supported promoting CSP use by individuals with specific demographic characteristics, particulary women over 35 who had never been screened.

CONCEPTUAL FRAMEWORK

In approaching the problem of how to motivate hard-to-reach women to use a CSP, it was apparent that the situation necessitated an adaptation of the Health Education Planning Model (Green et al. 1980). A community educational diagnostic survey was not feasible. Why individuals were using or were not using this service, their level of acceptability and satisfaction (predisposing factors), cost to access, convenience of place and time of service (enabling factors), and/or the perceptions of staff toward CSP users (reinforcing factors) could not be ascertained. Although it is preferable to systematically gather information on such questions by interviewing a sample of users in selected counties as well as CSP staff, I was unable to do so and had to rely on secondary sources: (1) previous cancer

Table 1
Selected Demographic Characteristics of Hale County and the State of Alabama

Location	Est. Pop. (1977)	% Black	% Rural	Pop. per Physician	% below Poverty Line	% without Adequate Plumbing	Socioeconomic Status Index
Hale County	15,500	63	79	3,972	55	51	50
Alabama	3,600,000	26	42	1,860	25	16	100

Sources: Southern Regional Council (1974); U.S. Department of Agriculture (1979).
Note: U.S. mean = 100; standard deviation = 20.

surveys and studies conducted under my direction in other areas of the state (Kronenfeld et al. 1980; Windsor et al. 1981), (2) published literature germane to cancer screening, and (3) consensus derived from discussions with experienced staff of the public health consortium. Although it is preferable to conduct a community educational diagnosis, often a program does not have the resources (i.e., staff, time, and money) to conduct such activities. In such cases, a reasonable response is to rely on the evidence derived from sources like those noted. In simpler terms, in the absence of empirical evidence about how best to approach a given problem, staff experienced in a program area, who are familiar with the literature and who have discussed the problem and its various solutions with other equally experienced professionals, can and should rely on their judgment.

PROGRAM SETTING

With the exception of six metropolitan areas, Alabama is essentially a rural state, not unlike others in the Southeast. It is approximately 400 miles in length and 150 miles in width, and has 67 counties. Currently, it has some 3.9 million residents, approximately 26 percent of whom are Black (1980 census). As in any of the southeastern states in which access, availability, and low per capita income play a significant role in the use of preventive health services, Alabama has to deal with a continuing problem of reaching the hard-to-reach in rural areas.

The demographic characteristics of the unscreened female population in Alabama are in many ways similar to those of the unscreened female population in the rest of the United States. It is not surprising, then, that Alabama has a high cervical cancer rate, approximately 50 percent higher than the national average. About 50 percent of the population in the southern half of the state of Alabama is Black. Therefore it was my particular concern early on to identify a project in which we could develop, implement, and evaluate a community health education program of greatest need to a specific group of residents. A group of ten counties in the southwestern section of our state, all of which were identified as medically underserved, were at particularly high risk for cervical cancer.

Selected demographic data are presented in Tables 1 (above) and 2 (p. 276) on Hale County, which was selected as the site of our health education demonstration project. The Hale County Cancer Screening Program was chosen as the demonstration site because of its pool of high-risk females over 35 years of age, approximately 3,500, and because it had been fully operational since 1977. As indicated in Table 1, residents of this county are predominantly Black, poor, and rural, with limited availability of and access to primary health care services or personnel.

It was felt that if we could demonstrate a behavioral impact—that is, increased use of services by those who had never had a Pap smear before—then we would be able to support magnifying our efforts above and beyond what was being done to use this service throughout the state. Having selected the problem and performed a situational assessment, we set the following objectives:

Table 2
Hale County CSP Users by Race and Quarter, 1978–1980

	1978				1979				1980				
	Quarters				Quarters				Quarters				
Race	1	2	3	4	1	2	3	4	1	2	3	4	Totals
Black	19	26	20	20	26	78	35	32	31	70	32	33	422 (46%)
White	22	28	13	45	35	98	20	46	39	76	27	40	489 (54%)
Total	41	54	33	65	61	176	55	78	70	146	59	73	911 (100%)

Objective of the study: To determine the extent of behavioral impact of a community health education program (with interventions one year apart) on a rural county

Behavioral objective of the program: To increase the number of new and repeat users over 35 years old of the cervical cancer screening program in Hale County during the second quarter of 1979 and 1980

THE PROGRAM

As noted earlier, we were unable to conduct a community educational diagnostic survey of beliefs, perceptions, and health practices of residents in this county. Our alternative, then, and one frequently faced by health education specialists in a practice setting, was to rely on existing literature, reports, and experience to develop an appropriate public health intervention. In developing the elements of the health education program to be introduced into this demonstration county, we used guidelines and principles presenting literature in public health education, community organization, communications, and social psychology (Becker 1974; Cullen, Fox, and Isom 1976; Green et al. 1980; James and Lieberman 1979; McGuire 1973; Marshall 1977; Rogers and Shoemaker 1971; Union Internationale Contre le Cancer 1974, 1975; Wakefield 1976). The five elements of the community program are described in Table 3. Although we had little empirical evidence of the utility of any of these elements in Alabama, my experience and the literature confirmed that no single source or exposure could be expected to have an appreciable impact on a target group's behavior. To motivate behavior, combinations of messages from multiple and salient channels, particularly outreach and interpersonal sources, had to be applied at repeated intervals. As indicated in Table 3, this problem was approached in a comprehensive fashion. A process was set up whereby each of the elements could be created and applied throughout Hale County.

In setting up element 1—community organization—we identified the important lay and professional leadership in Hale County, including the Hale County health officer, the Cooperative Extension Service leader, the president of the Hale County Medical Society, local church leaders, and other key personnel in this county with whom we could collaborate to promote the acceptance and gain local support of this effort. As noted in Table 3, our concern was to demonstrate to Hale County residents that this program was supported by their leadership. We perceived a need to use multiple sources of health information. Although we were unable to do a survey to confirm principal sources of health information, our studies conducted in other rural areas of the state found that local sources of information were relied on by residents in Alabama. With this information, we identified and made personal contact with the available channels that could be used to increase resident awareness

Table 3
Elements, Channels, and Purposes of the Community Intervention

Element	Channel of Communication	Purpose
1. Community organization	Key local lay and professional leaders	Increase acceptance and support Demonstrate and increase program credibility
2. Mass media	Electronic and print media—radio, local newspaper, church and club newsletters, posters, and bulletin boards	Increase awareness of and interest in program message Reinforce program message
3. Lay leadership organization	Leadership training—standardized package for breast and cervical cancer education program	Increase assumption of responsibility by locals in community or group Decrease misinformation Increase acceptance by groups through peer participation and pressure Increase standardization of messages
4. Interpersonal group sessions	Group process—1- to 2-hour session	Increase efficiency of networking Increase adaptability to personal evaluation and responsibility Increase motivation and social support Increase personalization of messages Increase legitimacy of at-risk role
5. Interpersonal individual sessions	Individual word-of-mouth diffusion	Increase persuasion Increase efficiency of diffusion Increase saliency of messages and behavior Increase trial and adoption

and interest in our program, including local radio stations, newspapers, church pastors and wives, and club newsletters and other print media. Using this process we created element 2—mass media—to make women aware of our program and reinforce our purposes.

Having identified and set up the implementation process for these first two elements, we moved to a more interpersonal level of communications, namely, lay leadership in organization, element 3. Relying heavily on the Hale County Cooperative Extension Service for input and assistance, we recruited 39 female lay leaders, 21 white and 18 Black, from existing community groups. They were trained by the director of Project HELP and me to conduct cancer education programs for their women's groups throughout the county. (Project HELP [Health Extension Learning Program], under the direction of Linda Goodson, R.N., is a joint, statewide Community Health Education Service venture of the UAB's School of Public Health, the ACES in Auburn, and the ADPH in Montgomery.)

A standardized package, a flip chart with script, was provided to the lay leaders for use in presenting the breast and cervical cancer education programs. The content of the program was conceptually based on salient dimensions of the Health Belief Model (HBM) (Becker 1974; Kalmer 1974). The HBM, which emphasizes the importance of individuals perceiving the problem as serious and themselves as vulnerable, had been field-tested and revised for this initiative in a countywide demonstration project conducted in 1977–1978 in another area of the state (Kronenfeld et al. 1980). This peer group process—element 4—produced 45 meetings on breast and cervical cancer education, with approximately 15–20 participants each. A total of about 750 women were documented as having taken part in the program's outreach efforts, the peer group process.

As noted in Table 3, there were a number of specific purposes for each channel. For example, we were concerned about reducing misinformation. By providing a standardized package, we were able to reduce to some extent misinformation and control for consistency of messages presented by the lay leaders. We were able through this mechanism to dramatically increase acceptance of our program's purpose by women in this community. Because of peer participation and peer pressure, we were able to translate our focus into their focus. Beyond the lay leadership training, the implementation of the program produced considerable interpersonal impact. Using this method, we established a locally based network, setting up mechanisms for motivation, social support, and personalization of messages. In addition, through these media we were able to legitimize the concept of the "at-risk role" at the most basic level in this community.

Lastly, although we were unable to document the amount of word-of-mouth diffusion of the program—element 5—it was felt that through the face-to-face discussions by women in this group, some women in the community groups who were unable to attend the meeting, or who discussed the program with participants, were informed of what we were trying to do. Assuming a modest level of word-of-mouth diffusion (e.g., 10 to 15 percent), we estimated that an additional 100 women had the program messages communicated directly to them by a relative, friend, or personal acquaintance who had participated in the educational meetings.

In the aggregate, these channels helped generate community recognition of the problem, assisted in gaining acceptance of the program, and reinforced our behavioral objective. Through the combined efforts, either participative or supportive, of organizations such as the American Cancer Society, the Hale County Medical Society, and the Hale County Health Department, and of local churches, their pastors and wives, and the media (newspaper and radio), we were able to accomplish our program objective.

DESIGNING AN EVALUATION

Evaluating an ongoing public health education program is usually difficult. Irrespective of the difficulties, however, a major question faced by all programs is whether or not the public health education program produced a behavioral impact. The potential confounding factors that will weaken a program staff's ability to attribute an observed success to its program need to be considered. The central issue that health education specialists in practice and academic settings have to deal with is internal validity of results (Campbell and Stanley 1966; Cook and Campbell 1976; Windsor et al. 1980, 1983). Internal validity here is described as the extent to which an observed behavioral impact can be attributed to a planned intervention. In the light of resources, time, and the existing data base, several possible designs were considered in this project. A comparison of the strengths and weaknesses of three designs considered in planning the program evaluation in Hale County is presented in Table 4. These designs—a one-group pretest/posttest, a simple time series, and a multiple time series—have been used to evaluate community health programs.

The health education specialist must consider what factors may have independently caused an observed impact. In other words, assuming a change occurred, did your program cause the observed change, did some other factor cause it, or was it a combination of both? In our situation, a simple time series design was used because an existing data base of high quality was available to confirm service use, that is, the behavior. Although several other designs might have been used, the time series was selected because (1) the Hale County program had been in existence for several years, and therefore we were able to establish a pattern of CSP use by new users, and (2) we were able to collect service use data for this county for a significant period (one year), spanning from before to after the program's introduction.

It is important to stress to those in practice settings that each situation in which a data collection system exists that can be used to monitor a pattern of preventive health behavior, the time series design may be an appropriate method to determine whether or not a program has produced an ob-

Table 4
Threats to Internal Validity for Three Quasi-Experimental Designs

	\multicolumn{8}{c}{Threats to Internal Validity}
Designs	History	Maturation	Testing or observation	Instrumentation	Regression	Selection	Mortality	Interaction effects
1. One-group pretest/posttest O X O	−	−	−	−	?	+	+	−
2. Time series OOO X OOO	−	+	+	?	+	+	+	+
3. Multiple time series OOO X OOO OOO OOO	+	+	+	+	+	+	+	+

Note: O = observation points; X = intervention application; (−) = weakness; (+) = strength.

servable change. This design is particularly useful for evaluating ongoing service programs in which measurement is relatively unobtrusive, that is, service use. There are, however, a number of methodological and analytical issues considered in selecting this design. In applying a time series design, health education program staff need to (1) establish the pattern and degree of stability of the target behavior; (2) collect health behavior impact data unobtrusively; (3) collect multiple data points for a full cycle prior to and following an intervention for a specific period in an abrupt fashion (Campbell and Stanley 1966; Windsor et al. 1984).

PROGRAM IMPACT

The health education program was applied and withdrawn twice, with interventions one year apart, in Hale County. This method was used to provide an opportunity for generating more convincing evidence, if apparent, of program impact. The first intervention period was directed by me, the second by staff of the local Cooperative Extension Service, the Alabama Cancer Society, and the ADPH. The intervention quarters were the second quarters in 1979 and 1980. The first intervention period is referred to as X, and the second intervention period as Y. A time series design with repeated treatments was utilized to evaluate behavioral impact. This design was selected because it represented a rigorous, feasible method to evaluate a program in a field setting. This design is more powerful than a commonly used alternative, the one-group pretest/posttest design (Baker 1978; Campbell and Stanley 1966; Cook and Campbell 1976; Windsor and Cutter 1981; Windsor et al. 1980, 1981. A computerized user–monitoring system of the CPS was used to confirm by quarterly report the pattern of new and repeat users. These data were examined to determine the extent to which the two interventions affected the pattern of use by new and previous users beyond what one would normally expect in Hale County. Without the existence of the data base we would not have evaluated program impact.

Data reported in Figure 1 identify the number of new and repeat users by quarter for the three study years—1978, 1979, and 1980. The data for 1978, the baseline comparison year, reflect the relatively sta-

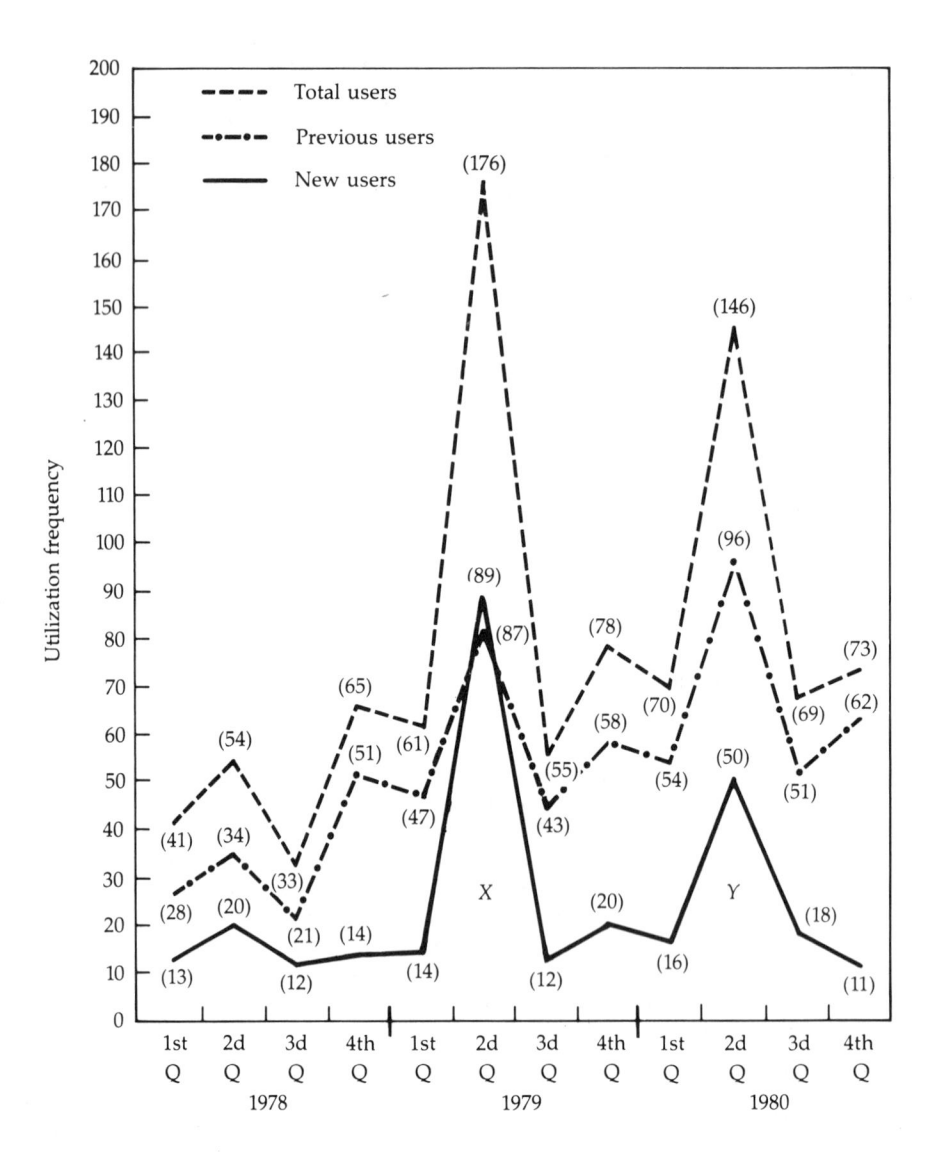

Figure 1
Frequency of New and Repeat CSP Users by Quarter and Year

ble level of use for new users and somewhat less stable use for repeat users. Data for the first intervention quarter (X) in the spring of 1979, when the five-element community health education program was introduced, confirmed that the new user data increased dramatically, about 345 percent. When compared to the average quarterly attendance in previous years, this clearly exceeded the observed pattern of use for all prior nonintervention quarters. A large increase was also noted for repeat CSP use for the intervention quarter, exceeding the observed pattern for the two immediately preceding high quarters by approximately 78 percent. Data in this figure confirmed that use during the period following the first intervention quarter in 1979 and 1980 reverted back to its nonintervention-period level for both new and repeat users (Windsor, Cutter, and Kronenfeld 1981; Windsor et al. 1981).

Another substantial increase, approximately 213 percent, was noted for new CSP users for the second intervention period, (Y) in the spring of 1980.

An examination of the repeat users also revealed another significant increase of approximately 85 percent. In the aggregate, approximately 100 more new users were motivated to use the CSP than would have been expected with the pattern observed during the nonintervention periods, had they remained uninterrupted.

Using a time series analysis, it was concluded that the two community health education programs had a significant behavioral impact on CSP use by new and repeat female clients. But the investigators could not have reached this conclusion without examining a number of methodological and analytical issues. The process that the investigators used to approach this problem is particularly pertinent to health education practice (Windsor and Cutter 1981). In other words, how do you determine whether an observed impact was due to the program or due to some other set of factors?

FACTORS AFFECTING INTERNAL VALIDITY—THEORY AND APPLICATION

Irrespective of the design used, a number of factors will influence the validity of an observed behavioral outcome. As noted in Table 4, at least eight factors may influence the internal validity of program outcome:

1. *History*—significant "unplanned" national, state, or local events occurring at the study location that result in exposure and/or actions by participants during the study period (e.g., Betty Ford's cancer surgery, change in the speed limit)
2. *Program or participant maturation*—natural biologic, social, or behavioral changes occurring among the study participants during the study period (e.g., growing older, becoming more skilled, program staff becoming more effective and efficient in program delivery)
3. *Testing or observation*—the effect of taking a test, being interviewed, or observed on the follow-up data derived from tests, interviews, or observations
4. *Instrumentation*—changes in the calibration of a measuring instrument, in observation methods, or in the data collection process, that is, validity and reliability of instruments and data
5. *Statistical regression-artifacts*—the selection of a study group on the basis of an unusually high or low level of a characteristic that yields apparent changes in subsequent measurements owing to biased sample selection
6. *Selection*—bias introduced in identifying for participation in a study a comparison or treatment group that is not equivalent to the treatment group because of demographic and/or psychosocial factors
7. *Experimental mortality*—nonrandom attrition of subjects from the study treatment or comparison groups
8. *Interactive effects*—any combination of the previous seven factors

Health education specialists need to become more familiar with the factors that may confound results. A graduate-trained health education specialist should be able to name, define, select, and apply a design that maximizes control over these and other factors. Health education professionals need to become much more appreciative of the issues involved in setting up an evaluation design.

Using the Hale County project data, we examined each factor identified in the previous discussion with regard to the plausibility of its having produced the reported results.

HISTORY

Although historical effects represent a main threat to internal validity of results in a time series design, the available evidence suggested little or no historical effect. No unplanned local, adjacent county, state, or national program or cancer screening event occurred during the three-year study period. In the target county all local program or organizational efforts that might have had an independent effect on CSP use were incorporated into the implementation plan of this project (e.g., Cancer Screening Month, American Cancer Society events). The control over such events is another benefit of a prospective design like the one employed. Therefore baseline data and anecdotal evidence of county-wide exposures or events that might have independently caused the impact do not support the plausibility of a unique force operating during the intervention periods.

In addition, though resources were unavailable to perform an extensive examination of utilization data from surrounding counties, no changes in CSP use of the magnitude noted were evident in two similar, adjacent counties. Although the seasonal variation of CSP use suggested a slight increase in the spring quarter of 1978, the seasonal variation was 3.5 times less (20 users versus 89) than the noted increases in 1979 and 1.50 times less (20 versus 50) than those in 1980. The small fluctuation seen in Figure 1 may have been caused by the ACS fund-raising and screening promotion efforts in May of each year in counties throughout Alabama, or it may just have been a seasonal artifact. As the principal investigator, I concluded from this evidence, combined with the supportive statistical analyses, that history represented an implausible explanation for the observed increases in CSP use by new users.

MATURATION

A maturation effect presents a highly implausible explanation for the noted behavioral impact. Participants in the CSP throughout the study were all adult females with similar socioeconomic characteristics. The age and racial characteristics of this county and of the CSP had a high degree of demographic stability. No major social, behavioral, or demographic transition occurred during the study period. It is unlikely that the observed change was due to any maturational characteristics of women utilizing the service or of the CSP itself. In addition, the Hale County CSP was selected because it had been operational for two years and was considered a "mature" program. No significant administrative or staffing changes occurred during the three-year study period.

TESTING OR OBSERVATION

Because the data points examined represent unobtrusive measures of behavioral impact, that is, use of service, neither testing nor observation could be a plausible explanation of the observed change during the intervention periods for new users. No direct contact between study personnel and subjects occurred. The time series design controlled for the effects of the multiple observations.

INSTRUMENTATION

An examination of the instruments and data collection procedures employed by the CSP suggested little evidence of instrumentation error. The instruments were identical during the three-year observation period. Procedures were standardized throughout the state and had been applied in a consistent fashion in Hale County since 1977. The impact variable was increased utilization, a relatively straightforward endpoint. As for data quality and accuracy, all service users were confirmed as Hale County residents. As previously noted, no significant administrative or staffing changes occurred during the study period in Hale County, suggesting a consistency in use of the instrument by CSP personnel and in client data collection. Instrumentation error did not seem to represent a plausible explanation for the observed increases.

STATISTICAL REGRESSION

One of our concerns was the extent to which an observed change was a statistical artifact. An examination of the demographic characteristics of users of the service for the three-year periods confirmed a stability of service user characteristics by quarter. Although more women used the service, those new users were not significantly different than previous users. As confirmed by the baseline data, the level and type of new CSP users were relatively stable during the nonintervention periods. Hale county was selected because it is generally comparable to a number of counties in the southwestern section of Alabama and not because of an extreme characteristic or screening problem. Therefore the evidence suggests that the observed impact was not a statistical artifact.

SELECTION

Selection as a source of main effect is ruled out because no comparison group was used in this study and because the demographic characteristics of women motivated to use the service were highly comparable to those of previous users. The age distributions and racial makeup of the new users were very stable.

EXPERIMENTAL MORTALITY

Since the dependent variable of this study was CSP use by new users, attrition by study participants was not an issue. Because of limited resources, the investigators were unable to determine repeat user attrition (missed appointments), during the course of the study period.

INTERPRETATION AND CONCLUSIONS ABOUT IMPACT

In the aggregate, the evidence supported the conclusion of the investigators that the observed behavior change in the spring quarter, 1979, in CSP use by new users was produced primarily by the community health education program. This conclusion was strengthened by the replication of the field experiment under local direction in spring 1980. The lack of temporal changes in new user frequency suggested that the seven factors cited had little effect on CSP use throughout the study period. The available evidence also indicated a gradual and understandable pattern of CSP repeat use during nonintervention quarters, plus significant increases in CSP repeat use during the periods when the health education efforts were applied in 1979 and 1980.

The evidence presented supported the interpretation that the increases in use of the CPS were due "primarily" to the two interventions. It was concluded that a community health education program grounded in public health education, community organization, communications, and behavioral science theory and practice literature can motivate a significant number of high-risk-profile females in sparsely populated rural counties to use available cancer screening programs.

RECOMMENDATIONS FOR FUTURE PROGRAM PLANNING AND EVALUATION

Although this experience was perceived as fruitful, it was apparent that improvements could be made. In conducting future studies of this type, other rural educational initiatives should build on this experience and on the methods we employed. Methodologically, the use of one or more matched control counties would have allowed for an even stronger degree of support for program impact than that observed. In addition, the inclusion of multiple counties would allow for data aggregation to such an extent that the data point would be a monthly, rather than quarterly, estimate of behavior patterns. This procedure would increase the number of data points and therefore increase the sensitivity of the time series analytical techniques applied in this study in determining the significance of an observed behavior pattern.

Singly or in combination, elements 1 through 5 of the intervention could be selectively applied or withheld for a longer period (e.g., six months) in matched pairs of rural counties with existing CSPs to more rigorously ascertain longer-term effects on CSP use of health education. Another weakness of this project was that we did not have data available to examine the reasons why some women were motivated to begin utilizing the service and why others, such as Black females, were not. In future work, a thorough characterization is needed of the predisposing, enabling, and reinforcing factors relating to utilization of the CSP by current nonusers and by new and repeat users in the community.

REFERENCES

Alabama Department of Public Health. Cancer Detection Division. Cervical Cancer Screening Program. 1980. *Annual Report.* Montgomery.

Anonymous. 1980. "Guidelines for the Cancer-Related Checkup; Recommendations and Rationale: Cancer of the Cervix." *Ca; Cancer Journal for Clinicians* 30(4)215–233.

Anonymous. 1981. "NIH Conferees Issue Pap Screening Recommendations; Conference Summary, Volume 3(4)." *Public Health Reports* 97(1):86.

Baker, S. 1978. "Multiple Time Series Evaluation of a Cervical Cancer Screening Program." Appendix in *Health Program Evaluation,* by S. Shortell and W. Richardson. St. Louis: Mosby.

Becker, M., ed. 1974. *The Health Belief Model and Personal Health Behavior.* Thorofare, N.J.: C. S. Slack.

Campbell, D., and Stanley, J. 1966. *Experimental and Quasi-*

experimental Designs for Research. Chicago: Rand McNally.

Clarke, E., and Anderson, T. 1979. "Does Screening by 'Pap' Smears Help Prevent Cervical Cancer?" *Lancet* 2(8132):1–4.

Cook, T., and Campbell, E. 1976. "The Design and Conduct of Quasi-experiments and True Experiments in Field Settings." In *Handbook of Industrial and Organizational Psychology,* edited by M. Dunnett. Chicago: Rand McNally.

Cullen, J., Fox, B., and Isom, R., eds. 1976. *Cancer: The Behavioral Dimensions.* New York: Raven Press.

Foltz, A., and Kelsey, J. 1978. "The Annual Pap Test: A Dubious Policy Success." *Milbank Memorial Fund Quarterly—Health and Society.* 56:425–462.

Fruchter, R.; Boyce, J; and Hunt, M. 1980. "Missed Opportunities for Early Diagnosis of Cancer of the Cervix." *American Journal of Public Health* 70:418–420.

Green, L. W.; Kreuter, M.; Deeds, S.; and Partridge, K. 1980. *Health Education Planning: A Diagnostic Approach.* Palo Alto, Calif.: Mayfield.

Guzick, D. 1978. "Efficacy of Screening for Cervical Cancer: A Review." *American Journal of Public Health* 68:125, 134.

James, W., and Lieberman, S. 1979. "What the American Public Knows and Does about Cancer and Cancer Tests." In *Public Education about Cancer: Recent Research and Current Programmes,* edited by P. Hobbs. UICC Technical Report Series, vol. 45. Geneva: Union Internationale Contre le Cancer.

Kalmer, H., ed. 1974. "Reviews of Research and Studies Related to Delay in Seeking Diagnosis of Cancer." *Health Education Monographs* 2(2):96–177.

Kleinman, J., and Kopstein, A. 1981. "Who Is Being Screened for Cervical Cancer?" *American Journal of Public Health* 71(1):73–76.

Kronenfeld, J.; Windsor, R.; Kilgo, J., and Wichers, D. 1980. "A Community Health Education Program on Breast and Uterine Cancer in Alabama." In *Public Education about Cancer: Recent Research and Current Programmes,* edited by P. Hobbs. UICC Technical Report Series, vol. 55. Geneva: Union Internationale Contre le Cancer.

Marshall, C. 1977. *Toward an Educated Health Consumer: Mass Communication and Quality in Medical Care.* Teaching of Preventive Medicine Monograph no. 7, DHEW Publication no. (NIH) 77–881. Washington, D.C.: Government Printing Office.

McGuire, W. 1973. "Persuasion, Resistance, and Attitude Change." In *Handbook of Communication,* edited by I. Pool, W. Schramm. Chicago: Rand McNally.

Rogers, E. and Shoemaker, F. 1971. *Communication of Innovations: A Cross-Cultural Approach.* 2d ed. New York: Free Press.

Rutstein, D. D.; Berenberg, W.; Chalmers, T. C.; Child's III, C. G.; Fishman, A. F.; and Perrin, E. B. 1976. "Measuring the Quality of Medical Care: A Clinical Approach." *New England Journal of Medicine* 294:582–588.

Silverberg, E. 1980. "Cancer Statistics—1980." *Ca; Cancer Journal for Clinicians* 30(1):23–44.

Southern Regional Council. 1974. *Health Care in the South: A Statistical Profile.* Atlanta, Ga.

Union Internationale Contre le Cancer. 1974. *Health Education Theory and Practice in Cancer Control.* UICC Technical Report Series, vol. 10. Geneva.

Union Internationale Contre le Cancer. 1975. *Summary Proceedings of the International Conference on Public Education about Cancer.* UICC Technical Report Series, vol. 18. Geneva.

U.S. Department of Agriculture. 1979. *Indicators of Social Well-Being for U.S. Counties.* USDA Rural Development Research Report no. 10. Washington, D.C.: Government Printing Office.

Wakefield, J., ed. 1976. *Public Education about Cancer: Recent Research and Current Programmes.* UICC Technical Report Series, vol. 24. Geneva: Union Internationale Contre le Cancer.

Windsor, R., and Cutter, G. 1981. "Methodological Issues in Using Time Series Designs and Analysis: Evaluating the Behavioral Impact of Health Communication Programs." In *Progress in Clinical and Biological Research,* vol. 83: *Issues in Screening and Communications,* edited by C. Mettlin and G. Murphy. New York: Alan R. Liss.

Windsor, R.; Baranowski, T.; Clark, N.; and Cutter, G. 1984. *Evaluation of Health Promotion and Education Programs: Principles, Methods, and Skills for the Practitioner.* Palo Alto, Calif.: Mayfield.

Windsor, R.; Cutter, G.; and Kronenfeld, J. 1981. "Communication Methods and Evaluation Designs for a Rural Cancer Screening Program." *American Journal of Rural Health* 7(3):37–45.

Windsor, R.; Kronenfeld, J.; Cain, M.; Cutter, G.; Goodson, L.; and Edwards, E. 1981. "Increasing Utilization of a Rural Cervical Cancer Detection Program." *American Journal of Public Health* 71:651–643.

Windsor, R.; Kronenfeld, J., and McCorkle, R. 1981. "Perceptions of Adults in Rural Alabama toward Skin Cancer/Melanoma: An Educational Diagnostic Survey." In *Public Education about Cancer: Recent Research and Current Programmes,* edited by P.

Hobbs. UICC Technical Report Series, vo. 62. Geneva: Union Internationale Contre le Cancer.

Windsor, R.; Kronenfeld, J.; Ory, M., and Kilgo, J. 1980. "Method and Design Issues in Evaluation of Community Health Education Programs: A Case Study in Breast and Cervical Cancer." *Health Education Quarterly* 7(3):208–218.

Analysis

This case discusses the implementation of a community health education program to increase utilization of cervical cancer screening services by high-risk women. The rural-based program was a joint effort of a state public health department, a university, and a cooperative extension service. If we look at this case from the standpoint of the components of the HE framework discussed in the introduction to this text, we see the health educator's role was primarily that of program consultant and evaluator. We also find an excellent example of the explicit use of a number of prominent theories now commonly encountered in health education practice. Program planning was based on the PRECEDE model (Green et al. 1980). However, as Windsor indicates, the community education diagnosis was not feasible. Often in a practice setting not all components of a model can be successfully implemented.

The content of the program was based on the health belief model, particularly the elements of perceived seriousness and perceived vulnerability (Rosenstock 1974). Adoption-diffusion (see glossary) appears to have provided the framework for the choice of methods of communication. Multiple methods of communication were chosen because evidence from earlier programs indicated that no single source would have the requisite impact. Adoption-diffusion also explains the utilization of services by women who did not attend group meetings. Community organization and group process strategies were widely used throughout this project. The selection and training of lay group leaders and their subsequent work in reaching the target population provide a good example of the use of these strategies concurrently.

Windsor illustrates the importance of undertaking a literature review during the planning phase. A thorough review, though it may take time at the outset, generally has long-range benefits, particularly in helping the health educator avoid mistakes or at least anticipate them. A thorough literature review goes beyond being an academic exercise because it may include direct contact with other practitioners whose names may be generated by other personal contacts or through the literature. Program planning should not be done in a professional vacuum. What have others done? How did they do it and what were the results? Is their experience applicable to your setting?

Over the past few years, evaluation has become increasingly important to health education practice. It is no longer possible simply to justify health education philosophically. In other words, positive results do not necessarily follow from good intentions. Just as health education is eclectic in drawing theory and methods from many disciplines, the practice of evaluation has roots in education, psychology, sociology, and other fields. Program evaluation can involve complex designs and analytical techniques that demand highly trained specialists. However, it can also be carried out by practitioners who have mastered some basics. More and more academic programs are providing their students with formal training in evaluation, and the focus of many continuing-education events and professional meetings has increasingly been on evaluation.

Windsor and his colleagues used a simple time series design to evaluate the program. This design is commonly used when program data can be collected at a number of points over time. As Windsor indicates, one's choice of design is often based on the design's ability to control threats to internal validity (those factors that, if uncontrolled or unaccounted for, make it difficult to attribute the results detected to the program). Evaluation should tell us not just what the results were, but whether the program did indeed cause the results.

Generally, as designs become more sophisticated, they provide better control over those ubiquitous threats to internal validity that Windsor catalogues. Here "sophisticated" means the use of control groups and randomization of program participants, which is often a difficult task in community settings. Moreover, as designs become more sophisticated, they become more expensive to implement. Decisions need to be made during program planning as to what percentage of available resources can be provided for evaluation.

Another issue of importance in this case was the linkage of a given health behavior to improved health status. Here the question was: Do routine Pap smears increase the cervical cancer survival rate? This question of linkage between behavior and health status is of vital importance to health educators. Since epidemiological links are often uncertain, health education programs should be held accountable, assuming there is sufficient time, resources, and personnel, for changes in behavior rather than for health status outcomes such as mortality and morbidity rates. For example, how strong is the link between cholesterol intake and coronary heart disease? Health education may persuade people to reduce their intake, but if the link between the behavior and health outcome turns out to be weak or nonexistent, one shouldn't fault health education if morbidity doesn't decrease. This issue has been examined at length by Green in a policy statement developed for the federal government (Green 1978). It is by no means an exaggeration to say that the credibility of health education may depend on programming being based on health behavior that is strongly linked to health outcome.

References/Select Resources

Cook, T. D., and Campbell, D. T. 1979. *Quasi-experimentation*. Chicago: Rand McNally.

The authors describe the time series design that Windsor used as well as many other evaluation designs. The book is a technical presentation that on occasion requires a fairly sophisticated background in statistics.

Green, L. W. 1977. "Evaluation and Measurement: Some Dilemmas for Health Education." *American Journal of Public Health* 67(2):155–161.

Green describes here many of the problems that may be encountered when vigorous evaluations of health education programs are attempted.

Green, L. W. 1978. "Determining the Impact and Effectiveness of Health Education as It Is Related to Federal Policy." *Health Education Monographs* 6 (suppl. 1, Spring):28–66.

This major policy paper by one of the leaders in health education provides a systematic review of recent research and discusses how it should influence future federal policy decisions.

Green, L. W.; Kreuter, M. W.; Deeds, S. G.; and Partridge, K. B. 1980. *Health Education Planning: A Diagnostic Approach.* Palo Alto, Calif.: Mayfield.

This seminal work in health education provides a description of the health education planning model known as PRECEDE, which is an acronym for "predisposing, reinforcing, and enabling causes in educational diagnosis and evaluation." The Windsor case illustrates how very often a planning model must be adapted to local conditions while still retaining the underlying conceptual framework.

Rosenstock, I. M. 1974. "The Health Belief Model and Preventive Health Behavior." In *The Health Belief Model and Personal Health Behavior,* edited by M. H. Becker. Thorofare, N.J.: Charles B. Slack.

Rosenstock, who was one of the original group that developed the health belief model, describes the components of the model and reviews the research up to 1974 on the model's ability to explain and predict preventive health behavior.

Windsor, R.; Baranowski, T.; Clark, N.; and Cutter, G. 1984. *Evaluation of Health Promotion and Education Programs.* Palo Alto, Calif.: Mayfield.

This is the first book-length treatment of evaluation methodology for health education. It provides the practitioner as well as the academician with the necessary tools to become skilled in evaluating programs ranging from the simple to the complex.

Discussion Questions

1. What are the strengths and weaknesses of using secondary sources versus a community survey for completing a community educational diagnosis?

2. What other designs could have been used to evaluate this project?

3. What differences would you have encountered in community organizing if the setting for the project had been a large urban area?

4. Contrast the methods employed in this case with those used in the case by Rosenberg (p. 216).

5. Identify some areas where the epidemiological link between health behavior and health status may be tenuous.

Prevention Through Consumer Education

Miriam M. Campbell, M.P.H., and Phyllis S. Williams, R.N.M.S.

This case study will describe the evolution of a Maternal and Child Health Council (MCHC) in the Bangor area of Maine from 1965 to 1981. The authors worked together in guiding the council during most of this period, albeit with very loose reins.

We will first describe how the council evolved, what it did, and its impact on Maine; then we'll tell you about our role in that evolution. It would be impossible to describe everything we did—16 years is a long time. But we will cite a few examples to illustrate our activities.

The Bangor-Brewer Tuberculosis and Health Association (THA) provided a "home" and basic resources for the MCHC. The linkage with the MCHC requires explanation. The THA was organized in 1909. Because of scarce resources in a rural state, it was always concerned with "health" issues as well as tuberculosis issues. With the advent of chemotherapy and ambulatory care as the preferred method of treatment of persons with tuberculosis, the THA placed even greater emphasis on "health" issues.

From the beginning, concern with the total health needs of the community dictated agency policy. And so it was that the THA sponsored such diverse programs and services as child health conferences, an adult medical clinic, interfaith clergymen's institutes, an Ostomy Association, and other patient support groups, plus an Information and Referral Center, telelectures for education of health professionals, and the first homemaker service in Maine.

Often the THA developed and/or participated in innovative health programs on a demonstration basis, turning responsibility for a program over to an appropriate agency once the need had been documented and acceptance of the program manifested.

It is important to note, however, that the THA's board of directors put no time restriction on demonstrations. Hence the THA was involved in direct health services on an ongoing basis until such time as a responsible, appropriate agency could be identified, or, in some cases, developed.

It was this concern with the totality of community health problems and the emphasis on providing direct services when needed that led to the disaffiliation of the THA from the National Respiratory Disease Association (now the American Lung Association). The disaffiliation came about as a response to the national association's narrowing of focus and its mandate that local affiliates give up their participation in direct community health services. This change in emphasis was seen by the THA's board as counterproductive, especially since the major part of THA's budget was derived from an endowment built up over the years from bequests in support of its community-based programs and objectives.

In 1967 the THA constructed a building with meeting rooms and classrooms to be used by the public for any health-related activity. The association was seen by the community as a neutral third party with few axes to grind. Therefore when Phyllis Williams came to Miriam Campbell and asked for help with maternal and child health issues, the response was "Of course." This is how it happened.

HISTORY

Historically, until 1961 a couple living in the Bangor area and expecting a first child had only the library, a busy physician, or parents and friends to turn to

---

Miriam M. Campbell is a Health Education Consultant in Chilmark, Massachusetts, and Phyllis S. Williams is a Health Education Consultant in Bangor, Maine.

for information. The labor room in the general hospital (now the medical center) was a drab four-bed unit. Consistent with traditional obstetric practices of the time, fathers were not allowed in the labor and delivery rooms, and medications and general anesthesia were used routinely.

An instructor in maternal and newborn nursing from the University of Maine School of Nursing set up a series of classes at the hospital for prenatal clinic patients. Though the clinic patients failed to attend, these classes were immediately popular. With the physician's approval, they were opened to private patients. Attendance increased from 4 at the first class to 64 at the fourth class—all through word of mouth.

As time passed, the hospital's original stipulations of no publicity and of no men in attendance were relaxed. Local radio stations and the newspaper provided publicity, and notices were sent to all prospective parents. In response to public demand, the classes were opened to husbands.

By 1965 a new obstetric unit was being planned for the area to supplement the three units already in existence—one at the air force base hospital, one at the osteopathic hospital, and one at the general hospital (now the medical center). The opening of this new unit, combined with plans by the regional Red Cross chapter to conduct childbirth classes, threatened to fragment efforts, a situation that, with the limited number of resource people available, could have resulted in the demise of all classes.

MATERNAL AND CHILD HEALTH COUNCIL OF GREATER BANGOR

The University of Maine instructor (Phyllis Williams) approached the executive director of the THA (Miriam Campbell), who, with the backing of her agency, agreed to cosponsor a community-based organization to continue to provide classes.

Phyllis played the role of convener and set up a meeting at the general hospital with Red Cross representatives, the chief of obstetrics, the director of nursing service, the director of the health department, the director of the Tuberculosis and Health Center, the director of public health nursing, and the instructor. The community-based organization was proposed. The idea was accepted as feasible for offering ongoing classes geared to the needs of the local population *rather than classes prescribed by a national organization*. The Red Cross generously agreed to bow out.

The need was apparent and the time was right. Each of the agencies contacted agreed to provide representation and financial support to the fledgling organization. And so, the MCHC of the Greater Bangor Area was born.

Though in many ways the MCHC and its programs paralleled what was happening in parent education across the country, it was unique in its organization.

With constructive guidance from Miriam, the council adopted a constitution that broadly defined its purposes, the chief one being the promotion of maternal and child health in the community, both directly and in cooperation with other groups, agencies, and individuals. When the Tuberculosis and Health Center's new memorial facility became available, the classes were transferred from the medical center to that neutral site.

Initially, a series of six classes were held four times yearly. The council sent out an evaluation questionnaire at the end of each series to use as a base for data accumulation and program planning. Phyllis developed a curriculum guide and recruited and trained more volunteer nurse-instructors.

Through the efforts of a young mother who had moved to the area, Lamaze training was added. Workshops were held to train nurses and others as Lamaze instructors. These were the first "lay" teachers in the council. The instruction was undertaken as a team effort, each team composed of a registered nurse and a lay instructor.

From the beginning, the council had *representation* from the National Foundation/March of Dimes, the classes having been promoted on their posters. The young mother of a child born with birth defects, frustrated by the confusion and lack of skill she and other such parents felt in following physicians' orders, appealed to the council for help. The MCHC turned to the National Foundation, which responded by (1) underwriting a *parenting course* stressing child health, safety, and emergency measures for infants and children; and (2) establishing a parent-to-parent referral network that provided support for parents facing similar problems and encouraged the sharing of parenting skills.

Though the classes were successful initially, after approximately three series attendance dimin-

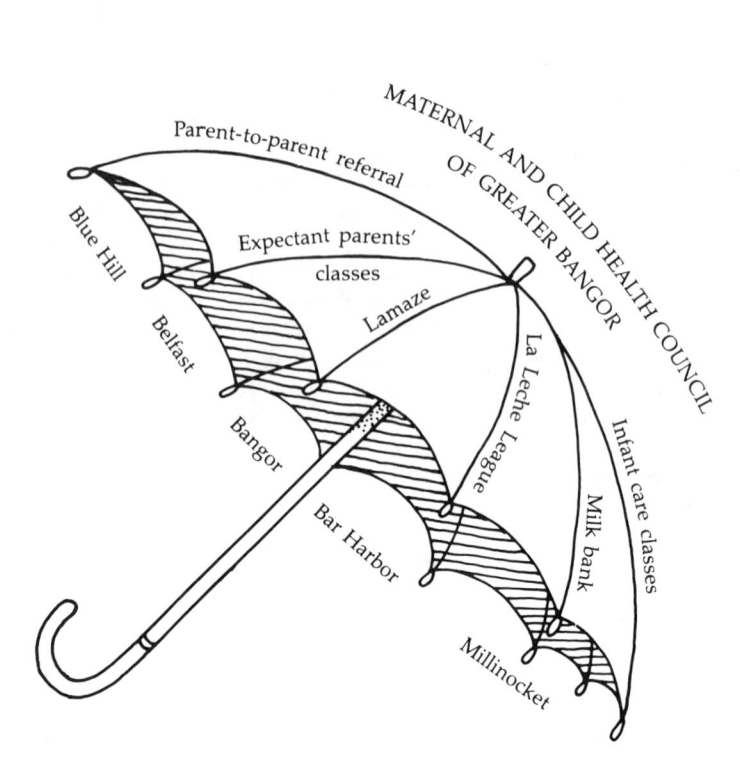

Figure 1
The Umbrella Concept of the MCHC

ished to a level where it was no longer feasible to hold them, possibly because the population was saturated. At that time, new parents seemed far more interested in the birth experience and expected child care to evolve naturally. They were interested in breast feeding, however, and La Leche League meetings fulfilled these needs.

The MCHC had always promoted breast feeding. Consequently, when a young mother organized a local chapter of the La Leche League, she was invited to join the council and to participate in the classes.

Through the council, speakers and instructors were provided for classes in babysitting. Members took part in television and radio programs and were guest lecturers in classes on sexuality, human development, and health education at the University of Maine at Orono.

A number of groups and individuals from communities up to 100 miles away approached the council for assistance in setting up parents' classes. Some of these referrals came as a result of membership in the International Childbirth Education Association, and some as a result of newspaper, radio, or television publicity. Though time and funds were limited, copies of the constitution, course outlines, and a few guidelines were always shared, and interested individuals were invited to attend classes, meetings, workshops, and teacher training sessions. At least six active parent education organizations in four different counties were nurtured into existence in this manner.

As these and other needs surfaced and were addressed, the unique organization of the MCHC, by now incorporated as not-for-profit, began to emerge. This framework has been described as the umbrella concept (Figure 1).

EVALUATION

Evaluation of programs and activities conducted under the umbrella of the MCHC through questionnaires and through interviews with medical and hospital personnel documented a number of changes.

Soon after the inception of the council, delivery room personnel and physicians stated that, on average, mothers who attended classes were better informed, less fearful, and more responsive and consequently needed less medication and anesthesia. After Lamaze classes had begun, fathers were admitted to labor and delivery rooms in all three hospitals (the air force base hospital was closed by then). Rooming-in was made available for mothers who chose to have their infants with them.

With the patient's increased interest and responsiveness and the interaction between the doctor and nurse and the couple, labor had become a positive activity rather than a lonely ordeal.

Mothers reported that they felt much better, less tired, and more alert than after previous births, when they had had much more medication and anesthesia. It was obvious, too, that infants born of mothers who had had minimal medication were more responsive and alert and tended to nurse better. There was an increase in the number of mothers who breast-fed.

The same increase in breast feeding had not been observed among low-income mothers, and their lack of attendance at childbirth classes was a matter of concern in the early days. A possible explanation lay in the stricter role definition among low-income families and the commonly held belief that childbearing was woman's work. However, their attitudes gradually changed. Attendance increased and eventually, with professional support, nearly three quarters of all mothers nursed for at least a period of time.

One further benefit of the changes in obstetrical and nursing practice was that nursing students at the Eastern Maine Medical Center were provided with a positive observation experience.

As one looks at the first two decades of the MCHC, one sees a volunteer organization shaped by the attitudes and needs of the times. However, the council has not only been shaped, it has been responsible for some of the shaping. Largely as a result of its efforts, the Bangor area has been responsive to positive change in the field of maternal and child health. And the council's influence has been felt over much of the state, either directly, through the nurturing of new groups, or indirectly, through the diffusion of its ideas by former council members who have moved.

Infant and neonatal mortality statistics for the country and for Maine are presented in Table 1. The infant mortality rate declined 55.5 percent in Maine from 1970 to 1980. Although there was a parallel decline nationwide, it was 10 percent less than the Maine figure. For the last two years for which data are available (1979–1980), Maine's infant mortality rate was among the five lowest in the 50 states. Neonatal mortality has also shown a sharp decline in Maine. From 1975 to 1980 the rate dropped 30 percent more than in the rest of the country. Maine's neonatal mortality for 1979 and 1980 was the lowest in the United States.

Infant and neonatal mortality data for the three counties most heavily influenced by the council's activities are presented in Table 2 on the following page. Washington County is the poorest in the state and has the largest number of nonwhite births (Indian). Waldo County has the largest number of out-of-hospital births. Waldo and Washington Counties had approximately 500 live births and Penobscot County about 2,000 live births for each year in the period 1974–1980.

The data in Tables 1 and 2 are interesting. Did the MCHC's activities influence infant and neonatal mortality in the three counties and in Maine as a whole? The answer to that question awaits the type of evaluation that is not possible in an ongoing service program without resources beyond those available to the council. We believe it is a question worthy of investigation.

Table 1

Infant and Neonatal Mortality Rate, Maine and United States, 1970–1980

Date	Under 1 Year U.S.	Under 1 Year Maine	Under 28 Days U.S.	Under 28 Days Maine
1970	20.0	20.9	15.1	16.1
1971	19.1	18.1	14.2	13.3
1972	18.5	17.7	13.6	12.8
1973	17.7	16.1	13.0	11.6
1974	16.7	16.1	12.3	12.6
1975	16.1	13.2	11.6	9.0
1976	15.2	11.0	10.9	7.6
1977	14.1	9.4	9.9	6.1
1978	13.8	10.2	9.5	6.0
1979	13.0	9.7	8.7	5.8
1980	12.5	9.3	8.4	5.9

Source: National Center for Health Statistics, *Annual Summary of Births, Deaths, Marriages, and Divorces: United States, 1980*, NCHS Monthly Vital Statistics Report 29, no. 13 (Washington, D.C.: Government Printing Office, September 17, 1981).

Table 2
*Infant and Neonatal Deaths,
Washington, Penobscot, and Waldo Counties, Maine, Selected Years*

	Under 1 Year			Under 28 Days		
Date	Washington	Penobscot	Waldo	Washington	Penobscot	Waldo
1974	16.5	20.3	20.9	10.3	17.1	18.3
1975	24.8	15.0	7.3	16.6	13.4	4.9
1976	9.2	10.9	17.8	7.3	9.8	13.4
1977	13.4	9.8	11.7	10.1	7.2	7.0
1979	10.5	9.8	6.7	5.3	6.2	2.2
1980	7.4	8.7	4.6	3.7	5.1	0

Source: Maine Department of Human Services, Division of Research and Vital Records, *Maine Vital Statistics, 1970–1980* (Augusta, 1982).

PROBLEMS

The MCHC has had, and continues to have, its growing pains and developmental difficulties. In the early days before "natural childbirth" had gained wide acceptance, there was considerable resistance to change on the part of a few obstetricians. The assertiveness of some council members was hard for the physicians to deal with. These physicians saw what they regarded as an overzealous promotion of natural childbirth as causing feelings of guilt and inadequacy among women who "failed" or had abnormalities of pregnancy that required intervention such as a caesarean section.

Another problem was that some obstetricians substituted one form of intervention or control for another. General anesthesia was abandoned, but paracervical anesthesia, along with pudendal and local infiltration, was substituted. Demerol and scopolomine were replaced by nisentil and various tranquilizers and antihistamines; routine induction of labor became common; and women were confined to bed on their backs with the fetal monitor in place. These interventions introduced new hazards into the birth process.

In 1975, with the help of funding by the National Foundation, a series of dinners was held at which the teachers and officers of the MCHC could meet with the obstetricians and pediatricians. These meetings promoted dialogue to mitigate some of the problems and misunderstandings. After these meetings, the chief of pediatrics at the medical center organized with the council an interdisciplinary group called the Maternal-Infant Health Committee. As a result of a series of forums presented by that group, a number of changes took place. Statistics were compiled concerning infant outcomes in a comparison of induced labor with natural labor. When those statistics clearly showed the hazards of elective inductions, such inductions were no longer sanctioned at the medical center.

Other issues tackled by the committee included the pros and cons of abortion for genetic reasons; patients' rights versus doctors' rights; and the value of consolidating obstetric services in one hospital. The forum on this last issue resulted in the closing of the obstetric unit in one hospital and the concentration of all allopathic maternal and infant health services at the medical center, the site of the neonatal intensive care unit. The only other obstetric unit remaining in the city is at the osteopathic hospital.

Home birth became a divisive issue in the late seventies. The first planned, unattended out-of-hospital birth in the area was in 1970. The couple involved attended MCHC classes. Gradually more young couples chose to deliver their babies at home. Owing to the increasing demand for home birth, a young woman living outside of Bangor began attending births. The daughter of a physician, she had had some previous knowledge of birth techniques and had studied further with the alternative birth organizations that were by then nationwide.

She also worked with physicians who were willing to acknowledge that home births were a reality with or without them.

She had joined the MCHC and attended meetings. However, the council members, for the most part, were hostile toward home birth, and most couples who were planning home births felt uncomfortable in the classes. A few teachers, recognizing the educational needs of these couples, set up classes outside of the council, focusing intensively on promoting a healthy pregnancy and a natural birth, but dealing openly with the hazards of out-of-hospital birth, the need to use the hospital should abnormalities develop, and ways of attaining alternatives in the hospital.

At about this same time, the umbrella concept began to diminish. Because in Maine the home-birth movement was predominant among educated young people seeking a simple life, the rural organizations were, admittedly, more involved in birth alternatives. The relatively conservative stance of the council frustrated them; it was seen as "establishment-oriented." At the same time, however, council classes were enjoying unparalleled popularity, and the officers felt it was impossible to administer the large night classes and to worry about the needs of groups in other areas.

Locally, however, birth alternatives were still in demand both because couples were seeking a more personal birth experience and because the costs associated with hospital birth were prohibitive.

The Maternal-Infant Health Committee held a forum on home birth, with advocates for both sides presenting the pros and cons. A birthing room is now available at the medical center; sibling visitation is allowed; and, as a means of cutting costs and attempting to combine the emergency capabilities of the hospital with the freedom of the home, some physicians may discharge healthy mothers and infants within hours after delivery.

Another response to the demand for birth alternatives has been the practice of certified nurse midwives in the area. Midwives had not been allowed to attend births at the medical center, but finally, in response to consumer demand via the council, criteria for their acceptance were instituted in December 1981.

As a result of the rising number of caesarean sections, a support group has been organized within the council to provide information in childbirth classes and conduct separate classes and support meetings for parents facing caesarean birth. The group has also worked for acceptance of the father's presence in the operating room for the birth of his child. The osteopathic hospital has made this option available, with the result that repeat caesarean sections are sometimes scheduled there by allopathic obstetricians.

The old saying "Once a C-section always a C-section" no longer applies in Bangor. A forum presented by the Maternal-Infant Health Committee, supplemented by a one-day workshop sponsored by the council, released data indicating that vaginal delivery was, in fact, safe following caesarean section for other than cephalopelvic disproportion. Thanks to thorough scholarship on the part of the chief of obstetrics and two council members, a woman is no longer assured that a repeat caesarean section is the only option.

As the result of an upsurge of interest in parenting, the parenting classes have been restarted. Responsive to the times, the classes are less formal than they were in the earlier series, and the focus is more on parenting skills, discussion, and support and less on the health and safety aspects.

Council members had worked with the prenatal clinic in attempting to supplement information given at clinics by the public health nurses. But the timing and clinic structure was such that the classes did not work out. Thanks to a sliding fee scale, clinic patients now attend the regular council classes. There are also classes for single women, sponsored by the health department and taught by a public health nurse who is an active member of the MCHC.

POSTSCRIPT

What of the future of the council? In a volunteer organization, the future is not easy to assess. For its first 15 years, the MCHC had no paid workers. There is now one part-time paid employee who is available to keep the office organized, and the teachers are paid a small stipend to cover expenses for child care and transportation. With this type of arrangement, the council is vulnerable to the political intrigue of better-funded organizations that might use the council to gain their own purposes or to quiet its activity.

In 1981 a grant for training childbirth educators was administered by the medical center. The training program was implemented by council members and former members who had remained available. But the potential for medical center control remained. Up to now, despite the attempts of other organizations to take over, the MCHC has remained an independent community-based organization. If that independence is forfeited in what is perceived by the board of directors as an expedient move, then the council, originally conceived as a group involved in a communitywide effort, will die.

On August 16, 1982, a new maternity unit was opened at the Eastern Maine Medical Center. The unit was the result of cooperative planning with input from council members and other professionals in the community. It includes nine private rooms and five semiprivate rooms. The isolation, transitional, and normal-newborn nurseries are internally located, as are the three delivery/operating rooms. The latter have the capacity for fathers to be present for caesarean birth. Their combination use also offers greater safety when previous caesarean mothers plan to deliver vaginally.

Doris Haire, a past president of International Childbirth Education Association and author of numerous articles on family-centered childbirth, gave Phyllis one specific recommendation—that the labor/birthing rooms have windows. In visiting hospital maternity units throughout the country, she had discovered that it was difficult for physicians and nurses to remain with patients if there were no windows in the units.

The labor/birthing rooms not only have windows, they also have a breathtaking east view, as does the Level II Neonatal Intensive Care Unit and the Maternity Unit. The decor contributes to a homey, warm environment.

Although the council's original purpose has been achieved, the process is an ongoing one. It has been largely through the activity and education of consumer groups—especially well illustrated by the MCHC—that medicine has become more responsive to the desires and needs of consumers. We are emerging from an era in which childbirth practices instituted to deal with the abnormal were applied to the normal, often for the convenience of the physician rather than for the ultimate health and safety of the consumer (McKay 1981). Although a volunteer organization with the freedom to respond to the times and the needs must be allowed to die by virtue of that freedom, another with renewed energy and purpose can rise from the ashes. An organization like the MCHC reaches many crossroads. It can choose the life and struggle of the community or die within an institution that promises to nurture and legitimize it.

ROLE OF HEALTH EDUCATION SPECIALISTS

Each of us brought to the task common as well as unique skills and knowledge. Miriam, the health educator/executive of the THA, functioned for the most part as the facilitator for the council. Phyllis, the nursing instructor at the University of Maine at Orono, was more involved in curriculum development, teaching, and teacher training. We worked together very closely planning strategies.

The convener role was easier than the facilitator role. As conveners, we organized meetings, bringing people together to discuss specific issues. This required defining the purpose of the meeting; deciding who should be invited (i.e., selecting the decision makers and those involved or interested in the issues); developing a tentative agenda; collecting agenda items whenever possible from those who were to attend; setting the time and place; and so on. Early on, we made these decisions; later, others were involved in making them. The convener *set* the tone of the meeting. That is, she identified the purpose and the issues; guided the discussion, allowing people to talk but keeping them on the track; periodically summarized the discussion, getting closure on issues if appropriate; and so on. You will recognize these as group process skills.

The use of committees for issue identification and problem solving was one of our major educational strategies. When feelings ran high on an issue, as they did many times, we had to constantly remind ourselves that the purpose of the committee discussion was to throw light on an issue so that informed decisions could be made. Therefore it was the convener's job to keep the group focused on an *objective* view of the situation. It was important that she not allow herself to get involved in the emotion or the politics of an issue. When traditional ways of doing things are questioned, emotions do run high. Power struggles and turf battles are inevitable. We had both during the history of the council. Careful planning and objectivity did not eliminate these obstacles, but they helped the council survive them.

The very first meeting at which the idea of the council was proposed is a good example. Unless the Red Cross decided not to run childbirth classes, the idea of the council was defeated before it started. Therefore the discussion focused on the needs of the target population, scarce resources, existing services, the growing interest in maternal and child health issues, the need to target resources appropriately, and the like. It was clear that there was much to do and enough credit to go around; so it was relatively easy for the Red Cross to bow out graciously, that is, decide not to offer childbirth classes. The door was wide open for its members to do something else or to participate in decisions about childbirth classes as members of the council.

The facilitator role was closely allied with the convener role but was not as easy. In the 16 years of the council's history, major changes ocurred in the behavior of the consumer and the professional regarding maternal and child health practices. Most of these changes were considerably more traumatic for the professional than for the consumer. The obstetrician was forced to change his or her role in childbirth from technician-in-charge to partner. Role change is difficult, especially when the change appears to threaten your livelihood. Many obstetricians were supportive of the new childbirth practices, but some were not. Some felt that the consumer was beginning to have far too much to say about the provision of medical care.

One example of the facilitator's role is the way she had to steer the council on a middle course between obstetricians who thought the consumer had too much to say and the layman who "demanded" to make *all* decisions regarding medical care. There were several real confrontations on this issue. The job of facilitator was made more difficult because some of our lay teachers did not understand how sensitive this issue was for some doctors. These laypersons were quite outspoken—to the point of criticizing individual physicians for practices they considered to be hazardous to their health!

We dealt with this situation by direct confrontation of both parties involved. The consumer's right to an opinion was acknowledged but so was the obstetrician's. Although there was evidence to support the consumer's perception, the obstetricians produced evidence to support theirs as well. We suggested that public criticism of individuals was not in the best interest of the council. The missionary spirit had taken hold of some of the interested consumers. We tried to show them that their goal would be more effectively reached if women found the methods they advocated better than the methods in more common practice—that is, the product would sell itself. Not only was public criticism not needed, it could be destructive. In fact, it did turn some women away from the childbirth classes.

We used a similar strategy with the obstetricians: apologizing for the public criticism, but at the same time holding our ground for the right to promote alternative childbirth methods. The issue cooled down, but a slow fire continued to burn. We were constantly aware of this as we dealt with related issues.

Community organization was of course our major strategy. Our goal was to bring into the council all organizations and individuals interested in childbirth, child care, and parenting issues. To this end, we kept up a constant stream of publicity through the media, but we aimed the promotion particularly at the target groups (parents and expectant parents) and at organizations with whom the target group might be in contact. Our strategy of using ad hoc, issue-oriented committees, as described earlier, worked well. The need for the committees was clear; there was a task to be done.

As time went on, new members of the council assumed leadership roles. We were still involved, but we no longer carried full responsibility for organizing council activities. Today many others have assumed this responsibility. However, regardless of who is involved in the council, the need for sound community-based planning continues.

REFERENCES

McKay, S. R. 1981. "Second Stage Labor—Has Tradition Replaced Safety?" *American Journal of Nursing* 81:1016–1019.

Williams, P. S., and Campbell, M. 1971. "A Community Approach to Maternal-Child Health." *Nursing Outlook* 19(1):44–46.

Analysis

This case focuses on the health educator as a community organizer (Barry 1982). It describes the organization and activities of a Maternal and Child Health Council. The health educator collaborated with a nurse educator in guiding the activities of the council for 16 years until her retirement. Although they conferred on all aspects of council activity, they divided the responsibilities: the nurse educator handled teacher training and curriculum development, and the health educator handled the community organization tasks. Although the case discusses the community organization aspects of the council, this does not mean that this strategy alone was responsible for the council's accomplishments. The preparation of teachers and the development of a curriculum that met the needs of the public played an equally important role.

The case illustrates that people learn over time as the result of a number of different learning experiences. The MCHC provided parents and professionals with several different learning experiences and gave them time to learn. A key ingredient in this process was the continuity of staff and the stability and credibility of the organizations that employed them.

Diffusion of innovation is the theroretical stance that explains the council's development (Rogers 1983). Classes relating to all types of maternal and child health issues were offered, and those members of the community who were interested took advantage of the classes. Other theoretical perspectives, however, are helpful in understanding how the consumer and professional recognized the innovation as useful to them. For example, diffusion theory does not include concepts about dealing with controversy, and there were a number of controversial issues, such as home birth and the elective induction issue.

The council's strategy for both these issues was the collection and presentation of the facts. The Maternal-Infant Health Committee collected data on induced versus natural labor and let the facts speak for themselves. However, knowledge often has little relationship to behavior. Did the facts persuade obstetricians to support a policy that did not sanction elective inductions? The case does not tell us. It is clear that some physicians were convinced by the facts. In Lewinian terms, their cognitive field regarding childbirth was restructured. Others may have gone along with it because their peers believed in it and they wanted to be part of that circle of peers. Again, Lewin (Lewin and Grabbe 1945) tells us that we accept the behaviors acceptable to our group. Some may have been forced to comply because they had no choice (Lewin 1951).

The elective induction issue, therefore, was resolved through the learning process. We can only speculate as to the effect of consumer pressure on this issue. Clearly, some consumers wanted a change in physician behavior with regard to elective inductions and made their feelings known through the council. This move probably forced the physicians to look at the issue, which they might not otherwise have done. Once they did, reason prevailed with a sufficient number to change the medical center's policy.

The home birth issue was different. The MCHC did not deal with it until it had continued to be an issue for a number of years. Initially it was too controversial. If the council had plowed into it, other council activities might have suffered. When it did not go away, the MCHC chose the objective factual approach. The final results of facing this issue were the acceptance of deliveries by nurse midwives at the medical center and the availability of a birthing room at the hospital. Consumer pressure did much of the convincing on this issue. Unlike the induction of labor issue, in which the "scientific facts" argued against induction, the home birth issue was scientifically more ambiguous. And from the physician's perspective, admitting nurse midwives to the hospital for deliveries made no sense economically.

It is important to note the distinction between these two controversial issues; their solution required different strategies. Zaltman and Duncan (1977:9) summarize this difference. They state that change occurs when a person defines a situation differently and that this redefinition can occur at two levels: "The individual may change his or her values or beliefs [i.e., there may be learning, a restructuring of the cognitive field]. Or change may also occur in response to pressure at the systems and social environmental level. Other persons in the environment with whom the individual interacts who are dependent on the individual . . . [can] exert pressure on him to conform to their expectations."

The concept of role (Baumgartel 1961) offers an alternative explanation for the difficulty some obstetricians and nurses had in changing their role in the birthing process. One's role in life carries with it a complex set of variables related to sense of self, status with peers and family, feelings of usefulness and belongingness, and so on. Acceptance of a changed role is therefore not easily accomplished. It is in fact very traumatic for many. The adjustment of the traditional technical roles of the nurse and physician in childbirth to include emotional support and education allowed for holding the technical role in reserve, if needed. Therefore they would keep a foot in both camps, as it were. For some people too much change too quickly can be harmful.

As we've seen, some physicians and nurses learned, believed in, and accepted the new birthing process because they saw it as a better practice than the previous procedures. In diffusion theory, they were the innovators or early adopters. Others complied because of consumer pressure and in some cases peer pressure. In diffusion theory, these would be the late adopters or the stragglers; it took them longer to accept the new practice as meaningful and useful. In Lewinian terms, "learning was imposed." Because they were forced to comply, by being exposed to the new practice some learned that it did work, and so they adopted it.

The principal strategy used in the case was community organization. Barry (1982) lists five ingredients in the "community organization potpourri":

1. There is the community itself, a society with its physical, social and economic structure. . . .
2. There are the needs of people, the problems of the community, . . . which call for solution, action, change or support.
3. There are the resources, human and material. . . .
4. There are the dynamic forces, overt and covert, which affect orderly processes of change.
5. There is the professional direction, the conscious use of knowledge and skill, utilized to bring these ingredients into harmony so that within the community setting, in the climate created by all the forces at play, the community resources are brought to bear to meet community needs in a dynamic movement toward society's goals.

To mix these ingredients so as to bring about one or more of "society's goals" requires skill in interpersonal relations, group process, and problem solving. It also requires an understanding of the structure and function of the community and its organizations. And in this case there was, in addition, a need for knowledge of maternal and child health issues as well as an understanding of one's own professional skills required to bring about the desired change. As the case illustrates, the community organizer helps the community solve problems. As in the Robinson case (p. 68), the complexity of the issues and the number and variety of personalities and organizations involved demanded a high level of knowledge and skill. This was not a task for a beginner; it required a seasoned professional.

If the health educator is to bring diverse groups in the community together, it is critical to steer an objective course. That does not mean the health educator does not have an opinion, but rather that the opinion should not control the decisions. If the purpose of education is to help people make informed decisions, the climate must allow for presentation of all sides of the question no matter how absurd or out of tune some may be. This demands objectivity by the facilitator (see the Semura case, p. 301).

The council's activities were sponsored by a stable organization, one that was valued by the community and was operated by staff who stayed with the project for 10–15 years. We are not aware of any studies that demonstrate that these two variables make a difference in goal attainment. But our collective experience suggests that they do.

The Bangor-Brewer Tuberculosis and Health Association was supported by the community both when it was part of the National Tuberculosis Association (now the American Lung Association) network and when it decided not to be part of that network. It is clear that the community of Bangor-Brewer wanted the THA. Other cases (Nybo, p. 54, and Semura, p. 301) also demonstrate that activities generated by and involving the community are more likely to meet their goals than activities generated by agency staff.

Because the THA had been in the community for over 50 years, it had stability. Both professional staff members who assumed major responsibility for the council had been in the community for a number of years. The council began with a stable staff and a stable agency; both staff and agency had earned credibility in the community. Because of this, as in the Robinson case (p. 68), they were able to concentrate total energy on the task at hand.

The key ingredients in the council's success were time, skill, and community involvement in meeting a need perceived by the community as important.

The data the authors present on infant and neonatal mortality for Maine are, as they say, "interesting." What role did the MCHC have in lowering these two measures of mortality? Maine is a poor state and has limited medical care resources. How come it has the lowest neonatal mortality rate in the country? Like the authors, we'd like to see an answer to that question.

References/Select Resources

Barry, M. C. 1982. "A Theoretical Framework for Community Organization." In *SOPHE Heritage Collection of Health Education Monographs*, vol. 1: *The Philosophical, Behavioral, and Professional Bases for Health Education,* edited by S. K. Simonds. Oakland, Calif.: Third Party Publishing.

This article gives a clear picture of the major concepts in community organization, with examples of how these are applied. The role of the community organizer—that is, the staff person, whether a health educator, a social worker, or a recreation worker—is described realistically and in detail. The use of community organization at the level discussed in this article is not a task for the novice. Nonetheless, the beginner can learn from Barry's thoughtful presentation of the issues. The beginner however, should function as a community organizer only under the supervision of an experienced health educator.

Baumgartel, H. 1961. "The Concept of Role." In *The Planning of Change,* edited by W. G. Bennis, K. D. Benne, and R. Chin. New York: Holt, Rinehart & Winston.

This is a short, clear description of the concept of "role." The author identifies ways in which this concept can be useful in analyzing human problems. He points out that most social change can be viewed as changing role relations. This is a good article for the beginner.

Bean, C. A. 1982. *Methods of Childbirth.* Garden City, N.Y.: Doubleday.

This is a basic text for those interested in methods of childbirth. An advocate for "natural" childbirth, the author describes the benefits of this method and presents in detail the preparations for it. She also offers the reader guidance in discussing one's preferred childbirth method with the obstetrician. In addition to this basic text on childbirth, there are several personal and community health texts that include a section on childbirth, such as *Health Today,* edited by L. K. Olson (New York: Macmillan, 1983).

Lewin, K. 1951. *Field Theory in Social Science.* New York: Harper.

In chapter 4 of this book, Lewin distinguishes between different types of learning and between learning and compliance. He says there are two ways to bring about change. One way is by inducing a change in an individual's needs or interests, that is, learning; the other is by compelling "the individual to do the undesired action either by direct force or by setting up a constellation where other stronger needs overbalance the effect of this first need." In the case of the MCHC, the need to be part of the group was stronger with some physicians than the need to continue specific childbirth practices. Like the next reference, this one may be difficult for the beginner. Benne has reviewed both references in chapter 8 of *The Planning of Change,* edited by W. G. Bennis, K. D. Benne, R. Chin and K. E. Corey (New York: Holt, Rinehart & Winston, 1976). The novice will find Bennis's discussion much easier to understand.

Lewin, K., and Grabbe, P. 1945. "Conduct, Knowledge, and Acceptance of New Values." *Journal of Social Issues* 1(1):53–65.

Lewin focuses here on reeducation, which, he says, "arises when an individual or group is out of step with society at large." Much of the community health educator's work is reeducation. One of the ten hypotheses Lewin formulates about reeducation deals with acceptance of new beliefs and values by accepting membership in a group. This principle is illustrated in the Campbell/Williams case. The article is rich with gems of insight into the process of reeducation. It is, however, a sophisticated treatment of the subject and therefore may be difficult for beginners unless they have some background in psychology.

Rogers, E. M. 1983. *Diffusion of Innovations.* 3d ed. New York: Free Press.

Diffusion research has greatly increased since Rogers published his first work on diffusion in 1962, when he reported on 405 studies; for this edition, he reviewed 3,085 studies.

Rogers has now extended diffusion theory to include factors that antecede and follow the adoption process. Several questions thus arise: Where did the diffusion come from? Which comes first, the need or the innovation? What kinds of problems are encountered, and how are they solved as the innovation is implemented?

The Campbell/Williams case offers a classic example of the diffusion of an innovation through a community. The stages in the process—knowledge (awareness, interest), persuasion (evaluation, trial), decision and implementation (adoption), and confirmation—can be traced for several of the innovations described (e.g., the acceptance of "natural childbirth"). The terms in parentheses after each stage in the process are those used by Rogers in his original formulation of the diffusion theory (*Diffusion of Innovations,* Free Press, Glencoe, Ill. 1962). Because these terms may be more familiar to some readers, they are used in this analysis.

Zaltman, G., and Duncan, R. 1977. *Strategies for Planned Change,* New York: Wiley.

In this book, which is basic reading for the health educator as change agent, the authors define and describe the steps in the process of change. Part 3, which deals with the change agent and the target population, offers an excellent description of the roles and "qualifications" of each. The Campbell/Williams case illustrates many of the skills described.

Discussion Questions

1. Assume you have just accepted a new position as a health educator for a community council. Maternal and child health have been major issues for this council. What is the first step you would take in this position before meeting with the council?

2. As a member of the council, you have been assigned the task of meeting with a hospital administrator to invite him to serve on a committee that is to consider admitting midwives to deliver babies in the community's hospitals. What would you say to him?

3. Identify the steps you would take to develop a curriculum for a class in parenting for parents who may be interested in taking the course.

4. Write down what you would say if you were facilitating a meeting on the home birthing issue during which an obstetrician and a consumer diverted the meeting from the agenda by shouting at each other because of divergent points of view.

5. Identify what you perceive to be the essential reasons why the MCHC survived for so many years and was successful in attaining many of its goals.

Establishing a Primary Care Clinic in a Traditional Public Health Organization

Jeanne I. Semura, M.P.H.

INTRODUCTION

This case describes a health educator's role in an effort to change a county's traditional mode of providing public health services (the names of persons and places are fictitious). The change modified existing public health services that aimed to prevent the spread of communicable diseases and provide preventive health services by establishing a county-funded clinic focusing on sick care.

The case occurred in 1971–1972 in a large, complex public health organization in a densely populated urban area. Serving a population of 7.5 million people living in a 4,000-square-mile area, the public health organization provided services through 23 geographical districts, one of which was the primary location for this case.

This county-operated organization, employing about 2,200 persons, was in the process of merging with hospitals and mental health facilities into a superorganization that would eventually employ about 23,000 persons. Concerned about this impending merger, administrators of the public health department began to seek community support for its services. One of their strategies was to send to the health officers of the service districts a directive requesting that community advisory councils be created. Figure 1 on page 302 shows the organizational relationships of key participants.

Jeanne I. Semura is a doctoral candidate at the University of Washington and a Health Education Specialist with the Group Health Cooperative of Puget Sound in Seattle, Washington.

Cast of Characters

Ms. Jane Samson Professionally trained as a community development specialist and public health educator. She worked in the community for three years prior to being delegated primary responsibility to organize the District Health Advisory Council (DHAC).

Mrs. Primera A community outreach worker in the Workington office of the community action agency, which was being dismantled. She frequently transported children and families from Workington to the district's clinic seven miles away in another city. She often expressed frustration when a sick or injured child was turned away by the public health clinic.

Mr. Pierce A retired Caucasian operating a small part-time business with variable work schedule. He was president of the League of United Latin American Citizens when the DHAC was created. A longtime resident of Workington, he became the spokesman for the Workington Health Task Force and eventually its president. On several occasions he was approached about running for public office but felt that elected office would coopt him and force him to compromise his values.

Dr. Warner A retired medical director of a research medical facility. He had held several administrative jobs at the central headquarters of the health department (which had a shortage of physicians and a more liberal retirement age policy than the research facility)

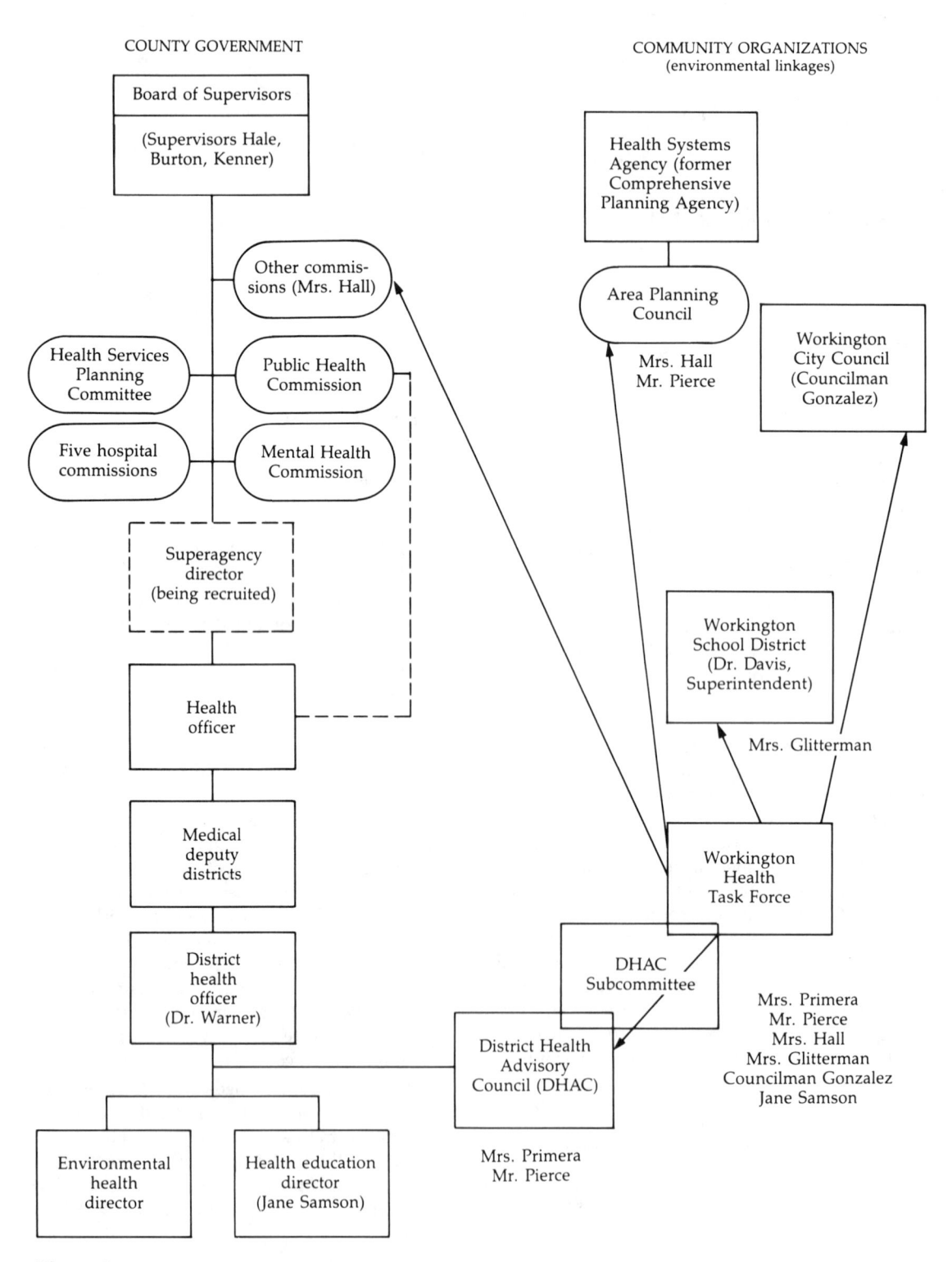

Figure 1
Organizational Relationships of Key Actors

before being named health officer for the district. He announced that he requested the position because he wanted to be of service to the poor.

Mrs. Glitterman President of the Workington PTA for many years and served in county, state, and national PTA offices. Active in school affairs and school board activities, she knew almost everyone in the community. She became interested in services for the elderly and said that she joined the Workington Health Task Force because she felt that services were needed by schoolchildren and by senior citizens who could not afford health insurance or fee for services.

Supervisor Burton Long-established member of the county's board of supervisors. Although he was currently running for reelection, his campaign was considered a mere formality because he had a strong base of support and a well-organized staff. The city of Workington was located in the area he represented. He was killed in an automobile accident three months before the election.

Mrs. Hall Ran a small upholstery business with her paraplegic husband in a neighboring city outside of the health district, a city that was also in Supervisor Burton's district. Active in local politics, she had been appointed by Supervisor Burton to a number of county commissions in the health and human services area. She was an officer on the new Comprehensive Health Planning board, which included the city of Workington in its planning area. A strong advocate of community-controlled health services, she was interested in assuring that government dollars go to needy white families as well as to minority groups.

Councilman Gonzalez A newly elected councilman of Mexican American descent who operated a small grocery store in Workington. He was the first member of a minority group elected to the city council in the city's history.

Supervisor Kenner A longtime member of the board of supervisors representing the south central area of the county. Known to be spontaneous in what he supported, he had a history of supporting and developing health and human service programs, especially since his district was a high-minority and middle-to-low-income area in the county. Three of the five cities in the health district, including the area where the King Hospital was being constructed, fell under his jurisdiction. He had the strong support of the Black community, which represented the majority group in his district.

Environmental Health Director Known to be innovative and broad in his interpretation of the traditional environmental health functions. During his five years of work in the district he built his staff from 6 to 12 people through bargaining and negotiating new functions and responsibilities. An energetic person, he was always in the center of or close to any new activity that was occurring in the various communities in the district.

Dr. Davis Superintendent of the Workington School District. He frequently received notifications about children being turned away by county clinics and about other problems in accessing health services for children. He had been in his position for several years and felt that the increase in minority enrollment was a major problem in the community.

Supervisor Hale Politically appointed to Supervisor Burton's position by the governor of the state, three months before elections. He agreed to keep Supervisor Burton's political appointments and staff intact. He was not well known to the city of Workington, although prior to his appointment he had served as state representative for the area.

THE CASE

FORMATION OF THE DISTRICT HEALTH ADVISORY COUNCIL

Responding to the directive, Jane Samson, health educator, was assigned by the district health officer to organize an advisory council. The central administrators did not attempt to clarify the directive beyond the statement that health educators should know how to do it.

Since the directive was unclear about the function and purpose of the advisory council, Jane Samson chose to allocate time on the initial agenda for the participants to determine their own interests and functions. After soliciting names of leaders of all the district's known community and health organizations from department heads in the health center and other organizations, she sent invitations to an organizational meeting.

At the DHAC's first meeting, the participants identified two areas of concern: (1) the need for more community education about the services offered by health agencies in the area, and (2) the need for current services to be more responsive to users and the community. Jane Samson suggested that two working committees be created so that each participant could select the area of his or her choice. One committee addressed *community education needs* to increase community awareness about the services offered by the new King Hospital and the health department and about the need for immunizations. The other committee addressed *consumer grievances*—the problems people had in obtaining health care, especially sick care for low-income families.

Conferring separately, the consumer grievance committee chose to develop a survey to measure consumer satisfaction. The community education committee recommended that the DHAC organize a series of community meetings in various locations in the district to discuss services of the public health department and King Hospital. At the second DHAC meeting the suggestions for community meetings was approved. The city of Workington was selected as the initial site for a meeting when Mrs. Primera and Mr. Pierce volunteered to organize and publicize the meeting.

The third meeting of the DHAC was energized when Mrs. Primera and Mr. Pierce reported on the success of the meeting in Workington, which was attended by 65 residents. The major concern raised was the lack of medical care facilities for low-income families who had no transportation to the Campton clinic. The DHAC had an enthusiastic discussion on ways to capitalize on the interest in health issues demonstrated by the Workington community. Jane Samson suggested that the DHAC consider establishing a subcouncil in Workington to work on the issues identified in the meeting. This model would be available to the five other distinct community areas in the Campton District if they desired. The DHAC adopted the idea when Mrs. Primera volunteered to organize a group in Workington, with Mr. Pierce and Jane Samson volunteering to help her.

The DHAC continued to work in both areas for another year until participation and interest in the DHAC waned.

CREATION OF THE WORKINGTON HEALTH TASK FORCE

Within a few weeks, after the third DHAC meeting, Mrs. Primera and Mr. Pierce invited their friends, local community organizations, and community leaders in Workington to attend a follow-up meeting. About 20 people from a variety of community and church organizations attended the meeting, chaired by Mr. Pierce. Mrs. Glitterman was among them. Tentatively defining the problem as the lack of public transportation to the main Campton District clinic and King Hospital, the group decided to meet with Supervisor Burton's chief deputy to explore ways to improve accessibility to the county's health services for the city residents. At that meeting, the deputy suggested several avenues that could be explored in the Workington community to obtain public transportation. The group decided to approach city officials in Workington with the suggestions.

Mrs. Primera, Mrs. Glitterman, and Mr. Pierce met with the Workington city manager to discuss various possibilities for transporting people to the public health clinic in Campton. They became aware of the many political and planning jurisdictions that must cooperate—regional and county areas, other cities, and state licensing agencies. This choice was abandoned when the complexity and red tape became obvious. The group began more seriously to discuss the goal of getting a clinic established within Workington.

In the meantime, Jane Samson suggested that the group find out whether local medical groups might be willing to provide low-cost medical care services. At its third meeting, the group met with the administrator of a newly opened proprietary (privately owned, profit-making) hospital in the city to discuss what services the hospital offered to low-income residents. The hospital administrator spoke of the hospital's plan for a private medical office building to be constructed sometime in the future, but he said there were no plans for an outpatient service beyond what currently existed, which was already busy. He offered to sponsor community education meetings with the hospital's house staff physicians as speakers and to send his volunteer coordinator to future meetings. His representative to the meetings was welcomed.

At their next meeting, the group named itself the Workington Health Task Force (WHTF) and decided that its main goal was to obtain a health clinic in Workington for low-income residents. The local newspaper, in a feature article on the WHTF meeting, described the desired services as "health services on a family basis, a well and sick baby clinic, and a youth clinic to fight drug abuse." Services for senior citizens were added after Mrs. Glitterman expressed the need at a subsequent meeting. Mrs. Primera was elected president, and Mr. Pierce, spokesman. Jane Samson continued to serve in a staffing support role that included planning agendas, coordinating and guiding activities and communications among group members, and assuring that minutes, agendas, and letters were typed and distributed. She chose to function unobtrusively, whereas Mrs. Primera, Mr. Pierce, and other members gave regular interviews with the local newspapers.

Each WHTF member contacted all known community organizations, schools, churches, and politicians to advocate for these services. Jane Samson was invited to speak at several community meetings about the services offered by the county, new programs such as King Hospital, and the Model Cities–funded primary care clinic. Mrs. Hall, who had heard about the WHTF, joined the group to support the need for services in the area. Councilman Gonzalez joined when urged by several of the Mexican American members of the WHTF. The president of the local Mexican American Scholarship Association, the head school nurse of the Workington Unified School District, a prominent Mexican American restaurant owner and businesswoman, and the wife of a local minister also joined the group.

ESTABLISHMENT OF A CLINIC IN WORKINGTON

Workington, a predominantly low- to middle-class white community had a population of 35,000 people, 40 percent of whom were estimated to be undocumented migrant workers and Hispanic Americans. It was believed that most of this group were of Mexican or Mexican American descent. In addition, there was a sizable senior citizen population.

The WHTF met with Dr. Warner to present their findings and to explore the probability that the public health department might establish a satellite clinic in Workington. Dr. Warner indicated that he had talked with his superiors, who were interested in such a clinic, but that the board of supervisors determined where funds for such services should go. At Councilman Gonzalez's request for statistical evidence of need, Jane Samson collected data on morbidity, mortality, and service utilization patterns and some testimonial descriptions of problems that Workington residents had in obtaining existing services.

Councilman Gonzalez combined this statistical information with information about projected tax revenues collected by the county from the city of Workington and presented his findings to Supervisor Burton. Concomitantly, the WHTF formally asked the city council to pass a motion requesting the establishment of a county health clinic in Workington. After the motion passed, the council asked Supervisor Burton to place its request on the board agenda. During the meeting of the board of supervisors, a 2–2 tie for a clinic occurred when, because of Supervisor Kenner's absence, his tie-breaking vote was not cast.

Representatives of the WHTF who attended the board meeting reported this discouraging information to the rest of the group. The members of the WHTF disagreed about their next steps: Some wanted to give up; some wanted to collect more information about the needs; some wanted to get more community support. Jane Samson helped to focus the discussion on ways to get wider support for the clinic. Finally, because Mrs. Hall and Mr. Pierce knew several key leaders in the Black community, they suggested that other WHTF members contact any leaders or groups they knew in Supervisor Kenner's area to gain support for the clinic. Mrs. Hall reminded the task force that much of the taxpayers' monies for health services had been going into Black communities and that services should be shared with other needy people, such as those in Workington. The members agreed to continue their quest.

At the next city council meeting, the councilmen discussed whether to resubmit the clinic proposal on the board's agenda. Although the WHTF members attending the meeting urged resubmission, the council decided to take no action without a vote on the issue. At the next WHTF meeting, the general feeling of despair was evident. But most members felt that the goal was still worth pursuing. They continued to talk with health planning groups, voluntary agencies, and other health groups throughout the county about their need and goal.

The headline "Supervisor Burton Killed in Automobile Accident" appeared on the front pages of the major newspapers a few weeks after the city council meeting had been held. The WHTF members, concerned over the loss of a supporter, discussed whether they should continue with the meetings they had already scheduled. It was decided that they would persist despite the uncertainty about Supervisor Burton's successor.

The WHTF had previously requested a meeting with Dr. Warner, his staff, and the city council to discuss whether services could be offered without establishing a clinic located in Workington. During this meeting, the district's environmental health director described the need to look at housing and environmental health problems as well as clinical ones. The council offered to provide federally funded staff to carry out a house-to-house survey of needs. Dr. Davis, superintendent of schools, voiced concern about the county's ability to operate services for sick children in the community since past services were nonexistent. One councilman announced that he had talked with staff at the local proprietary hospital and that they were accelerating the development of a fee-for-service medical clinic to serve the residents of Workington. Dr. Warner advocated a clinic funded and operated by the county.

After discussing the mixed responses it received at the joint meeting, the WHTF decided to approach Supervisor Hale, who had just been appointed to replace Supervisor Burton, to support the clinic. However, Supervisor Hale began immediately to campaign for reelection. Although he was not well known in all areas of the district, including Workington, Supervisor Hale was reluctant to spend much time there because the number of registered voters in the city was small as compared with other areas in the district, areas that served 1.5 million residents in the county.

When they encountered difficulty in establishing a meeting date with Supervisor Hale or members of his staff, the WHTF members decided to invite his opponent to meet with them. The meeting was well attended, and the local newspaper covered the meeting in a column written by a member of the WHTF. In the discussion about the clinic, Supervisor Hale's opponent publicly supported the establishment of the clinic. At a subsequent meeting, the WHTF members were not sure what their next steps should be, because there appeared to be a general lack of interest among city and county officials in continuing their support for a clinic in Workington. Jane Samson asked the members if their goal for establishing a clinic was still considered to be a worthwhile one. They answered affirmatively.

During these events, a number of meetings that were unplanned and unanticipated by the WHTF were occurring. Councilman Gonzalez, at a cocktail party for Supervisor Hale in a neighboring community, reminded Hale that the Hispanic community in Workington, when combined with those who, encouraged by Mrs. Glitterman, supported health services for schoolchildren and senior citizens, made for an effective block of voters. On another occasion, Supervisor Hale met Mrs. Hall, whom he continued to meet at a number of subsequent political meetings. On each occasion she explained the need for a clinic in Workington. She later confided to some of the members of the WHTF that she had offered to resign from her commission assignments if Supervisor Hale would promise to establish a clinic. She explained that she was a carryover appointee from Supervisor Burton's administration and that Supervisor Hale could therefore replace her with one of his own supporters. As Supervisor Hale's campaign progressed, he continued to meet various members of the WHTF and citizens of Workington who wanted his support for a clinic.

After much debate, the WHTF decided to push for a clinic before the November 3 election. They asked Councilman Gonzalez to resubmit the request for funds for a clinic to Supervisor Hale. Councilman Gonzalez made the motion at the city council meeting. The council appeared reluctant to approve the motion. Councilman Gonzalez reminded the two councilmen running for reelection that the Hispanic community, joined with supporters of health services for schoolchildren and the elderly, constituted a major block of voters in the city. After further debate, the council voted

3–2 to request the clinic. The two "no" votes were from councilmen who supported a fee-for-service medical office building being proposed by the private hospital.

The council requested that Supervisor Hale resubmit the clinic funding on the board of supervisor's agenda. On September 19, the board approved $109,397 on a 4–1 vote, with the contingency that a suitable building be found in the city. Mr. Pierce thanked the members of the board and offered to find the appropriate space. The board, incidentally, also announced the appointment of the new director of the superagency, which made the reorganization of the hospitals, mental health, and public health departments official.

During the next two months, Mr. Pierce, Mrs. Glitterman, Mrs. Hall, Councilman Gonzalez, and Dr. Warner inspected many vacant buildings in the Workington area. None was found to be suitable. The WHTF and Dr. Warner preferred a new building designed for clinic use rather than an old renovated library.

The WHTF met to discuss the problem. After considering some strategies, they decided not to wait until after the election for a more suitable building but to accept the renovated library with the understanding that Supervisor Hale, if elected, would help them obtain a more appropriate building.

On October 15, the board of supervisors approved the lease of the old library. Dr. Warner and the district staff were instructed to prepare for the opening of the clinic on October 24. Jane Samson was assigned to be responsible for decorating the clinic, preparing handout information on services to be offered, and coordinating the invitations and physical arrangements for the open house held after the opening ceremonies. As part of the celebration, the new superagency director welcomed the audience, and Supervisor Hale and each city councilman described his role in supporting the establishment of the clinic.

ANALYSIS

The political model of organizational change (Baldridge 1977; Estler 1982) explains the successful establishment of the clinic. Some of the assumptions of this model applicable to this case are as follows:

1. Special interest groups identify issues from the general social context.
2. The legislative process is used as an action channel.
3. Outcomes are determined by bargaining, influence, and trade-offs.
4. Participants are fluid according to the stakes and stands involved.
5. Power and personal influence affect outcomes.
6. Decisions are made when deadlines force the issue.
7. The changing nature of coalitions creates opportunities for foul-up.

These assumptions suggest a number of strategies. For example:

1. Gain the support of persons known to have power and influence.
2. Establish and legitimize support through official sanction and coalitions or by using the rules of the system (Estler 1962).
3. Find out which bargaining games are being played and who the players are (Allison 1971; Baldridge 1977).
4. Choose the right time and place to confront the opposition.
5. Establish coalitions with groups having similar interests.
6. Set deadlines for reaching a decision about an issue.
7. Concentrate on one goal and refuse to be coopted in adding new goals.

Although the political model explains the success of the WHTF's efforts, it does not explain the loose threads or the streams of events and participants that interacted briefly with the change effort and then disappeared. "Organized anarchy" (March and Olsen 1976) describes an organization characterized by:

- Problematic goals
- Unclear technologies
- Fluid participation

The public health organization manifested these three characteristics. In an "organized anarchy," decisions are made via the "garbage can" model (Cohen, March, and Olsen 1972; Estler 1982; March and Olsen 1976). Figures 2 and 3 on the following pages identify the stream of problems, solutions, participants, and choice opportunities and what happened to them over time.

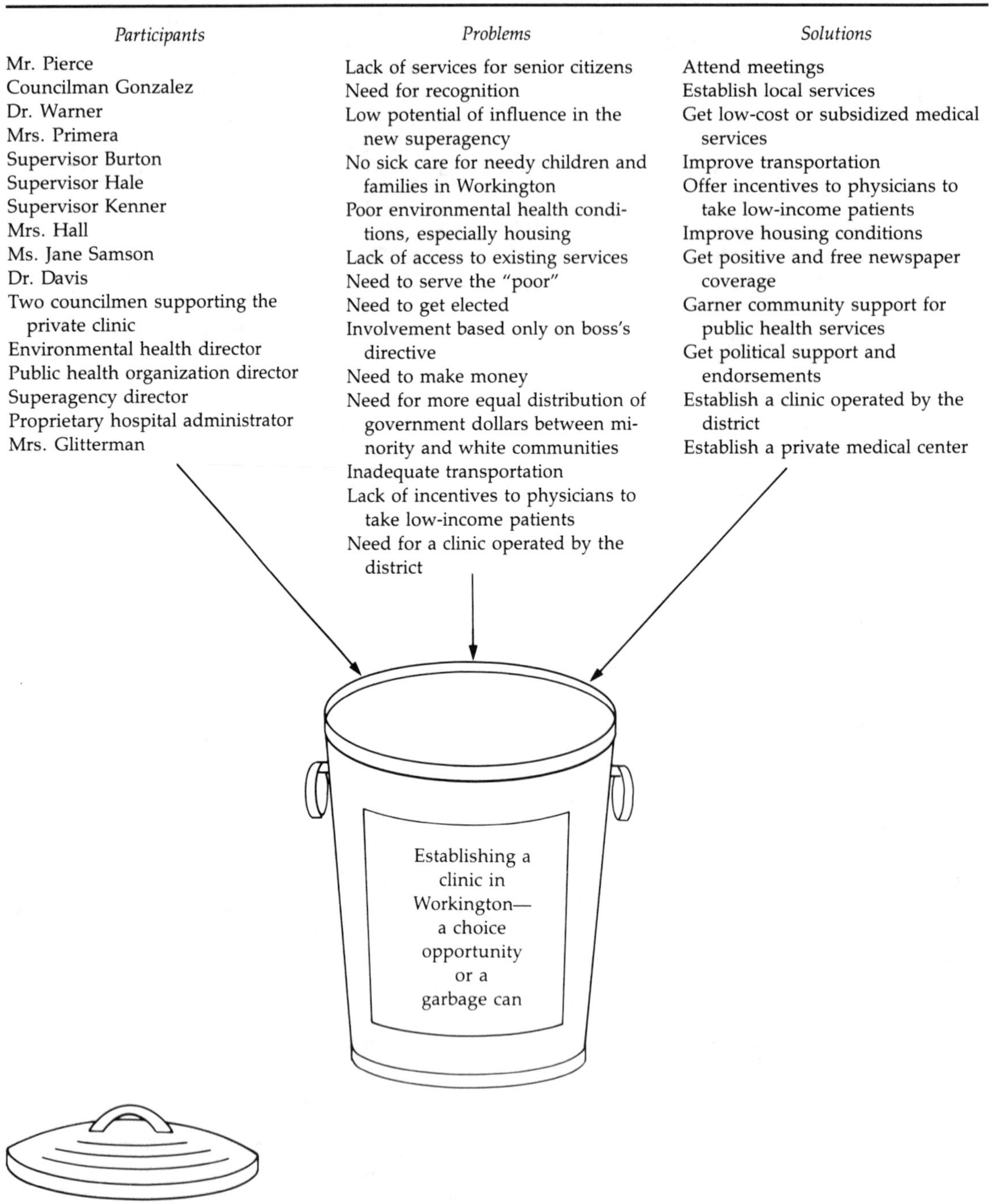

Participants	Problems	Solutions
Mr. Pierce	Lack of services for senior citizens	Attend meetings
Councilman Gonzalez	Need for recognition	Establish local services
Dr. Warner	Low potential of influence in the new superagency	Get low-cost or subsidized medical services
Mrs. Primera		
Supervisor Burton	No sick care for needy children and families in Workington	Improve transportation
Supervisor Hale		Offer incentives to physicians to take low-income patients
Supervisor Kenner	Poor environmental health conditions, especially housing	
Mrs. Hall		Improve housing conditions
Ms. Jane Samson	Lack of access to existing services	Get positive and free newspaper coverage
Dr. Davis	Need to serve the "poor"	
Two councilmen supporting the private clinic	Need to get elected	Garner community support for public health services
	Involvement based only on boss's directive	
Environmental health director		Get political support and endorsements
Public health organization director	Need to make money	
Superagency director	Need for more equal distribution of government dollars between minority and white communities	Establish a clinic operated by the district
Proprietary hospital administrator		Establish a private medical center
Mrs. Glitterman		
	Inadequate transportation	
	Lack of incentives to physicians to take low-income patients	
	Need for a clinic operated by the district	

Establishing a clinic in Workington—a choice opportunity or a garbage can

Figure 2
Streams of Problems, Solutions, Participants, and Choice Opportunities

A NEW CLINIC

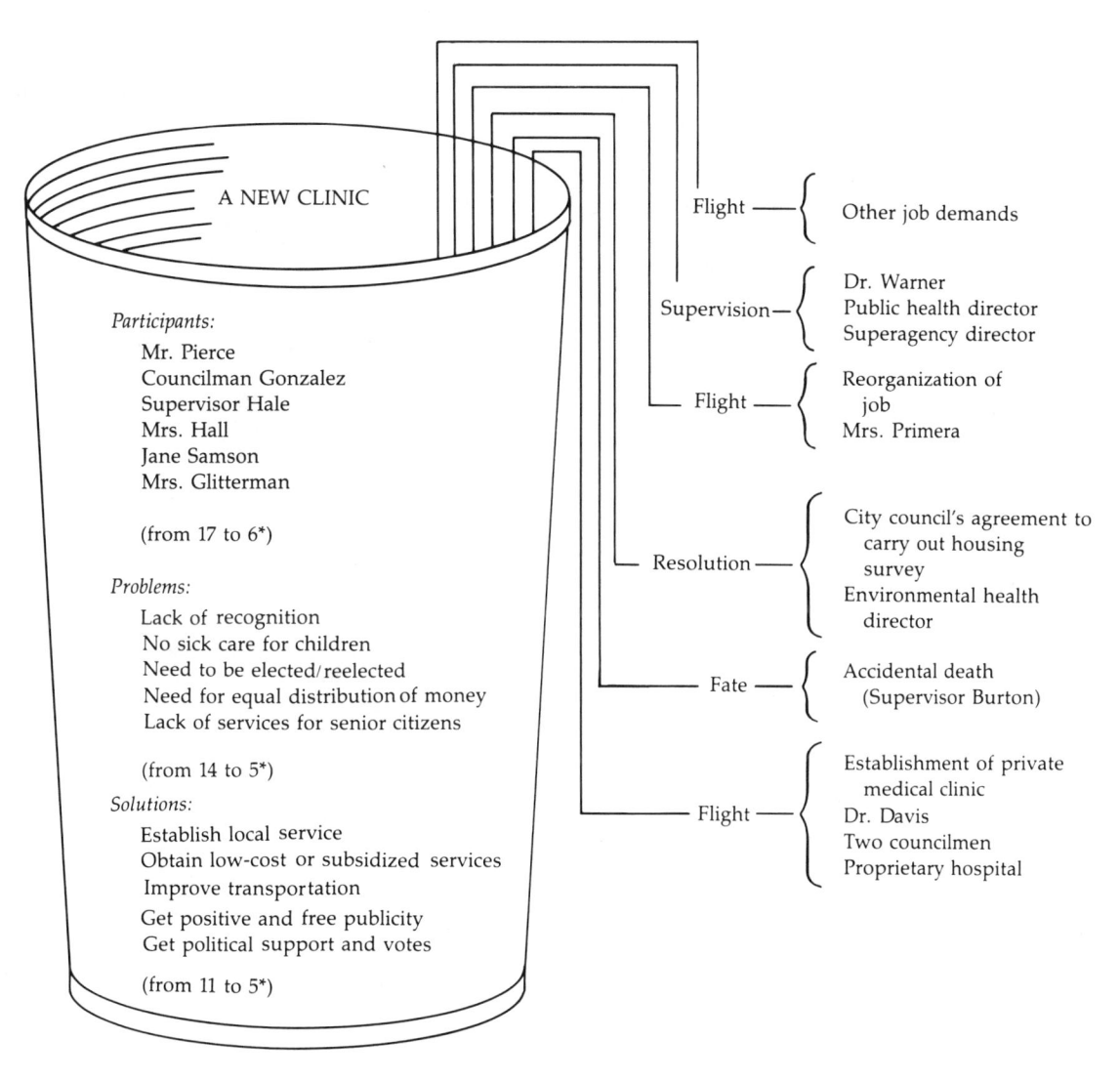

Participants:
- Mr. Pierce
- Councilman Gonzalez
- Supervisor Hale
- Mrs. Hall
- Jane Samson
- Mrs. Glitterman

(from 17 to 6*)

Problems:
- Lack of recognition
- No sick care for children
- Need to be elected/reelected
- Need for equal distribution of money
- Lack of services for senior citizens

(from 14 to 5*)

Solutions:
- Establish local service
- Obtain low-cost or subsidized services
- Improve transportation
- Get positive and free publicity
- Get political support and votes

(from 11 to 5*)

Flight — Other job demands

Supervision — Dr. Warner / Public health director / Superagency director

Flight — Reorganization of job / Mrs. Primera

Resolution — City council's agreement to carry out housing survey / Environmental health director

Fate — Accidental death (Supervisor Burton)

Flight — Establishment of private medical clinic / Dr. Davis / Two councilmen / Proprietary hospital

*Original number in garbage can and remaining number over time.

Figure 3
Competing Demands and Shifting Participation over Time

The garbage can model of decision making describes loosely coupled solutions, problems, and participants. It offers a useful means of describing the unforeseen and unplanned changes that occurred concomitantly with the planned-change effort. Cohen and March (1974) suggest strategies that help deal with unplanned change: for example, spend time, persist, exchange status for substance, facilitate opposition participation, overload the system, provide garbage cans, function unobtrusively, and interpret history.

All events cannot, of course, be controlled, and so there are always exciting challenges for the change agent/health educator.

POSTSCRIPT

The Workington Health Clinic is still in operation despite budget cuts that closed 13 clinics in the county. It is servicing an average of 700 patients per month. As of April 1982, further cutbacks were imminent, with the Workington Health Clinic remaining prominent on the list of services to be eliminated. A county official felt, however, that there was some hope that it would survive this new threat for, as she said, "The clinic has a lot of community support."

Mr. Pierce said: "I don't know what is going to happen, but the clinic continues to be busy and should bring in a fair amount of income for the county, since they are charging a $20 fee per visit." He thought that the clinic would be close to paying for itself if all fees could be collected.

Although the active membership has dropped to several persons and some founding members express concern that the bylaws requiring the presidential term to be limited to two years has not been followed, the WHTF continues to meet to raise funds for health scholarships and to act as patient advocates in the clinic.

REFERENCES

Alinsky, S. D. 1971. *Rules for Radicals*. New York: Random House.

Allison, G. T. 1971. *Essence of Decision*. Boston: Little, Brown. 1971.

Baldridge, J. V., et al. 1977. "Alternative Models of Governance in Higher Education." In *Governing Academic Organizations*, edited by G. Riley and J. V. Baldridge. Berkeley: McCutchan.

Cohen, J. D., and March, J. G. 1974. *Leadership and Ambiguity—The American College President*. New York: McGraw-Hill.

Cohen, J. D.; March, J. G.; and Olsen, J. P. 1972. "A Garbage Can Model of Organizational Choice." *Administrative Science Quarterly* 17(7):1–25.

Emery, R. E., and Trist, E. I. 1965. "The Causal Texture of Organizational Environments." *Human Relations*, 18(1):21–32.

Estler, S. E. n.d. "A Contextual Theory of Choice: Study Guide to March and Olsen." Typescript, University of Washington.

Estler, S. E. 1982. "Perspectives on Organizational Change." Typescript, University of Washington.

March, J. G., and Olsen, J. P. 1976. *Ambiguity and Choice in Organizations*. Bergen, Norway: Universitetsfjforlaget.

Pfeffer, J., and Salancik, G. 1978. *The External Control of Organizations*. New York: Harper & Row.

Analysis

This case focuses on the health educator as a community organizer. It describes the organization of a primary care clinic, accomplished through the political, not the learning, process. Semura (the health educator identified as Jane Samson) describes her role as "staffing support." Her job involved organizing agendas with the chairman, taking and mailing minutes of the meetings, seeing that letters were written, arranging for between-meeting appointments, and handling similar housekeeping details. Note that the appropriate handling of housekeeping details and the identification and continued involvement of key people who should not be overlooked were critical to the functioning of the Workington Health Task Force.

Guiding and focusing discussions at meetings was an equally important function. The health educator's skill in carrying out these functions, and especially her ability to stick with her objective (i.e., to help the members of the WHTF make their own decisions), provided the support the WHTF needed to accomplish its goal.

Semura explains the behavior of the principal actors in the case with two theories. The first is a political theory of organizational behavior based on power and the negotiations and compromises that occur between two parties when one wants something the other has or can get for him or her. This theory, as Semura points out, has implications for the kind of decisions that are made. These decisions are often not rational and are usually self-serving. They are not necessarily made because someone believes in a cause, but because that cause meets someone's needs.

The second theory, the "garbage can theory of decision making," offers an explanation for the numerous unplanned events that occur during planned change. Decisions in "organized anarchies" are made for a variety of reasons, none of which have much to do with a rational process. These theories do explain how the task force accomplished its goal. Lewin's "imposed learning" theory also explains this. The board of supervisors approved the funds for the clinic because this action gave them the reward they wanted: votes. However, Lewin's theory does not include concepts that explain how all the issues relate to the results.

Semura refers to several meetings not directly related to the task force that occurred between the principal actors. These meetings are akin to the informal lobbying referred to in the Robinson case (p. 68). The lesson, of course, is never to lose an opportunity to promote your cause with anyone who can help, regardless of where you may meet him or her. It should be noted that "unplanned" meetings may also be planned.

This case raises several issues relevant to the practice of health education. The first is that of agency-generated versus community-generated needs. The demise of the District Health Advisory Committee was not surprising. It was generated by the public health department to meet that department's needs. The WHTF, on the other hand, was generated by the people to meet their needs. The fact that the latter thrived and the former did not is consonant with the basic principle of learning: People will learn/do those things that are meaningful and useful to them.

This case and others (Nybo, Robinson, and Campbell/Williams, pp. 54, 68, and 288) illustrate that a contributing factor to successful goal attainment is an objective perspective by the health educator. This does not mean the health educator cannot care about an issue, but rather that she or he must not get caught up in the emotion of the issue. The ability to listen to a discussion, sort out extraneous issues, and bring the discussants back to the central issue is a skill all health educators should develop as expertly as possible.

Semura says she functioned "unobtrusively," yet her contribution was hardly unobtrusive. When a health educator works with community groups, the goal is usually to help them confront some type of community health issue. Community people will work on these issues if they see them as important—and as their own. Therefore *they* should be the spokespersons for the project; *they* should be interviewed and have their names in the paper, not the professional staff.

However, this situation presents a dilemma for the health educator. If he or she does a good job of facilitating, guiding, and keeping a group focused on its goal, and is truly unobtrusive about it, some people (possibly even personnel in the agency employing the health educator) will wonder what the health educator really does. This problem is, unfortunately, a built-in barrier to the recognition and appreciation of the skills of the health educator.

References/Select Resources

Arnold, M. 1982. "Ambiguity in the Role of the Health Educator." In *SOPHE Heritage Collection of Health Education Monographs*, vol 1: *The Philosophical, Behavioral, and Professional Bases for Health Education*, edited by S. K. Simonds. Oakland, Calif.: Third Party Publishing.

In this paper, originally published in 1962, Arnold distinguishes between the health educator's external and internal roles in his/her organization. What Arnold describes as the internal integrative role represents many of the functions carried out by the health educator in the Semura case. In the early 1960s, as Arnold notes, this role needed to be made more explicit because there was considerable disagreement and misunderstanding concerning the health educator's role versus that of other health professionals. Without evidence to the contrary, this situation may still be true over 20 years later.

Cohen, J. D.; March, J. G.; and Olsen J. P. 1972. "A Garbage Can Model of Organizational Choice." *Administrative Science Quarterly* 17(7):1–25.

This article explains how decision making takes place in what the authors describe as an organized anarchy. They have termed their model the garbage can model, because it is rapidly filled with choices, problems, solutions, and the energy of participants. Although the authors have used universities as an example of organized anarchy, it is important to consider, as Semura does, that health educators will encounter organized anarchies in community settings. Small as well as large organizations may fit the garbage can model.

Discussion Questions

1. What were some of the obstacles the health educator faced in maintaining objectivity in this case?

2. Identify ethical issues with which the health educator had to deal in this case.

3. Assume you are the health educator at a meeting with WHTF members at which the discussion degenerates into lamentations over how difficult it will be to get the clinic in their community. You ask if they still want the clinic; the answer is yes. How would you structure the discussion to get the members back on target?

4. Given the discussion of the WHTF's activities provided in the case, write the minutes of its meeting after Supervisor Burton was killed. Use your imagination to fill in some details.

5. Assume the WHTF was not politically sophisticated. When it was clear that getting the clinic would be a political issue, what were the task force's options?

6. Given the assumptions of the political model of organizational change and of the "organized anarchy" model, identify the events in the case that fit those assumptions.

PART FOUR

Case Studies in Worksite Settings

Most Americans receive hospital and health insurance coverage for themselves and their families from their employers (Health Insurance Institute of America 1982: 13). As a result, business has become the main purchaser of medical care through third-party payment insurance. The cost to business in the early 1980s was $80 billion annually (Williams 1983). Therefore public health and business leaders have begun to look at work organizations as places for promoting health (Anonymous 1983; Richmond 1980) and potentially saving costs.

Any workplace is a possible site for the practice of health education. One case (Donnelly) in Part Four is set in a medical center, another (Falck) in a school system. Health educators have worked in these settings for some time, but they have been concerned with the patients or students, not the employees. Some companies have employed health educators for 40 years, but the workplace as a site for comprehensive health education is relatively new.

A great deal of activity is now occurring at the worksite in regard to health education. Much of this activity is centered in large corporations, where resources are more available (Parkinson et al. 1982). Many of the numerous smaller firms that are now beginning to seek assistance in developing program components have begun to work with local health institutions such as hospitals and voluntary organizations.

Part Four does not present cases that are representative of the great diversity of programs now occurring at the worksite. Rather it offers a selected sampling of programs. However, the issues presented in these cases typify those that arise at most worksites.

ISSUES

REDUCING EMPLOYEE HEALTH CARE COSTS

Health promotion programs are only one way to reduce employee health costs (Cordello, Lebo, and Kenegan 1980). Two other alternatives are cost-sharing and reimbursement for unused health services (Anonymous 1983; Williams 1983). The cost-sharing plan is based on the assumption that if employees pay a greater share of costs, they will use medical care more judiciously than if everything is covered by insurance. Under the reimbursement plan, if employees do not use health services, the company will reward them for being healthy by refunding a part of the unused money set aside for medical care. The assumption here is that employees will be motivated to use the services judiciously.

Proponents of these plans cite the cost savings to the employer. Opponents regard as false the assumption that people use medical services needlessly. They also regard as false the assumption that there can be an economic motivation to stay healthy. In their view, employees are likely not to practice better health habits without appropriate instruction.

They are concerned, further, that employees will delay going to a doctor for "minor" symptoms in order to get an insurance rebate. By not catching serious conditions through the early examination of symptoms (early cancer detection, for example), employees may jeopardize their health. The reimbursement plan might then lead to higher costs because services will be sought mainly for severe and costly conditions. Another complication is the likely discrimination between younger and older workers. The older worker is more likely to be a user of medical services than is the younger one.

Many people have looked toward workplace health promotion as a quick solution for decreasing the costs of health benefits. However, though some costs are controlled by changes in employee health habits (Chadwick 1982a, 1982b), legally regulated costs, third-party policies and procedures, and employer policies are not affected. Today we are experiencing a large increase in employee health benefits. Combined with unbridled medical costs, spiraling inflation, and other macroeconomic factors, health benefits are out of control (Williams 1983).

THE CHANGING BUSINESS WORLD

While public health officials are beginning to look at the workplace as an ideal setting for intervention and for establishing new health habits, business leaders are also starting to reorganize and reconceptualize the structure of industry and employer-employee relations.

Pressure from foreign markets and new technological developments are forcing American business and labor leaders to examine their own roles and their relationship (Shortell 1982). As new patterns of work and management evolve, there is the opportunity to include health promotion in the workplace. The McCauley case, which describes the development of a program for AT&T, is an excellent example of how changing circumstances within an organization can provide the opportunity for developing a health promotion program.

Another issue is change among employees. Employees often change jobs during their working years, whereas the leading causes of death and disability are not evident until an employee is in the mid-years or has retired. How, then, does an employer benefit from current expenditures on health promotion?

Basic issues such as these need to be addressed by the health educator when marketing health promotion programs to employers. The immediate and long-term benefits must be identified. Specific health behaviors, their benefits, and costs must be isolated. Cost factors related to life and disability insurance rates and to workmen's compensation must be calculated, as was done in both the Cantlon and the McCauley cases. For example, preferred rates to groups with employees demonstrating lowered risks and good health habits (e.g., using seat belts, not smoking) are one avenue to explore for direct cost reduction. This approach would be consistent with Green's PRECEDE model, which deals with the reinforcing and enabling factors affecting the desired behavior (Green et al. 1980).

INTRODUCING HEALTH PROMOTION TO BUSINESS AND INDUSTRY

It is important to consider that cost control usually implies omitting some input to increase profits. But in employee health promotion, we are asking for a business investment with little guarantee that it will reduce costs or yield a profit. Studies describing cost savings are sparse (Parkinson et al. 1982:3). However, both the McCauley and the Cantlon cases illustrate that the management of some organizations is willing to invest resources in health promotion if the advocates for the program are able to provide strong enough justification (potential cost savings) and if the organization itself has a history of innovation and a strong commitment to human resource development.

But it is understandable why some employers are wary of new ideas about employee health promotion and reluctant to implement large programs. For example, annual physical examinations, chest X rays, and even multiphasic screening, which have been popular, have not yielded the payoff they promised.

To date, most health promotion programs have been conducted by large companies (U.S. DHHS 1980). However, most companies have fewer than 100 employees and cannot afford the costs of comprehensive health promotion programs (U.S. Bureau of the Census 1977).

When introducing health promotion into the workplace, health educators are trying to implement change in the current modes of activity. Resistance is to be expected. Certain roles may be affected by change: the role of management in personal health promotion, of corporate medical personnel, of the personnel administrator, and of the local medical and hospital community. Also affected are voluntary agencies and community hospitals with employee outreach programs. The point is that introducing health promotion into industry is a complex matter affecting many levels of activity (Lippitt, Watson, and Westley 1958).

As the Cantlon, McCauley, and Donnelly cases illustrate, health educators need to understand the system or corporate culture. Corporate culture is defined as the basic values that set a pattern for an organization's activities, opinions, and actions. "That pattern is instilled in employees by managers' examples and passed down to succeeding generations of workers" (Anonymous 1980:148). Of course, health educators may find themselves in a tenuous position if their activities threaten the corporate culture. This can happen if the health educator is unaware of or does not accurately understand the organization's culture. But with an accurate understanding, one can *influence* corporate culture, as exemplified both in the McCauley case, where an active effort was made to integrate health promotion into the corporate culture to provide support and continued reinforcement for programming efforts, and in the Ware case (an industrial setting). The challenge to the health educator is to integrate health promotion with existing services and, where possible, to efficiently utilize corporate and community resources (Katz and Fielding 1980).

THE ROLE OF THE HEALTH EDUCATOR

The role of the health educator in the worksite is potentially multifaceted, just as it is in other settings, such as communities and medical care facilities. The health educator (1) may be responsible only for directly providing programs for employees; (2) may, as a staff person, also act as an administrator whose primary role is to manage the implementation of a program; or (3) may serve as a consultant or facilitator who assists many firms in developing and implementing programs. The Lindemann case is an excellent example of this third function.

The Ware case suggests that the role in the worksite can be fragmented, depending on the other players on the scene and their interest in and responsibility for the program. The same is true of practice in the medical care setting.

The cases illustrate issues relevant to the practice of health education in general, such as the issue of responsibility versus authority. The Donnelly case raises the issue of developing personal support systems for health education. Squyres (1982) refers to this same need in medical care settings. All the cases in Part Four demonstrate the importance of knowing the system in which you are working.

Falck illustrates how resources found within the workplace can serve as vehicles for health promotion. She offers two examples of tailoring the program to existing systems: the use of employees as promoters of health and the plan to build on social relationships within the school system to establish peer group support for health promotion activities. The same idea is seen in Donnelly's case study. Silversin and Coombs (1981) emphasize the value of using social relationships in promoting dental health, and this approach is applicable to health promotion in general.

The Donnelly case is set in a nonprofit human service organization, but the costs were of as much concern there as in a profit-making organization. After all, if employers invest in their employees, they expect a return on their investment. As Donnelly illustrates, that expectation is not necessarily based on a concern with profit: management perceives it as a matter of survival.

CONCLUSION

In the past few years some health educators have been involved with programs in a variety of workplaces. With the growing interest by management and labor in health issues, especially the cost of medical care, it is likely that this area will present increasing opportunities for health educators. To take advantage of these opportunities, health educators need to advocate for education and promotion programs, using accurate and strong supporting data. The Estabrook case (p. 117) demonstrates how research can be used to communicate the value of health education.

Knowledge of corporate structures and the ability to analyze the decision-making process are essential. The specialized knowledge needed, in addition to professional and administrative skills, includes an ample comprehension of employee benefits, workmen's compensation, insurance, state regulations, union issues, and basic marketing principles.

REFERENCES

Anonymous. 1980. "Corporate Culture: The Hard-to-Change Values That Spell Success or Failure." *Business Week,* October 27:148–160.

Anonymous. 1983a. "Paying Employees Not to Go to the Doctor." 1983 *Business Week,* March 21:146, 150.

Anonymous. 1983b. "Response in Depth: Company Wellness Programs Highlight New Directions in Health Care." *Response* (Washington, D.C.) 12(2):4, 20.

Chadwick, J. H. 1982a. "Cost-Effective Health Promotion at the Worksite?" In *Managing Health Promotion in the Workplace: Guidelines for Implementation and Evaluation,* edited by R. S. Parkinson and Associates. Palo Alto, Calif.: Mayfield.

Chadwick, J. H. 1982b. "Health Behavior Change at the Worksite: A Problem Oriented Analysis." In *Managing Health Promotion in the Workplace: Guidelines for Implementation and Evaluation,* edited by R. S. Parkinson and Associates. Palo Alto, Calif.: Mayfield.

Collen, M. F., ed. 1973. Special Issue on the Status of Multiphasic Health Testing. *Preventive Medicine* 2 (June).

Cordello, D.; Lebo, J.; and Kenegan, A. 1980. "An HMO Brings Health Education to the Workplace: A Strategy to Help Reduce Health Care Costs." In *Proceedings of the 30th Annual Group Health Institute Boston, May 4–7, 1980.* Washington, D.C.: Group Health Association of America.

Green, L.; Kreuter, N. W.; Deeds, S. G.; and Partridge, K. B. 1980. *Health Education Planning: A Diagnostic Approach.* Palo Alto, Calif.: Mayfield.

Health Insurance Institute of America. 1982. *Source Book of Health Insurance Data, 1981–1982.* Washington, D.C.

Katz, H. J., and Fielding, J. E., eds. 1980. "Health Education and Promotion: Agenda for the Eighties." Summary report of an Insurance Industry Conference on Health Education and Promotion, Atlanta, Georgia, March 16–18, 1980 (sponsored by the Health Insurance Association of America).

Lippitt, R.; Watson, J.; and Westley, B. 1958. *The Dynamics of Planned Change.* New York: Harcourt Brace Jovanovich.

Parkinson, R. S.; Beck, R. N.; Collings, G. H.; Eriksen, M.; Green, L. W.; McGill, A. M.; Merwin, D.; Pearson, C. E.; and Ware, B. G. 1982. *Managing Health Promotion in the Workplace: Guidelines for Implementing and Evaluation.* Palo Alto, Calif.: Mayfield.

Richmond, J. B. 1980. "Health Promotion at the Worksite." *Public Health Reports* 95(2): cover 2.

Shortell, S. M. 1982. "Theory Z: Implications and Relevance for Health Care Management." *Health Care Management Review* 7(4):7–21.

Silversin, J. B., and Coombs, J. A. 1981. "Institutions and Oral Health Behavior." *Journal of Applied Behavioral Medicine* 4(3):297–320.

Squyres, W. 1982. "The Professional Health Educator in HMOs: Implications for Training and Our Future in Medical Care." *Health Education Quarterly* 9(1):67–80.

U.S. Bureau of the Census. 1977. *Statistical Abstract of the United States.* 98th annual ed. Washington, D.C.: Government Printing Office.

U.S. Department of Health and Human Services. National Institute for Occupational Safety and Health. Division of Technical Service. 1980. *Symposium on Health Education and Health Promotion in the Workplace.* DHHS Publication no. (PHS CDC) 210–79–0045–0000. Cincinnati.

Warner, K. E. 1978. "Health Maintenance Insurance: Toward an Optimal HMO." *Policy Sciences* 10:121–131.

Williams, L. S. 1983. "Rx Needed: Fast Aid for Rising Health Care Costs." *PPG Products Magazine* (Pittsburgh, Pa.), p. 2.

Occupational Health Education: A Nontraditional Role for a Health Educator

Beverly G. Ware, Dr.P.H.

BACKGROUND

Model making and pattern making are intrinsic parts of the automobile industry. Handcrafted wood models are the foundation of all new cars, and the patterns are essential to the development of the car components. Model and pattern makers are craftsmen, practicing two of the few remaining skills learned only through years of apprenticeship. In late 1979 the first of three epidemiological investigations documenting for the first time potential excess cancer deaths among woodworkers was released by the Michigan Cancer Foundation (Swanson and Belle 1982). This study analyzed the 39 cancer deaths noted among wood pattern makers in one major auto manufacturer's wood shops between January 1970 and December 1978. The incidence of colon and rectal cancers and, in one location, of bladder cancer was greater than expected.

A second study, by the Memorial Sloan-Kettering Cancer Center (1979), covered the wood shops in 14 plants of a major auto manufacturer. Analysis of cancer deaths among workers in these shops indicated that colon and bladder cancer rates were higher than expected. The third study was conducted by the National Institute of Occupational Safety and Health (NIOSH) (Robinson, Waxweiler, and McCammon 1980). Broader in scope, it focused on cancer deaths among members of the Pattern Makers' League (PML), a union affiliated with the AFL-CIO, to which the majority of pattern makers in the United States belong. The NIOSH findings revealed a disproportionate number of deaths from brain tumors and colon cancer among pattern and model makers in general and from leukemia among those who worked predominately in wood shops. In contrast to the earlier studies, the NIOSH investigation indicated that the potential problem may not be restricted to workers in wood shops, but may also involve pattern makers working with metal.

These studies generated considerable news coverage in the Detroit area, especially because the workers at one wood shop sought out the media to assist in their efforts to highlight the excess cancer deaths at their location.

RESPONSE TO THE PROBLEM BY ONE AUTO MANUFACTURER

The internal response to the widely publicized findings was reflected in the actions of one company. First, a brief review was undertaken of all existing epidemiologic information relating cancer to any woodworking process. Findings indicated a strong association between furniture making and nasopharyngeal cancer, and a possible association between other types of woodworking and both stomach and hematopoietic cancers (Acheson 1976; Milham 1976). In addition, medical records of the company's active woodworkers were examined for evidence of cancer, revealing no unusual findings.

Concurrently, a series of meetings was initiated by the corporate Employee Health Services with NIOSH personnel and with the PML's national leadership to review findings and chart future directions. In these meetings, NIOSH recommended

---

Beverly G. Ware is a Corporate Health Education Programs Coordinator at Ford Motor Company in Dearborn, Michigan.

that several general work practices be immediately implemented and that workers in the wood shops be informed of the results of the three studies conducted to date. The initial meeting with the PML addressed the NIOSH report and recommendations, particularly focusing on how to inform the workers of the studies' results. It was agreed that the PML would develop written information to be used in one of its newsletters. This material would be reviewed with the company before publication. The possibility of a medical examination for the wood pattern makers was also discussed. The necessity for employee education was identified as an essential component of any medical testing efforts to be undertaken.

ENTER THE HEALTH EDUCATOR

The Employee Health Services of this automobile manufacturing company had, a few years earlier, employed a professionally trained, experienced health educator. She had been hired to develop and implement a pilot Cardiovascular Risk Intervention Program for salaried employees at the company's world headquarters complex. This position, although unique because there were no other health educators employed in the "private sector," was in reality a rather traditional health education activity. What made it different was (1) the organization itself, a very large and complex hierarchy that was not health-related and whose reason for being was to make a profit, and (2) the expectation that health education would achieve health behavior change as a result of programs implemented.

By a rather chance occurrence, the health educator had become involved with assisting in the form and content of informational programs being written and implemented to meet Occupational Safety and Health Administration (OSHA) standards. These standards, which regulated exposure and work practices to protect workers from specific occupational hazards known to be harmful to health, contained requirements for delivering specific information to workers and for training them. The health educator became a helpful source for translating the technical jargon of toxicologists, industrial hygienists, and physicians into wording a worker might easily understand. In subsequent projects, it became possible for the health educator to design the informational intervention itself.

When it came to informing the pattern makers about the results of the studies to date, the health educator was requested to join in the planning activities. She became a member of the Employee Health Services team working on this project, expressly to develop the informational program for employees.

In spring 1980, the company appointed a medical advisory committee of experts in cancer research, oncology, and occupational health from state universities, medical centers, and the state health department to examine the existing evidence concerning the situation and make recommendations for future company directions. An initial medical examination program was suggested as one of the activities to be implemented. Specific testing and data-gathering protocols were detailed in later meetings of this group.

This committee also emphasized the need to educate employees about the examination program prior to the examinations. To provide a better background for this educational effort, the health educator was appointed as the company's representative to the first conference called by the Worker's Institute on Safety and Health (WISH) for national and regional representatives of the PML. WISH, a newly formed organization, had received an OSHA "New Directions" grant to conduct training and educational activities. OSHA had requested WISH to assist the PML in developing an educational/medical surveillance program for union members. At that first conference the issues discussed concerning the education of pattern makers dealt primarily with the medical surveillance program, focusing on the following:

1. The scope of the information that workers should have in regard to health risks and work hazards: that is, how detailed and how technical the material should be.
2. Necessary information on the medical surveillance itself: the need for examinations, the nature of the testing, an explanation of procedures, and so on.

The two-day WISH meeting for regional presidents and representatives of the PML was held on a university campus. Also in attendance were medical, education, and labor consultants employed by WISH, along with representatives from the automobile industry. The primary purposes of the meeting were to discuss the history and current state of the cancer problem among pattern makers, to determine the needs to be met, and to introduce future program directions to be undertaken by WISH and the PML.

During the sessions it was emphasized that the education of the pattern makers was central to their understanding the need for and accepting the multiprocedure examinations. Because educational activities were thus seen as critical to alerting PML members of a potential threat to health and to gaining participation in the examinations, the health educator had a ready-made focus for the development of a program in the company. A series of meetings with company "team" members from the medical, industrial hygiene, toxicology, labor relations staffs, as well as local and national pattern makers' management staff, led to establishing the format and content for future sessions with the workers. The agreed primary purpose of the educational activity was to gain voluntary participation for the medical surveillance activities. To this end, workers would be provided with specific information on the events to date leading to this session. The industrial hygiene efforts underway would be discussed, but emphasis was to be given to the forthcoming medical examination. As a starting point, a comprehensive document would be prepared for employees and handed out at the information session so that workers could take it home and share it with their families. Timing of the informational program was a critical factor. The educational sessions were to be scheduled a week before the exams were to begin, so as to not lose the effect of the education as a motivating factor for participation. Each session, scheduled on work time, was to be limited to no more than 30 employees.

THE EDUCATIONAL INTERVENTION

Preparation for the educational sessions with employees included developing a detailed outline for the content and process of the meeting, designing a flip chart for use at the session, and synthesizing and editing the material to be included in the handout given to employees. Further, staff members participating in the sessions met together once to review their roles. Supervisory personnel, in concert with union representatives, arranged the scheduling of attendance for the 150 employees of the wood model shop at the company's Design Center. Because of the importance of the project and the attention it was receiving, it was decided that corporate staff members of the "team" would provide the primary staffing for the meetings, with staff from the center's medical department participating on a limited basis.

As planned, 6 one-hour sessions were conducted over a two-day period for all 150 employees, along with a number of company supervisory and local union personnel. A physician introduced the program. The health educator offered the initial information on intervention. She was followed by an industrial hygienist who discussed industrial hygiene activities, and by a physician who presented the concept of medical surveillance. The question-and-answer period of about 30 minutes resulted in lively discussions. To end the meeting, a nurse from the center gave brief instructions concerning the procedures to be followed for the guaiac test, and the health educator summarized the proceedings.

As mentioned previously, the main function of educational intervention was to stimulate motivation for voluntary employee participation in the medical screening activities, some of which would be rather unpleasant and uncomfortable. The procedures included pulmonary function testing, a sigmoidoscopy to 60 cm into the lower bowel with the use of a flexible tube instrument, and, for those over 50, a barium enema.

Although there is little evidence that information alone achieves behavior change (Mendelsohn 1973), considerable evidence exists to indicate that, in some kinds of situations, information is all that is needed to provide behavior change (Green et al. 1980: chap. 6; Hecht 1974). This was such a case. Even after the initial publicity, front-page newspaper articles on the subject appeared at least once a week for some time. Union representatives were knowledgeable about the problem and actively supported the medical surveillance program for PML members. Pattern makers were talking among themselves. One employee who had just returned to work after having a polyp removed was convinced of the importance of screening. Moreover, the company was scheduling free examinations at the worksite, on company time, with the colonoscopy being performed by specialists from a local hospital. Each employee would receive a report on the results of his or her exam by the physician at the location.

A total of 90 percent of the employees of the wood model shop had a complete medical examination. Those not participating were on medical leave or chose to have the test done by their own physician.

ROLE OF THE HEALTH EDUCATOR

It is important to remember that the health educator had already demonstrated her abilities in the company prior to this project by designing and implementing a successful and popular Cardiovascular Risk Intervention Program. Further, she already had considerable familiarity with OSHA standards and with information programs for employees concerning occupational health hazards. Her function was enhanced by an adequate diagnosis-and-needs assessment indicating that an educational effort was essential to a program's success. Because the issue was new and revealed that employees were potentially at considerable risk, it was necessary to proceed with recommendations having a sound scientific base and consonant with the interests of the union and the company.

The planning also included designing the educational program around the known constraints. There was, for example, the constraint of time: A one-session group intervention could take no more than one hour because employees were to be paid at overtime rates for attending before or after their work shifts. Content was dictated not only by the expressed purpose of achieving voluntary participation in the screening, but also by the information that various company and outside experts deemed essential.

Perhaps the most important role that a health educator has in such a situation is to construct an educational activity that will meet the objectives yet be based on sound theoretical principles, despite existing limitations. Although an unstructured group discussion or question-and-answer format would not be feasible or acceptable, a *structured* group meeting in which a question period is provided is suitable. Employees are accustomed both to formal methods of relating to supervisory and management personnel and to formal training activities.

A well-designed educational program effort, even as limited in scope as a meeting with a handout, is based on scientific principles. Skillful use of theories such as the health belief model (Rosenstock 1974), fear in seeking medical treatment (Leventhal, Singer, and Jones 1965), changing attitudes (Fishbein 1967), and the cognitive processing model (McGuire 1978) provide ample evidence to support the provision of a wide range of information programs.

In a large company, where only one health educator is employed, initial development of an educational activity that others will eventually use is a primary role for the educator. Thus, in designing an educational intervention, the educator must take into account that other staff, many of whom will have no background in health education, will be conducting the program and that every detail must therefore be as explicit as possible. The health educator will usually be able to undertake initial implementation of the program to test it out and to train staff to conduct the educational activity. This was true of the program for the workers in the wood model shop. And in this case the health educator's effort was but one of many educational activities being directed toward the employees. Attendance at the medical exams was the result of a variety of influences. Many people provided reinforcement and support. Employees were also exposed to messages from several sources. The overriding concern about the threat of cancer was apparent in all communications. To ease that concern, the company offered an examination that was specifically directed toward looking for potential or existing problems needing attention.

IMPACT OF THE PROGRAM

After the woodworkers in the initial group were screened, the company decided to offer screening to additional groups of employees: those who had prior work experience in the wood shops and were now in supervisory positions or in other departments, and other wood and metal pattern makers in the company. The educational activity was undertaken by physicians and nurses in the medical facilities of the unit responsible for the screening. The informational material, including the flip chart presentation, was used, being modified as necessary for a specific group. The health educator ceased being active in the program, except for consultation.

Not surprisingly, the rate of participation began to dwindle to about 55 percent of those eligible for screening as time went by. Two factors appeared to be responsible for the decline: lack of front-page coverage on the topic by newspapers, and no dramatic occurrence (i.e., newly discovered cancer in the initial group of examinees) to spur action. Perhaps the realization, now dawning, that the problem was not as widespread as first thought and feared also had some effect in reducing the urgency for the exam.

As for the health educator, more of her time was now devoted to educational efforts in the area of potential and existing health hazards. New kinds of programs were developed, spanning a wide range of audiovisual methods and materials.

From this experience, it was possible to draw the following conclusions:

1. The health educator in a corporate setting must work within the constraints of the organization and the particular presenting situation. Learning to live with one-shot information programs may be a requisite.
2. The health educator must build credibility in demonstrating the need for the content and process of health education. Knowledge of scientific literature to provide support for his or her recommendations is essential for the successful conduct of programs.
3. Complex problems do not yield to simple solutions. Education will usually be only one of the many interventions being tried. It may be that the specific contribution of the educational activity will not or cannot be measured.
4. The health educator must learn to effectively use resources existing in the corporation, and, further, to coordinate separate entities toward a common purpose in which all have an interest.
5. Though responsible for developing educational activities, the health educator will likely have little control over any other aspect of the program, even that which will affect the provision of the educational component.

REFERENCES

Acheson, E. D. 1976. "Nasal Cancer in the Furniture and Boot and Shoe Manufacturing Industries." *Preventive Medicine* 5:295–315.

Fishbein, M. 1967. "Attitudes and the Prediction of Behavior." In *Readings in Attitude Theory and Measurement*, edited by M. Fishbein. New York: Wiley.

Green, L. W.; Kreuter, M. W.; Deeds, S. G.; and Partridge, K. B. 1980. *Health Education Planning: A Diagnostic Approach*. Palo Alto, Calif.: Mayfield.

Hecht, A. B. 1974. "Improving Medication Compliance by Teaching Outpatients." *Nursing Forum* 13:112–129.

Leventhal, H.; Singer, R.; and Jones, S. 1965. "Effect of Fear and Specificity of Recommendation upon Attitudes and Behavior." *Journal of Personality and Social Psychology* 2(1):20–29.

McGuire, W. J. 1978. "An Information-Processing Model of Advertising Effectiveness." In *Behavioral and Management Science in Marketing*, edited by H. L. Davis and A. J. Silk. New York: Wiley.

Memorial Sloan-Kettering Cancer Center. 1979. "Report of Wood Shops in 14 Detroit Area Plants." Typescript, New York.

Mendelsohn, H. 1973. "Some Reasons Why Information Campaigns Can Succeed." *Public Opinion Quarterly* 37(1):50–61.

Milham, S. 1976. *Occupational Mortality in Washington State, 1950–1971*, vol. 1. NIOSH Research Report 76–175A. Washington, D.C.: U.S. Department of Health, Education, and Welfare, National Institute for Occupational Safety and Health.

Robinson, C.; Waxweiler, R. J.; and McCammon, C. 1980. "Pattern and Model Makers, Proportionate Mortality, 1972–1978." *American Journal of Industrial Medicine* 1:159–165.

Rosenstock, I. M. 1974. "The Health Belief Model and Preventive Health Behavior." *Health Education Monographs* 2:354–386.

Swanson, G. M., and Belle, S. H. 1982. "Cancer Morbidity among Woodworkers in the U.S. Automotive Industry." *Journal of Occupational Medicine* 24:315–319.

Analysis

This case documents the implementation of a program designed to stimulate voluntary participation in a cancer screening program for those who appeared to be at greater than expected risk for colon and rectal cancer. The health educator's role included assessing needs, designing materials, and presenting the program as part of a team to the employees. In addition to this explicit role, the health educator's activities should be considered in relation to her role as a representative of the company.

A number of theories are identified in the case as providing the basis for the design of the educational intervention. For example, the health belief model is cited. Although Ware does not state explicitly how it was used, we can assume that the educational sessions were intended to convince employees of the seriousness of rectal/colon cancer, their susceptibility to it, and the benefits of participating in the cancer surveillance (Becker 1974). It is important to note that, as Ware states, programs should be based on sound theoretical principles despite existing limitations. Here organizational structure and purpose put immediate limitations on how the program was to be implemented.

A basic strategy throughout this case was the use of multiple methods and multiple sources of information. When the latter are used, the message must be consistent, otherwise the target population may be confused and reject all messages (Green 1978). The health educator used a number of professional operating procedures that led to the success of the program (90 percent of employees were examined). These included meetings with the employees' union and the company "team" that was to carry out the program. She also employed basic principles of planning, such as performing both an educational and an organizational needs assessment. The latter was conducted to determine the constraints that could affect the program. The program needed a sound scientific base but also had to reflect both company and union interests.

There are two compelling reasons for integrating health education into occupational settings. First, both formal and informal training are common at the worksite to improve job performance. The work setting provides a central place where education can be provided efficiently and effectively (Kassim 1983). Group dynamics can be readily used because natural groups are often a part of the work setting. "The working group is one of the major types of social groups, and social interaction at work is one of the main forms of social interaction" (Argyle 1972:104).

The second reason for integrating health education into occupational settings is that work and the work environment constitute a major determinant of well-being. Today, the effects of many industrial toxicants and hazardous conditions are well known. Less clear is how the occupational setting influences the development and outcome of diseases and illnesses that have traditionally been viewed as nonoccupational disorders.

Given the worksite as an appropriate setting for education as well as a possible source of disease, the role of the health educator employed in industry becomes crucial. As an employee of the organization, the health educator must work within the context of the organization. The educator's superiors either explicitly or implicitly demand that his or her prime allegiance be to the organization rather than to the employees. That can be an uncomfortable role. But this is not to say the health educator should not try to influence organization policy. Rather, it is a cautionary note that the health educator may well be an expendable commodity. The obvious task is to convince the organization that a healthy workforce is in the organization's best interest. This can be quite difficult, if not impossible, if an organization has a low investment in its employees.

In this case we might ask: Why didn't the health educator work to investigate the cause of cancer? It is likely that her options were limited.

Experience suggests that the dramatic gesture of sacrificing a job for principle rarely results in needed change. This does not mean that persons should not leave a position if they disagree with the policies or practices. It means that change is more likely to occur if one stays with a difficult situation and pecks away at the issues over time. The decision to stay or not to stay is a reality most health educators face more than once in their career.

References/Select Resources

Argyle, M. 1972. *The Social Psychology of Work.* Baltimore: Penguin.

This book, first published in Great Britain, discusses a variety of topics that would be of interest to health educators who either are employed by or serve as consultants to large industrial organizations. These topics include job satisfaction, group work, personality and work, the effects of technology, and worker motivation.

Becker, M. H. 1974. "The Health Belief Model and Personal Behavior." *Health Education Monographs* 2(4):409–419.

This paper outlines the health belief model and describes the research up to the early 1970s that has contributed to its modifications. The health belief model has been used to explain sick role behavior as well as preventive health behavior and still plays a prominent role in health education research.

Green, L. W. 1978. "Determining the Impact and Effectiveness of Health Education as It Relates to Federal Policy." *Health Education Monographs* 6 (suppl. 1):28–66.

This important policy paper presents a number of recommendations to support the development of health education policy. Green offers a concise review of past health education research that has helped formulate such principles as using multiple methods to achieve a single goal.

Kassim, K. 1983. "Genetic Testing and Chemical Hypersusceptibility in the Workplace." *Urban Health* 12(2):36–41.

Kassim explores the ethical and legal ramifications of using genetic testing of employees to identify workers who may be most at risk for occupationally related diseases. The discussion involves minorities, women, and job discrimination.

Miaoulis, G., and Bonaguro, J. 1980. "Marketing Strategies in Health Education." *Journal of Health Care Marketing* 1 (Winter):35–44.

The authors integrate planning models for health education with marketing planning models. Tables and figures illustrate how current methodology in health education may be augmented by the basic marketing principles. Clearly written, the article is valuable for both students and practitioners. It emphasizes needs assessment, the planning process, and the monitoring of consumer actions. It is particularly useful for those who may have responsibility for marketing health education programs to industry.

Parkinson, R. S.; Beck, R. N. Collings, G. H.; Eriksen, M.; Green, L. W.; McGill, A. M.; Merwin, D.; Pearson, C. E.; and Ware, B. G. 1982. *Managing Health Promotion in the Workplace: Guidelines for Implementation and Evaluation.* Palo Alto, Calif.: Mayfield.

This book provides guidelines for implementing and evaluating workplace health promotion programs generally, as well as background papers on specific content areas. Chapters 4–20 provide short descriptions of company programs, including the Ford Motor Company's Cardiovascular Risk Intervention Program.

Society for Public Health Education, Inc., and Association for the Advancement of Health Education. 1981. *Health Education of the Public in the 80's.* Reston, Va.

This joint offering of two professional associations provides an overview of the status of health and the problems associated with improving health. The gap between consumer knowledge and health practices is demonstrated with supporting research. The role of health education in bridging that gap is discussed, and programs in a variety of settings are described: medical care settings, work settings, and schools. Directions for the future are outlined for improved health education practice.

Discussion Questions

1. Assume you work for the Pattern Makers' League. Write an article for the union's newsletter, informing the members about the results of the NIOSH study.

2. Develop a flip chart, or other appropriate tool, to provide necessary information to the pattern makers about a screening examination for colon cancer. You will have their attention during 15 minutes at the lunch break.

3. Identify ways in which the company, through its policy and practices, cooperated with the health educator in planning and implementing the educational intervention in this case.

4. Ware states that in this case information was all that was "needed to provide behavior change." Identify the factors that made this situation possible.

5. Ware has identified several theories useful in designing the educational intervention in this case. Specify how you would use these theories in developing a similar educational intervention.

The Total Life Concept

Molly McCauley, R.N., B.A.

One of the great challenges for a workplace health promotion program is to develop solid support for the program within the culture of the organization. This backing should include not only a willingness to provide a variety of wellness and/or disease prevention programs but also a commitment to change within the organization itself to provide an environment conducive to individual change. The Total Life Concept Program (TLCP) of AT&T Communications began with this basic premise.

BEGINNINGS

For several years the Medical Department had been offering a number of individual wellness programs. But we had never focused enough on each component to evaluate it properly and thus justify our approach. Hence we began to put together what we hoped would be a total wellness program. At about the same time AT&T was beginning a process of massive change as a result of the divestiture taking place in the Bell System. Because we were now becoming a market-driven organization, we needed to be able to help employees step up to the corporate changes. Management, by recognizing the impact that these changes would have on employees, was now looking for ways to help employees through this transition. Although thoughts turned to the development of a stress management program, the Medical Department was inclined more toward a comprehensive integrated program.

Managers would have to be convinced not only that they needed to accept the health promotion issue in philosophy, but that we as a business and new organization would have to carry out health promotion as part of our culture. (We define *culture* as an integrated pattern of human behavior that develops over time. Culture formation involves a learning process and a sharing of common goals and activities.) That is, our business would have to support positive health practices through developing and maintaining environmental supports. Therefore one of the program components would be to build environmental support for the overall program.

Our corporate medical director was instrumental in getting management to understand the basic concept we were developing. The medical director presented the case for the program at a meeting with one of the vice-presidents, who then became an advocate for the program with upper management.

To support our case, we developed a Management of Change Approach proposal. This approach provided for (1) a wellness program, (2) corporate cultural support, and (3) integration of individual and organizational health. Our first step in the process was to document the scope of the problem facing AT&T Communications as of November 1982.

- In 1983, Communications medical insurance will increase 30 percent.
- During 1980, seven categories of largely preventable disease cost Communications 74.8 years of lost productivity and approximately $2.5 million due to disability.
- One third of the total disability days were due to stress-related illness during 1980.

Molly McCauley is a Staff Manager of Health Promotion/Health Education at AT&T Communications in Bedminster, New Jersey.

Table 1
Potential Cost Savings from the Total Life Concept Program

Disorder	Savings
Malignant neoplasms—colon, rectum, breast, and reproductive system	$2,477,980
Malignant neoplasms—respiratory	$ 239,635
Low back disorders	$ 677,126
Ischemic heart disease	$ 895,254
Neurotic and stress-related disorders	$ 597,190
Total savings/year	$4,887,200*
Total program cost/year	$2,202,500*
Net savings/year	$2,684,700*

*Rounded out.

Next we projected the cost savings potential of the program on the basis of conservative estimates of savings for health care and disability costs (Table 1).

We received the go-ahead for the development of a pilot program in late 1982. Four months elapsed between the approval by upper management and the monitoring of the program. Our program was offered at two sites: Bedminster, New Jersey, and Kansas City, Missouri. Our research design for each project site was as follows:

Group 1 (Study Group)
- Receives Health Risk Appraisal as a pretest
- Participates in program intervention
- Receives Health Risk Appraisal as a posttest

Group 2 (Control)
- Receives Health Risk Appraisal as a pretest
- Receives Health Risk Appraisal as a posttest

Group 3 (Control)
- Receives Health Risk Appraisal as a posttest

After a marketing campaign to attract employees, a three-hour orientation session was offered. At this session we discussed the development of the program and what would take place during the course of the program. A film entitled "Wellness Lifestyle" was also presented. At the end of that session employees completed a Health Risk Appraisal. However, before doing so, they were oriented to the purpose of the appraisal—that is, what it does and what it doesn't do, how it fits into the health care delivery system, what they would gain from completing it, and how it would be used for the program.

We used a commercially available Health Risk Appraisal to which we added a number of questions to explore health and job attitudes. For example: How do you feel about your job; about the company you work for; and about your supervisor and co-workers? Do you feel responsible for your health? How much do you feel in control of your health? Do you feel you can change things?

After the employees received a written report on their risk appraisal, they were invited back in large groups (150 employees per group) to receive a verbal presentation with slides, which explained in simple terms the written report. (In using the Health Risk Appraisal, it is important to clarify the longevity report because people tend to focus on when they are going to die rather than on ways to change so as to promote longevity.) The employees in the study groups then began the individualized programs that will be described in the next section. All the programs are done on company time, and the employees do not pay for any of them. However, for our final recommendations we will be looking at other options.

THE PROGRAM

The Health Risk Appraisal as a pretest and posttest instrument will provide medical and behavioral indicators to enable us to evaluate the impact of our program. After employees complete the pretest, they complete the Total Life Concept Wellness Orientation and Planning Booklet. This booklet allows the employee to develop an individualized program. There are five steps in the booklet:

1. *Assessment:* Here employees explore their knowledge and attitudes, their skills, their relation to their culture, and the support and reward systems available to them.
2. *Identification:* This step helps the employees determine where they need to be in relation to the assessment. The employees identify

specific goals for norms, skills, and support. These goals will represent their TLCP.

3. *Development:* In this step the employees choose where to begin, write a program for change, and make a commitment to success by signing a TLCP contract, if they so desire.
4. *Implementation:* This step provides the employees with the opportunity to sign up for programs, support groups, task forces, and leadership committees.
5. *Transfer:* The final step enables the employees to apply skills gained in one part of their TLCP to another area. This promotes the concept that the TLCP is not an isolated event but rather an ongoing process for realizing their potential.

Ten self-help courses are offered through the TLCP:

1. Exercise—for Fitness, for Fun, for Health
2. Taking the Ache out of Backache
3. Overweight? Reshape Your Shape
4. Cease Fire (Smoking Cessation)
5. High Blood Pressure—A Little Is Too Much
6. Cholesterol: Facts and Fancies
7. Catch Cancer Early
8. Coping with Stress: How to Climb out of the Pressure Cooker
9. Person-to-Person: The Art of Good Communication
10. Alcohol and Drugs—Have You Had Enough?

As an example, the exercise program consists of 3 one-hour sessions per week. An orientation session acquaints the employee with the goals, requirements, and benefits of the program. After the employee is tested and evaluated for exercise capacity and needs, a personal exercise program is designed. The employee then engages in exercise sessions three times a week, using the organization's fitness center. Periodic "knowledge" sessions are offered to sharpen understanding of the value of exercise and how to fit it into one's schedule. Exercise capacity is reevaluated, along with achievements and future needs. Finally, a plan is suggested to continue an exercise program outside of the course. Employees who enroll in the course are required to attend the orientation session, participate in at least 30 of 36 sessions, prearrange absences with the program leader, and attend two of the three "knowledge" sessions.

CLOSING THOUGHTS

At present the pilot phase of the TLCP is still going on and results are not yet available. But we are gratified by the high participation rate. About 600 employees have participated in the study groups at each site, with a total of 1,500 employees serving as controls. Management not only has been generous with company time but has visibly supported the program by providing space and facilities. In addition, changes have been made to support the program: for instance, the fare in the cafeteria and in vending machines has improved, and exercise breaks have been incorporated into meetings. Our program has had a strong start during its first year, and we believe that when the data are in, they will show we have met our goal: to motivate change that will result in healthy employees supported by a healthy organization.

Analysis

This case is an excellent demonstration of the necessity for developing a strong proposal to influence or persuade corporate management to support a health promotion program. If we look at the scope of the problem documented by McCauley, it is readily apparent that considerable work and cooperation were needed to develop this part of the proposal. Access to the requisite information is very important, and in this case information was needed on insurance costs and projections, the cost of disorders, and disability and productivity data. Obtaining this type of information requires the assistance of a number of departments in the organization besides the medical one. These other departments could possibly include those concerned with human resources and fiscal management. The health educator should develop linkages throughout the corporation not only to guarantee success of the program once it is operational but also to generate the data necessary to build a case for the program with the decision makers.

One of the most interesting concepts that emerges from this case is that of the organization's culture. For the health educator, understanding the culture is as important in a worksite setting as it is in an international setting. As we stated in the introduction to Part 4, culture sets the pattern for a company's activities, opinions, and actions. It also determines what is acceptable behavior among the various levels of employees. For example, is it acceptable for a health educator on the staff of a medical department to request an appointment with an executive vice-president to discuss ideas for a comprehensive health promotion program? In the McCauley case, we see that that would probably not have been acceptable. Rather, the medical director met with a vice-president who then promoted the project to upper management. Further, the health educator must attempt to determine what there is in the corporate culture that may either facilitate or hinder the development of the total program or some of its components.

The McCauley case also illustrates the importance of trying to incorporate the concepts of health promotion into the corporate culture. If this attempt succeeds, health-promoting activities become more than just a frill or an employee benefit; they become a corporate expectation. For example, at the upper management level at Pepsico, health promotion appears to have become part of the corporate culture. As *Business Week* notes, "Pepsi executives are expected to be physically fit as well as mentally alert: Pepsi employs four physical-fitness instructors at its headquarters, and a former executive says it is an unwritten rule that to get ahead in the company a manager must stay in shape" (Anonymous, 1980:154).

It is indeed a great task to influence or change corporate culture. But there was a unique opportunity at AT&T to influence culture just at the time health promotion was being developed. This corporation, as McCauley notes, was undergoing an upheaval as a result of the breakup of the Bell System. AT&T was now faced with becoming a market-driven company. This situation clearly necessitated a change in culture if the company was to successfully compete in the marketplace. The opportunity was at hand for new elements to become part of the corporate culture.

Two other issues that emerge in this case are the appropriate use of the Health Risk Appraisal and the question of time in planning and implementing a program. The Health Risk Appraisal was used very judiciously. It was well recognized that participants needed to be briefed before completing the appraisal and debriefed and counseled afterward. The appraisal was used appropriately as an evaluation tool and as an aid to assist employees in planning their own program.

In this case as well as the Cantlon case (p. 332), we see a program being rapidly implemented after approval. It is difficult to say whether there is greater pressure on a health educator to produce results in a corporate setting than in other settings. In a corporate setting, resources may often be marshaled very quickly, thus facilitating rapid implementation. Indeed, in regard to both the McCauley and the Cantlon case, it was probably a combination of the pressure for results and the available resources that contributed to the program's rapid development and implementation.

References/Select Resources

Anonymous. 1980. "Corporate Culture: The Hard-to-Change Values That Spell Success or Failure." *Business Week*, October 27:148–160.

This article was one of the first to legitimate the concept of corporate culture. Several vignettes demonstrate the effects of culture on an organization. Among these vignettes is one that points out the necessity for AT&T to adapt its culture to changing circumstances.

Peters, T. J., and Waterman, R. H. 1982. *In Search of Excellence*. New York: Harper & Row.

This best seller on what makes a successful corporation explores corporate culture in depth. In fact, the authors state that excellent companies are culturally driven and therefore function in accordance with rigidly shared values.

Discussion Questions

1. Why is the concept of corporate culture important in this case? How would you go about determining the corporate culture of an organization?

2. What are some other ways, besides those mentioned in this case, in which an organization could support healthful practices among its employees?

3. In addition to using the Health Risk Appraisal, how else would you evaluate this program's impact on the employees? How would you evaluate the impact on the organization?

4. Outline a marketing campaign to attract employees to a worksite health promotion program.

5. What additional self-help courses would you suggest be offered as part of a worksite health promotion program?

Reach Out for Health

Angelica Cantlon, B.S., M.S., R.D.

This case will describe the planning and the first-year implementation of a worksite health promotion program at Southern New England Telephone (SNET). The company employs 14,000 people in the state of Connecticut, 5,500 of whom work in the New Haven area, where the main office is located.

BACKGROUND

Most telephone companies make a sizable investment to train their employees. Training programs are given on company time, as are some educational programs not directly related to work. SNET is no exception to this general practice.

The leadership of SNET has a history of looking at issues from the long-term perspective. Therefore neither the notion of the company investing in a series of programs on health nor the idea of investing in a program with a long-term payoff was foreign to this administration.

In 1979 a new medical director was brought in who devised and instituted an overall Corporate Health Strategy that in the first two years saved the company approximately $3 million. The Health Promotion Program was preceded by three other major components of this strategy: the Medical Disability Monitoring System, the Safety Program, and the Alcohol Rehabilitation Program.

The purpose of the Medical Disability Monitoring System is to ensure that both ill and injured employees return to work as soon as they are able to safely perform some type of work. Introduced in late 1980, this system for monitoring and selectively challenging questionable disability cases resulted in a 22 percent decrease in benefit absence, which equates to a net savings to the company (after expenses) of over $1 million per year in disability wage payments.

The developers of the Safety Program took a close look at on-the-job accidents at SNET. In 1981 it was estimated that the total direct and indirect costs of such accidents were at least $4.8 million. In just the first six months of a well-designed comprehensive intervention program, occupational accidents were reduced by 27 percent. The program includes enforcing proper safety procedures and use of appropriate safety gear (hard hat, eye goggles, safety straps, etc.) during performance of specified jobs, instituting the use of safety belts in company motor vehicles, and providing an intensive Drivers' Education course for all employees who use company cars. The net savings to the company is nearly $1 million per year. Plans are now being developed for extending the program to prevent off-the-job accidents.

The Alcohol Rehabilitation Program offers counseling for employees with problems of alcoholism or drug abuse. It is estimated that the annual net savings to the company are over $1 million.

Each of these programs is oriented to monitoring, requires disciplinary action to some extent, and directly affects health costs to the company.

HEALTH PROMOTION PROGRAM

In January 1982 one of SNET's more progressive general managers, a person known for initiating and pioneering many innovative programs, ap-

---

Angelica Cantlon is Manager of Health Promotion/Cost Control at Southern New England Telephone in New Haven, Connecticut.

proached the medical director with a request for a pilot Health Promotion Program for his 400 Network Engineering employees. Once the program was approved, I was brought in as a health promotion consultant to design and implement the program in a timely fashion.

PILOT PROGRAM

Initially, we set up focus groups with various cross sections of the population to determine what their perceptions and expectations of a health promotion program were and what kinds of components would interest them. The information pointed to a program that would first assess their health status and then offer such components as fitness, nutrition, weight control, stress management, and smoking cessation. The focus groups also mentioned a need for cafeteria changes, specifically more low-calorie choices.

Armed with this information, we designed materials, formatted publicity campaigns, developed audiovisual presentations, and trained appropriate staff to screen employees and to provide the program. We also set up suitable locations; for instance, by using screens, we transformed a hall into the Health Screening Area and partitioned the open space for intervention programs.

During the early part of May, employees were exposed to a variety of posters and flyers announcing the upcoming program, which we dubbed "Health 80s." In orientation sessions given by the medical director to groups of 50–60 employees, the components of the program were fully explained in an upbeat and visually appealing manner. Employees took part in three-minute fitness breaks, were given apples and balloons, and were asked to turn in a sign-up card for a health screening appointment before leaving the orientation session.

Within one to three days each employee was called to set up an appointment for a 45-minute health screening (held on company time) to be conducted within two weeks. On the day of the screening appointment the employee came to the reception area, with a completed life-style questionnaire, and proceeded through seven screening stations to determine the following: height/weight, body fat, blood pressure, smoker's lung, lung capacity, fitness, and blood chemistry for a SMAC 24. Each measurement was performed by one of SNET's occupational nurses. After the last station the screenee received orange juice and a roll while his or her questionnaire was reviewed by an exit interviewer to ensure all tests had been done and the questionnaire was completed. At the exit interview, each screenee made a counseling appointment for the following week.

The individualized health counseling sessions were conducted by SNET's occupational nurses. During the 45-minute session (on company time), the employee was given a health risk profile that documented his/her clinical and life-style data; a catalogue of courses was reviewed, with the nurse suggesting which ones might be best on the basis of the risk profile; and the employee's questions were answered. On leaving the counseling room, the employee signed up and gave a deposit for courses that were recommended by the nurse and/or those that particularly interested the employee.

Screening and counseling were held from May through June, with risk reduction programs beginning the last week in June. These programs, on half company/half personal time, included Fitness (aerobic dance, walk/jog, running), Healthy Back, Nutrition Awareness, Weight Control, Basic Stress Management, Stop Smoking, and a film/lecture series given by community organizations (e.g., American Heart Association, American Cancer Society, American Lung Association).

An overwhelming number (78 percent) of the population participated in the program. There was a constant buzz throughout this particular work group about Health 80s. Walking with peers during the lunch hour became more popular then sitting in the cafeteria. Managers and staff were saying that attitude and morale were more positive, and there was an observable improvement in productivity. In general, employees were saying they never felt better and that Health 80s was the best thing SNET had ever done for them.

In six months' time 65 percent of this original group were retested. There were three outstanding findings:

- Fifty-one percent fewer smokers
- A loss of 0.3 tons of fat
- Eighty-one percent of the screened employees physically fit versus 19 percent during the first screening (data based on the step test)

Table 1
Screening Measurements

Focus of Screening	Procedure	Function of Procedure
Height/weight	Beam balance scale	Measures height/weight
Body fat	Large skinfold calipers	Measures three sites to determine fat and lean ratio
Blood pressure	Sphygmomanometer and cuff	Measures blood pressure systolic/diastolic
Smoker's lung	Co-Span Analyzer	Measures carbon monoxide present in the lung of a smoker
Lung capacity	DataMed Spirometer using an Apple Computer with screen and printer readout	Measures lung capacity
Fitness	Step test	Determines changes in pulse rate; pulse checked immediately before and after three-minute step test performed to a metered beat
	Sit and reach	Measures flexibility
Blood chemistry	Venipuncture	Evaluates fasting blood sugar, triglycerides, total cholesterol, HDL (high-density lipoprotein), LDL (low-density lipoprotein), and HDL:LDL ratio

However, the company did not wait for these six-month data in deciding to make this program corporatewide. The reasons: The Health Promotion Program was obviously benefiting these 400 SNET employees; SNET knows its employees are its best asset; and SNET believes its employees deserve programs to maintain their health. Accordingly, the company launched a corporatewide Health Promotion Program for all levels of management and nonmanagement. In addition, the program was another component established under the overall Corporate Health Strategy. The case was made that because the first three programs had led to such large cost savings, some of the money could be reinvested in a Health Promotion Program that offered an even greater potential for cost savings down the road.

September 1982 was a landmark month for SNET: Top management made a commitment to a comprehensive corporate-based program for the company's 14,000 employees. Having this commitment, plus strong financial support of $3 million over three years and a respected medical director who had an established track record, we launched our Reach Out for Health program. Although we had accomplished much of the groundwork during the pilot program, we needed time to reevaluate each phase of the program to ensure its viability on a broad-based scale.

PLANNING

January 1983 was chosen as the starting date for the program; so from August to December, planning was under way.

We decided to offer the program during the first year to our 5,500 employees in New Haven, because this was the site of corporate headquarters and had the largest number of employees in any given area. During the next two years we would introduce the program in all other areas of the state, with employee populations in any one area ranging from 50 to 2,000.

Having chosen our first site, we hired staff for operating and conducting the program. The operations staff comprised a manager, a publicity coordinator, a facilities planner, a registration assistant, and clerks. The technical staff, responsible for developing, marketing, and conducting the program, was composed of a clinical/counseling coordinator, a nutritionist, exercise physiologists, physical educators, and several health educators. Most members of the technical staff had master's degrees in their respective fields and work experience in the corporate environment. As the program grew, supervisory responsibility was required to oversee the per diem staff who provided the program throughout the state. All health promotion staff other than the manager of health promotion and the manager of operations were contracted staff.

With New Haven as the first site of the program and with staff in place, we were ready to get our program moving.

AWARENESS AND MARKETING

A massive publicity campaign was mounted to arouse interest, sell the concept of health promotion, and offer information about Reach Out for Health. All the resources available to SNET were used during this phase, including posters, flyers, bulletins, newswire (information via telephone number), in-house newspaper, closed circuit television, videos, and the local newspaper.

In addition, we conducted orientation sessions, as in the pilot program, for large groups (200–300 employees). We developed a highly animated slide presentation that not only offered information about the program but included motivational techniques. The presentation was humorous, yet serious, and it touched individuals in a personal manner by relating to real-life health issues of stress, overweight, and cigarette smoking. It let them know there were not only answers but a support system—their company itself and their co-workers—that would help them achieve a higher level of both mental and physical fitness. It gave them a chance to make a permanent, positive health behavior change. A short fitness break followed, to the music of "Rocky" and Olivia Newton-John's "Let's Get Physical." Employees were psyched up, involved, ready to do something.

At this meeting each employee was given a packet of information: a program overview, instructional pamphlet, life-style questionnaire, and screening appointment sign-up card. On completion of the sign-up card, the employees took their first step toward a healthier tomorrow and "earned an apple."

PERSONALIZING

As in the pilot program, employees were screened and counseled within three weeks after the orientation session. The only major change was that this time the lab analysis covered only FBS, triglyceride, total cholesterol, and HDL and LDL (see Table 1 for further explanation). The SMAC 24 was too comprehensive a set of measurements, given the prevention-oriented approach of this program. A Hemoccult test and a nutrition analysis were added to the screening and completed on each employee.

Both screening and counseling were again provided by SNET's 17 occupational nurses, who rotated on a weekly basis (only five nurses were required during any given week of screening).

Counseling has a threefold purpose:

1. To assess and review with the employee his/her health status on the basis of life-style information and clinical data.
2. To refer high-risk persons to a physician or other health care professional as deemed appropriate (e.g., a hypertensive to an M.D., an alcoholic to a professional in Employee Assistance).
3. To recommend the health education and/or fitness program (22 programs in total) most likely to maintain or improve the employee's health. In some cases a community resource might be suggested. On completion of counseling, the employee registers for the recommended program(s) and gives a deposit.

As in the pilot program, screening and counseling continue to sustain a high participation rate of 75 percent. Both components are on company time. Some 45 to 50 percent of the employees participate in company-based health education and fitness programs. These programs are held at the various company building sites, are held on the employees' own time (before or after work and during lunchtime), and cost from $10 to $35, a fee that is partially paid by the company (60 percent company expense, 40 percent employee expense).

Table 2
Courses Offered in Reach Out for Health Program

Title	Course Format	Course Description
Nutrition Awareness	6 weeks Module 1: 1 hr/wk Module 2: ½ hr twice a week	Didactic/participatory work on consumer issues, labels, purchase of vitamins; dietary guidelines
Keep It Off	8 weeks Module 1: 1 hr/wk Module 2: ½ hr twice a week	Techniques for modifying behavior, changing attitude, and generating motivation, as well as meal planning based on food preferences
Nutrition Potpourri Pressure Cooker Nutrition Nonsense	Each nutrition course meets 1 hr/wk over 2–3 weeks	Compilation of targeted subject matters in nutrition
Stop Smoking System	8 days	Variety of methods and techniques in a skill-oriented approach to the quitting process
Listen to Yourself	8 weeks 1 hr/wk	Variety of techniques to reduce stress: relaxation, biofeedback, visual imagery, assertiveness, communication skills
Joy	All fitness classes meet 2–3 times per week ongoing	Aerobic dance class, primarily for women
Stretch Out and Strengthen		Exercises for stretching and strengthening of major muscle groups; includes aerobic portion; not choreographed, but done to music
Peer Walking		Walks with peers on specified routes as an aerobic workout
Nautilus/Swimming		Fitness programs offered by YMCAs throughout the state

Most programs have a reward system of reimbursement for employees who attend 80 percent of the classes and meet their personal goals (e.g., a six-month cessation of smoking, an improved pulse rate during fitness training, a maintained weight loss at six months and one year). The reimbursement is one half the initial cost in the form of a Reach Out for Health gift certificate that can be reinvested in another course of their choice. The variety of courses offered is shown in Table 2.

In addition to the courses listed in the table, other programs have been specifically designed for target groups. For example, we have offered a Back Safety Program to certain work groups who have a high incidence of back disability and injury owing to the nature of their job (Line and Cable; Installation and Repair). The program has two aims:

1. To educate these employees about body mechanics; that is, how they use their body to perform a certain job.
2. To teach them particular exercises that stretch and strengthen the back and supporting muscles (e.g., abdominals).

Other work groups, such as Operator and Directory Assistance, are extremely sedentary in a

Table 2 *continued*

Title	Course Format	Course Description
Consumer Issues/ Self-Care	8 weeks 1 hr/wk	Guidance in using the medical system and in understanding medical benefits and self-care techniques (i.e., first aid, medications, etc.)
Dual Role: Working and Parenting	6 weeks 1 hr/wk	Techniques for helping the working parent manage time and stress—deal with priorities and make problem-solving decisions
Parenting	6 weeks 1 hr/wk	Strategies used in parenting, based on natural and logical situations, to avoid family conflicts and power struggles
Family Wellness	8 weeks 1 hr/wk	Discussion of health issues for the family, including stress, nutrition, self-care, dental health
Older Adult	6–8 weeks 1 hr/wk	Strategies for dealing with issues of aging, providing for the elderly parent, and similar issues

high-stress, productivity-measured job. Courses for them are designed to relieve lower back and neck strain as well as the tension that comes with the work. In addition, five-minute videos have been produced that promote overall relaxation. These are available for use in the lounge area.

Still other work groups, such as Sales Reps, are constantly on the road during the day. A self-help computerized fitness and diet program, based on their exercise and food preferences, designs a progressively advancing fitness plan and balanced-diet plan. They can use this program on their own time with co-workers and/or with their families.

Environmental support is also of extreme importance to reinforce and maintain changed behavior. To that end we have developed the following:

1. A Corporate Smoking Policy offers guidelines for smoking and nonsmoking areas within the company.
2. A Cafeteria Program highlights low-calorie, low-cholesterol, low-fat food choices while educating the employees about food and nutrition through posters and flyers distributed every week in the cafeterias.
3. A Family Wellness Program offers support at home, with spouse and children participating, in the areas of meals, communication, exercise, self-care, and dental health.

EFFECTS OF THE PROGRAM

What difference has this program made in the health habits and the health status of employees? For the latter we await long-term data about the participants. We are currently analyzing data on short-term gains of the program. We do have individual postdata that show lowering of pulse rates, of cholesterol and triglyceride levels, of blood pressures, and of weight. So there have been a number of immediate changes in clinical indicators of health status. We also know that during any given lunch hour, people are walking the streets of New Haven, dancing in a fitness group, meeting with their peers who have quit smoking, or simply enjoying shopping for clothes for their newfound figures. Such changes spur people to continue and to encourage others to begin to take action. Participants have shared their enthusiasm with co-workers who have not participated. At the one-year point we see the beginnings of the ripple effect of that sharing.

Participants have also given us targeted feedback to modify, add to, or simply improve components of the program to make them more relevant, more personal, more issue-oriented.

The true key to our success is maintenance. As we branch out to other parts of the state with our program and begin year two, we anticipate maintaining our top-management's support and our employees' enthusiasm.

We were aware from the beginning that hard and fast data would be five to ten years in coming, but if what we see today heralds what is to come, we are encouraged that we're heading in the right direction.

Analysis

A question very often asked is why health promotion at the worksite is so readily adopted in one organization but not in another. The Cantlon case to some extent provides an answer to this question by allowing us to examine the factors that appear as positive forces for initiating health promotion at a worksite. First, we see an organization that invests heavily in human resource development by the regular provision of training and educational programs. We also see a corporate management that looks at the world from a long-term perspective. As Cantlon notes, these two factors made it very acceptable for the organization to invest resources in health promotion. What we see here, then, is a corporate culture (see McCauley case analysis, p. 329) that is highly amenable to health promotion.

Beyond these factors we see a medical department with strong leadership that has developed a track record in producing results in the areas of safety and alcohol rehabilitation, thus saving the company a substantial sum of money. We also see as a catalyst a general manager, a known innovator, who recognized that a health promotion program would be of benefit to his section.

All these factors preceded the program. When the health educator arrived, she quickly assessed the needs of management and developed a well-defined pilot program that produced quantifiable results. The upshot was a corporatewide program for all employees. The company's commitment to this program is illustrated by the hefty dollar investment that enabled the medical department to hire a large staff with a variety of skills. This program would not suffer from what Green has labeled the cycle of poverty in health education, wherein programs that are initially underfunded do not produce the results they should, which leads to further underfunding (Green 1982).

The role of the health educator in this case was primarily that of program manager. However, she began as a consultant for the health program, with responsibility for the day-to-day operation of the pilot program. Role change and growth is certainly not uncommon in health education; it is usually desirable but rarely occurs as rapidly as it did in this case, in which the health educator first functioned alone and then made a transition to managing a staff of 22.

The strategies used in the case were promotional. The awareness and marketing campaign utilized all the company's media resources in combination with large-group orientation sessions designed to motivate employees to sign up. Multiple methods, whether used during the educational intervention or during the awareness phase of a program, generally will have greater impact on a greater number of people than will any single method (Green 1982).

Bruner's (1971:42–44) concepts of predispositions to learn are helpful in understanding the organization of these orientation sessions. He points out that learning depends on the exploration of alternatives, and therefore instruction must facilitate this exploration. Such instruction occurs in three phases: activation, maintenance, and direction. To activate the process, there must be some curiosity or level of uncertainty, which Mathews (1982) refers to as tension. To maintain the process, the learner must see that the benefits exceed the risks. And the direction depends on knowledge of the results of the exploration so that its value will be recognized. The orientation sessions were set up so as to pique curiosity, demonstrate the value of participation over nonparticipation, and provide participants with the means to know the results of participating.

The Reach Out for Health program is a good example of how health education is integrated with other program components such as screening and counseling. Considerable thought and planning went into developing programs to meet the needs of employees in specific job categories. This case thus points up the necessity of careful analysis of job functions and requirements. Without firsthand knowledge of the job, the health educator must either interview supervisors or directly observe workers. Tailoring a program directly to the employee needs, on the basis of job requirements, helps stimulate participation.

Finally, this case illustrates how much can be accomplished within a short time in planning a program, conducting it, and generating the interest of both the employees and management in it. As Cantlon notes, management has provided strong financial backing as well as a series of environmental supports. The challenge for this program is to maintain all this support in light of the delayed availability of outcome data. Although we are not privy to the thinking of management, it appears that the data available from the ongoing evaluations, in conjunction with management's interest in innovation, bode well for the continued support of this project.

References/Select Resources

Bruner, J. S. 1971. *Toward a Theory of Instruction.* Cambridge: Harvard University, Belknap Press.

Chapter 3, "Notes on a Theory of Instruction," offers several useful concepts about the process of helping individuals learn, or the process of instruction. The section headings in the chapter suggest the range of concepts covered: predispositions, structure and form of knowledge, sequence and its use, the form and pacing of reinforcement, activating problem solving, structure and sequence, and reinforcement and feedback.

Green, L. W. 1982. "Determining the Impact and Effectiveness of Health Education as It Relates to Federal Policy." In *SOPHE Heritage Collection of Health Education Monographs,* vol. 2: *The Practice of Health Education,* edited by B. P. Mathews. Oakland, Calif.: Third Party Publishing.

This work pulls together all data relevant to the practice of health education that have been gathered through research. From these data, Green derives several principles to guide federal policy for both research and practice in health education. However, these principles are applicable to health education in settings other than the federal government.

Mathews, B. P. 1982. "Administrative Climate: Its Implications for Health Education." In *SOPHE Heritage Collection of Health Education Monographs,* vol. 1: *The Philosophical, Behavioral, and Professional Bases for Health Education.* Oakland, Calif.: Third Party Publishing.

In this article Mathews offers a comprehensive view of the issues related to administrative support, or the lack of it, for the health educator. Among our case studies, the Cantlon case is one of the best examples of the value of strong administrative support.

Discussion Questions

1. Why did the employees of SNET respond so well to the health promotion program?
2. In your opinion, to what degree was the success of this program due to the competency of the health educator?
3. The objective of an orientation session is to motivate employees to enroll in a health promotion program. Design and describe an orientation session.
4. Cantlon describes a number of environmental supports developed to reinforce and maintain behavior change. Suggest additional environmental supports.
5. Cantlon describes several programs designed for specific work situations. Select two specific occupations (e.g., truck driver, teacher, waiter, state legislator), and design a health promotion program to meet their specific needs.

Promoting Worksite Wellness: A Community-Based Project

Brenda Lindemann, M.P.H.

In 1978, I was working for the North Shore Health Planning Council (NSHPC), the health systems agency for a large residential and industrial area north of Boston, including 27 cities and towns covering 289 square miles. The council had been challenged by the State Health Department's Division of Preventive Medicine to demonstrate an interest by local employers in worksite health promotion and to get a local committee organized within two months. The carrot held out to us for this effort was the promise of four-year funding for a demonstration worksite health promotion project. The state gave us funding for two months from monies that had been returned that year by other grantees. Following is an account of what we did in those two months and in the subsequent four years of the Employee Health Promotion Project (EHPP).

BEGINNINGS

Since the State Health Department wanted an expression of interest, I quickly put together a survey to determine interest. A brief questionnaire was sent to 280 "major" employers, including hospitals and municipal government agencies having 100 or more employees. The survey asked what their specific health promotion and risk reduction activities were, what they would like them to be, and whether they would be interested in being members of a regional committee committed to health promotion programs in worksites. One hundred of the 280 questionnaires were returned, after some follow-up by phone. A similar survey was conducted each of the four years of the program, but we did not continue to follow up after the first year because we learned that the time and energy invested in doing so was not worthwhile.

We organized an Advisory Committee that included representatives from employers, labor, voluntary and community health agencies, hospitals, physicians, local government, NSHPC volunteers, and interested consumers.

These tasks accomplished, we reported to the State Health Department and received the first-year appropriation from the proposed four-year grant. In each successive year we reapplied and received anticipated diminishing funds, which we supplemented from other sources. The NSHCP contributed increasing amounts each year; and in the two final years we received a grant from the risk reduction program of the Centers for Disease Control. The entire Project operated on a modest $30,000 a year. I was the only full-time employee assigned to direct the project.

THE EHPP

Once the EHPP committee was organized, we began to plan and to try out ways to interest employers in health promotion. As EHPP director, I served as a facilitator, educator, motivator, and trainer. The training was both formal and informal. An example of the informal training was my work in helping the Advisory Committee become familiar with health promotion issues and resources. In turn, the committee apprised me of the practical problems encountered at worksites in fostering the concept of and implementing health promotion activities.

Brenda Lindemann is the Assistant Coordinator for the Health Education Service at the Massachusetts Institute of Technology Medical Department. She was previously the Director of the Employee Health Promotion Project for the North Shore Health Planning Council, Inc.

Early on, we developed two working task forces from the Advisory Committee, one for the development of worksite programs and the other for general educational activities such as education and training workshops, public speaking engagements, and the compilation of a directory of health promotion programs available in the area.

The members of the committee agreed on its role in reaching the project's goal: to serve as a catalyst to increase awareness about and interest in health promotion activities and to assist employers in implementing or expanding those activities at their workplace. In accordance with that goal, the committee and I saw our function as linking interested employers with available community resources for health promotion. For example, if an employer was interested in a smoking cessation program, we would identify resources (always more than one) and recommend criteria for selecting a quality program while leaving the choice up to the employer. We aimed (1) to provide employers with information about health promotion in general and about specific screening programs, educational activities, and group programs for behavior modification; and (2) to assist or train some of the health program providers to develop their services so that they could offer quality programs to worksites. The following section elaborates on our activities, and the final section describes what we accomplished.

FOSTERING WORKSITE HEALTH PROMOTION

The EHPP functioned as a third party in helping employers and providers organize health promotion programs. Our goal the first year was to persuade and assist ten employers to undertake a program, defined as one screening or educational activity—for example, a blood pressure screening or a multisession, group weight control program.

Our first tasks were to acquaint employers and health care providers with the whys and hows of worksite health promotion, encourage and support cooperative efforts between employers and providers, organize committee and task force volunteers to assist the project, and develop support for and commitment to the project.

We used two approaches to make employers and providers more aware of the importance of worksite health promotion: an annual survey of employers and public information.

All major employers in the area were surveyed annually. The survey asked what worksite health promotion programs the employers had sponsored or would be interested in sponsoring. A cover letter explaining the purpose of the project and information flyers were included with the questionnaire. The survey was mailed to the chief executive officer unless he or she had identified a specific person within the company as the lead person for worksite health promotion.

Public information activities were carried on throughout the project year:

1. Project staff and volunteers spoke to professional groups such as personnel and service clubs (e.g., the Rotary or Kiwanis).
2. Press releases were issued to local newspapers.
3. The NSHPC's newsletter, which included articles about the EHPP, was sent to area employers and providers.

The EHPP did not conduct worksite health promotion programs. Serving as a liaison, it encouraged and supported cooperative efforts between employers and health care providers in the community. The goal was to assist employers and providers to engage in a productive relationship that would continue in the future without outside help. Consultation and technical assistance were based on the following considerations:

1. Employers needed help to do internal planning, select an appropriate provider, and work jointly with the provider to assure a quality program.
2. Providers needed some preparation to work within the contraints of a work setting and suggestions as to appropriate techniques for program implementation of quality programs.
3. Both groups needed to be reminded of meetings, program responsibilities, and other details.

The volunteers and I assumed a low-key, "enabler" role to keep the process moving. We were sufficiently competent to maintain the respect of both the employer and the provider, passive enough to assure ultimate responsibility would be taken by the employer and provider, and sensitive enough to individuals' feelings and internal politics to allow our ongoing third-party role.

Volunteers were an important, if not essential, resource to the EHPP. They served on the Advisory Committee and task forces and learned to work with employers and providers in implementing screening, behavioral change programs, and educational and training workshops. In time, the volunteers, by working with me, learned enough about facilitating the programs to handle these on their own—an example of my role in informal training.

Part of the EHPP strategy was to develop support for and commitment to the project by volunteers and employers who had taken part in any of its activities. We kept them informed of the project's progress—what programs were under way and how many people were taking part in the health promotion programs we helped organize and in the educational workshops we sponsored. Particular project-related accomplishments by volunteers and employers were acknowledged in press releases to local papers and articles in the NSHPC's newsletter. Volunteers and employers were asked to write letters of support for the project when grant applications were prepared.

IMPLEMENTING WORKSITE HEALTH PROMOTION PROGRAMS

Three models for facilitating the implementation of worksite health promotion were used: consultation teams, direct staff assistance, and indirect assistance that fostered the development of numerous spin-off programs.

The Consultation Team model is process-oriented, allowing for education of the employer, provider, and project staff and volunteers. As a first step, the program task force of the Advisory Committee and I developed criteria for selecting program sites. Criteria considered were type of employer (business, industry, municipal government, hospital), number of employees, work schedules of the employees, geographic location of the employer, sociodemographic characteristics of the employees, interest level and potential commitment of employer to future programs, and resources available from the employer for health promotion.

Program sites that met the criteria were then selected from among interested employers. A consultation team was formed for each site. The employer named a person responsible for program development. A preliminary meeting was held with this person, the project director, and a volunteer from the committee's program task force.

At the initial meeting(s), discussions focused on the type of program requested by the employer and the different types of providers who could be most helpful in implementing it. Information was given on what constituted a quality program and which provider might best meet the employer's needs. We encouraged employers to interview more than one provider. Once the provider was chosen by the employer, that person became a member of the consultation team.

The consultation team conducted all aspects of program planning, implementation, and evaluation. As the volunteers gained experience, I became less involved. The volunteers were able to assume primary responsibility for facilitating team meetings and maintaining liaison with the project committee.

In the Staff Technical Assistance model, I worked directly with the employer to select a provider. Then the provider, employer, and I planned, implemented, and evaluated the program. My role included offering advice, keeping the process moving—for instance, reminding others of deadlines and assisting in problem solving.

We found the Staff Technical Assistance model to be more effective when the employer and provider were knowledgeable about organizing programs and when employers preferred to work quickly rather than participate in an in-depth planning process with a consultation team.

During the first two years the EHPP typically worked with each employer to implement a single risk-factor program during a given year.

During the two years that the EHPP was funded primarily by the Centers for Disease Control, our focus shifted to working closely with two major employers to implement "comprehensive" programs. That is, each employer implemented a minimum of three worksite health promotion programs during the year and conducted a more extensive evaluation to assess their impact on the employees' knowledge, attitudes, and behavior. The Consultant Team model was used in the development of these two programs as well.

Spin-off programs serve as evidence of the effect the project had in raising the awareness of employers and motivating them to become involved in worksite health promotion efforts. Employers originally assisted by the project continued the programs on their own; and employers who had attended educational or training workshops sponsored by the project or who had asked for consultation planned and implemented programs independently.

EDUCATIONAL MODELS

Employers, employees, and providers learned about the worksite health promotion programs through general publicity and the experiences of their fellow employers, employees, and providers. It was clear, however, that employers needed more in-depth information about the hows and whys of worksite health promotion. Although this could be provided through consultation, many employers would not ask for consultation, either because they were not sufficiently interested or because they felt that such a request would involve a commitment they were not prepared to make at that time. Attending a workshop on the topic did not call for a commitment but simply offered an opportunity to learn. Therefore, we ran two orientation workshops for employers.

The first workshop, held during the first year (1978), provided an introduction to health promotion activities and explained why a company should sponsor them. The second was held at the beginning of the last year (1981) and placed emphasis on planning, implementing, and evaluating health promotion programs. These workshops included a panel of employers and providers who had experience with worksite wellness programs and who described to their peers the hows and the whys of the programs undertaken at their respective worksites. Small group discussions followed the panel discussions. Each workshop lasted half a day and was organized for maximum interaction among participants and for the provision of highly specific information.

A wrap-up workshop was held at the conclusion of the four EHPP years: "Worksite Health Promotion: The Next Step . . ." Some of the content of the guide we compiled (*Worksite Health Promotion: A Guide*) was the result of the work groups at this workshop.

As the project progressed, it became clear that many of the providers also needed assistance in developing or improving skills in planning, implementing, and evaluating health promotion programs. Since occupational health nurses (OHNs) play a key role in worksite health promotion, workshops for this group focused on providing them with skills to plan and implement worksite programs.

The EHPP sponsored OHN training workshops during the two middle years (1979 and 1980). During 1979 two related one-day workshops were held. In the first one, discussions covered (1) typical roles of the OHN, (2) strategies for starting or expanding health promotion activities, (3) identification of barriers and ways to overcome them, and (4) an overview of program planning. The nurses were asked to conduct, during the month between workshop sessions, an inventory of employee interest at their worksite and to bring back the results to the follow-up workshop. This session focused on (1) the nurses' experience since the first workshop, (2) principles of adult education and health education, (3) additional points in program planning, (4) levels of program activity appropriate to various settings, and (5) recognition of constraints and use of available resources. The workshop in 1980 was based on a needs assessment of OHNs. This more specific workshop included information on how to implement exercise/fitness and stress management programs.

One significant consequence of the North Shore OHN training was the formation of a North-of-Boston Chapter of the American Association of Occupational Health Nurses. This group continues to meet and now organizes and conducts its own training programs.

To further facilitate information exchange, Resource Tables displayed health education materials and promotional information for program providers at each education and training workshop. The

EHPP resource directory was available for purchase at these tables.

Because committee members were in need of specific information if they were to promote the concept of worksite programs, we held short educational sessions before project committee meetings. Each session dealt with a particular type of worksite health promotion program.

Finally, the resource directory we developed was updated once during the course of the project. To persons outside of the health care system the array of health providers and services can be intimidating and confusing. The directory served as a reference for employers on agencies, organizations, and private consultants who offer worksite health promotion programs. The information was organized according to the type of health promotion program—for example, cancer education and screening services, employee assistance programs, exercise programs, and hypertension screening services. Included in the directory were "guidelines for selecting quality programs," prepared by the Education Task Force volunteers. They were developed especially to assist employers who might purchase and use the directory without direct assistance from the EHPP. The guidelines were helpful to program providers who wished to implement their programs through the EHPP. Over 200 copies were purchased by company managers, OHNs, and other health care providers.

As a concluding component of the project, a self-help guide was developed for area businesses, health care providers, and other groups interested in developing health promotion programs at the worksite. This too was made available to all employers in the area.

EVALUATION

The EHPP had five main goals:

1. To establish and/or expand health promotion programs among 3 percent of major employers on the North Shore.
2. To develop ongoing mechanisms to foster health promotion at the worksite.
3. To establish and/or expand worksite health promotion programs.
4. To survey all major employers to determine what programs were underway and where there was interest.
5. To conduct educational activities

The data collected for the EHPP (Table 1, pp. 346–347) have been used to demonstrate the effectiveness of the project in achieving these goals.

Another level of evaluation was a "Performance Evaluation Program," which was conducted in 1981 by the U.S. Department of Health and Human Services Bureau of Health Planning (U.S. DHHS 1981). The EHPP was one of the two health promotion projects in the country selected as especially useful examples of a successful health planning program. A case study was prepared for national distribution.

REFERENCES

North Shore Health Planning Council. 1982. *Worksite Health Promotion: A Guide.* Peabody, Mass.

U.S. Department of Health and Human Services. 1981. *Performance Evaluation Program,* Study III. Health Promotion and Disease Prevention, Contract no. HRA 232-79-0128. Washington, D.C.: Government Printing Office.

Table 1
Evaluation Data Compiled by the EHPP (Four-Year Summary)

A. Survey of all major employers to determine what programs are under way and/or which employers show an interest:

Year	Surveys Returned	Employers Interested in Assistance
1	42	29
2	39	25
3	40	21
4	36	11
	157	86

B. Employers establishing or expanding worksite health promotion programs: 64 (23 percent of North Shore's major employers)

C. Types of employers participating in EHPP programs:

	Direct Assistance	Spin-off
Business/industry	8	31
Municipal	5	4
Health/social service	8	8
	21	43

D. Number of EHPP programs:
    Direct assistance: 44
    Spin-off: 130
    174

E. Average total number of employees of employers participating in EHPP programs:
    Direct assistance: 446
    Spin-off: 905
    1,351

F. Number of program participants:
    Direct assistance: 2,200
    Spin-off: 12,500
    14,700

G. Estimated total number of individuals participating in EHPP programs (nonduplicated count): 7,000

H. Number of employers not reporting programs in 1978 but beginning programs with EHPP assistance: 41

Table 1 *continued*

I. Types and numbers of EHPP programs (direct assistance) and numbers of clients reached:

	Number of Programs	Number of Clients
Smoking cessation	3	78
Weight control	6	371
Employee assistance program	3	38
CPR (cardiopulmonary resuscitation)	5	76
Stress management	5	133
Hypertension	9	932
Exercise	2	131
Breast cancer	4	92
Other	7	335
	44	2,186

J. Mechanisms developed to foster health promotion at the worksite:
   1. Employee Health Promotion Committee
   2. North-of-Boston Chapter, American Association of Occupational Health Nurses

K. Educational activities:
   1. Technical assistance workshops:
      Number of workshops   3
      Total attendees   241
      Employers represented   65
   2. Occupational health nurse workshops:
      Number of workshops   3
      Total attendees   46
      Employers represented   22
   3. Resource directories distributed (updated once):   220
   4. EHPP public addresses:
      Number of groups addressed   25
      Estimated number of attendees   500
   5. *Worksite Health Promotion: A Guide:*
      Copies distributed to persons attending the last EHPP workshop   75
      (Additional copies were printed for general distribution.)

Analysis

This case illustrates, perhaps more clearly than any other in this book, the responsibilities of the health educator as defined and verified by the Role Delineation Project (U.S. Department of Commerce 1982). The health educator's activities flow from one step to another in the project with apparent ease.

Lindemann's first task was the needs assessment. This task was carried out by mailing a survey to the executive officers of the major employers (business, industry, municipal government) in the area. Information from the survey was used in planning the project that Lindemann, the health educator/project director, coordinated, or for which, as she describes it, she was the enabler/facilitator. She provided direct health education services to companies that did not want to deal with in-depth planning, and she evaluated the efforts of the project. That is exactly the order of activity specified in the verified role, although the process does not always—nor does it have to—occur in that order.

All planning models relevant to the practice of health education are a composite of a number of theories that explain the process of learning/social change or predict behavior; the combined theories in a model provide a guide for developing programs on the basis of these explanations or predictions. Several planning models could apply to this case. The one that fits best is "Steps in Health Education Planning, Operation, and Evaluation," developed by D. Sullivan and adapted by Ross and Mico (1980:208–209). The steps are as follows: Involve people, set goals, define the problems, design the plan, conduct activities, and evaluate the results.

The theory that explains how companies became involved in worksite health promotion is diffusion of innovations (Rogers 1983). The goal of the Advisory Committee was to act as a catalyst in spurring employers' interest in participating in health promotion programs. Lindemann and the committee depended on diffusion of an innovation to spread the word about, and persuade employers to become involved in, worksite health promotion. They helped the process along with publicity and workshops.

A basic principle of learning applied throughout this project was the involvement of the learner. Lindemann involved relevant individuals and groups in the Advisory Committee, in the public speaking program, in consultation teams, and in workshop planning, implementation, and evaluation.

Lindemann's communication skills are worthy of note. She indicates that both volunteers and employers who participated in the project became its advocates. This advocacy would not have been possible had they not seen beyond their own involvement to that of others and to the broader issues the project addressed. Committee meetings and EHPP articles in the NSHPC's newsletter were the tools for informing them of the project's progress: who was participating, what they were doing, what was going on elsewhere in worksite health promotion, and what issues were of particular interest and needed clarification. Sharing this information with employers and volunteers made them feel part of the effort so that they were motivated to advocate for the project. Too often, we forget to communicate with people we hope will advocate for us.

Lindemann's skill in training was also important to the success of the program. The volunteers on the Advisory Committee and on the consultation teams needed to learn how to function in their new roles. They had to learn skills in negotiating with employers and providers. They also needed knowledge about specific health promotion programs and health promotion issues. In learning skills, volunteers simply followed the lead of the health educator, who consciously used modeling as an educational method. The knowledge was provided through the mini-educational sessions prior to Advisory Committee meetings and through articles in the NSHPC's newsletter. These training methods required little or no extra time or effort by the volunteers. Time and effort are issues of prime consideration in training volunteers.

Volunteers properly trained and involved in any health education project can be an invaluable aid. This case offers a good example of how to prepare them for their role. And here the health educator requires maturity: not only must she or he be able to judge when volunteers are ready to go off on their own, but also she or he must be able to allow them to do so.

One professional operating procedure worthy of note in this case was the mailing of the surveys to the chief executive officers of the companies. Making the initial approach to the head of an organization is a sine qua non in trying to get entrée to an organization. She or he may turn your request over to someone else in the company, but that is a help because the person to whom the buck is passed has a directive from the boss to get involved.

The record-keeping that had to be done to evaluate the project was not inconsiderable. It illustrates the importance of beginning on the first day of the project to set up a record system that will allow for evaluation of the project's main objective.

The temptation in any program that involved screening is to ask how many were screened, how many new cases were found, and how many were followed up. And although these data were compiled, we need to keep in mind that the goals and objectives of this project were not to screen a given number of persons but rather to interest employers in engaging in health promotion activities at the worksite. That's the objective that was evaluated.

References/Select Resources

Rogers, E. M. 1983. *Diffusion of Innovations.* 3d ed. New York: Free Press.

For this third edition of his work on diffusion, Rogers notes the tremendous increase in diffusion research since the first edition in 1962, when he reported on 405 studies on diffusion. For this edition, he reviewed 3,085 studies.

Rogers here extends diffusion theory to include factors that antecede and follow the adoption process and thus poses new questions. For example: Where did the diffusion come from? Which comes first, the need or the innovation? What kinds of problems are encountered, and how are they solved as the innovation is implemented?

This case illustrates the diffusion process in its simplest form. An idea is floated in a community; people become aware of it; some try it out and like it; then others decide to try it. The adoption of health promotion programs by some of the spin-offs in this case was a direct result of diffusion.

Ross, H. S., and Mico, P. R. 1980. *Theory and Practice in Health Education.* Palo Alto, Calif.: Mayfield.

Chapter 11 of this text for the entry-level health educator deals with planning. Several planning models are discussed. The student can compare their similarities and differences and get practical experience by identifying the usefulness of one model over another in specific settings.

U.S. Department of Commerce. National Technical Information Service. 1982. *The Refined and Verified Role for Entry Level Health Educators.* Access no. HRP–09–04273. Springfield, VA.

This is the second report in the Role Delineation Project series. The first defines the role, and the third is a curriculum guide for entry-level health educators.

This report describes the study that verified the defined role. The sample of health educators, surveyed to determine whether or not they carried out the functions described in the defined role, included health educators in schools, communities, and medical care facilities. The survey findings indicate that the same knowledge and skills are required in all settings, though they are used more in some settings than in others. The difference among settings is one of emphasis. This report is a must reading for anyone interested in the profession of health education.

This case offers a mini-verification of the defined role because the health educator's responsibilities fit the role as described.

Discussion Questions

1. Assume you were the health educator in this case. Suggest means other than the survey by which you could have determined the interest of employers in health education.

2. What do you perceive to be the major function of the Advisory Committee?

3. Put together a short education session to be held just before the Advisory Committee meets. Include objectives, methodology, and evaluation; indicate how much time you think the session should take.

4. What would you teach a volunteer about how to approach an employer who has requested information about a health promotion program?
5. Identify a similarity between this case and the McCauley and Cantlon cases (pp. 327 and 332).

Organizing a Health Promotion Program at a University Medical Center

Gary J. Donnelly, M.P.H.

This case study describes the planning and organization of a work site Health Promotion Program at a state university medical center. Diffusion-adoption theory provided a conceptual framework for program development. The case represents my own perceptions of the forces that impinged on the program during its first year. There are, of course, limitations on this type of analysis, but it is hoped that the discussion will provide valuable insight into the role of a health education practitioner working in a medical care setting.

INCEPTION OF THE HEALTH PROMOTION PROGRAM

The Health Promotion Program was developed as a result of the efforts of a few persons who believed the medical center had a responsibility to promote healthy life-styles as well as to respond to disease. Conceived as an educational intervention, the program is singularly focused on the concept of wellness. The process of learning to "feel well," in this instance, is facilitated by participation in physical fitness, recreational, and awareness-raising activities. Accent is always on the positive benefits of engaging in these activities. In fact, fun and personal enjoyment have become the most important program themes.

The University of Massachusetts Medical Center comprises a medical school and a tertiary-care hospital facility. A diverse population of nearly 4,000 employees, medical students, interns, and residents (house officers) make up this "community." The center is situated on a 135-acre campus with recreation facilities, including showers and locker rooms. Other health and recreation resources are close by. Prior to the development of the Health Promotion Program, students and employees had organized softball leagues, bowling leagues, yoga classes, jogging clubs, and the like. It was anticipated that through an organized approach many additional activities could be initiated and existing activities could be better publicized and utilized.

ROLE OF THE HEALTH EDUCATOR IN DEVELOPING THE HEALTH PROMOTION PROGRAM

My position is health educator for the hospital's Ambulatory Services Department in the medical center. During all phases of organizing the Health Promotion Program, I worked very closely with two persons from the Medical School: an associate professor in the Department of Family and Community Medicine and a program coordinator for the Office of Continuing Education. This "gang of three," as we will be referred to, consulted with one another every Monday morning to plan the development of the program. The following discussion traces the development stages during the first year.

PROBLEM DIAGNOSIS STAGE

The health-related needs of the population were identified primarily through informal assessment procedures. The first step was to identify individuals with an interest in health promotion from a

---

Gary J. Donnelly is a Health Educator for Ambulatory Services at the University of Massachusetts Medical Center in Worcester.

spectrum of medical center departments. Those who were already involved in activities were approached, and they led to others. The resulting network was eventually formalized into an ad hoc Advisory Committee. My nonthreatening status within the medical center community, knowledge of most of the "major actors" whose resources and support would be needed for the program, and understanding of the political climate of the organization facilitated the development of the Advisory Committee. In addition, because my department was mandated to provide ancillary and supportive services for the medical center, I was able to adjust my schedule so as to devote a major portion of my time to staff the Health Promotion Program.

My first task was to develop a needs assessment instrument to determine the current health practices and interests of the population. With the help of committee members, I modified a life-style assessment questionnaire and pretested it on department heads and members of the Department of Family and Community Medicine. The questionnaire reflected the program's philosophy, that is, wellness. There were no queries about disease; all questions related to life-style issues.

The information from the pretest was fed back to those who took it during a large meeting of department heads. This strategy proved useful in gaining the cooperation of this group and enabled the Advisory Committee to devise a more effective questionnaire.

PLANNING STAGE

The gang of three made a series of presentations about the concept of a health promotion program to formal groups I had identified in the center's hierarchy: the Faculty Council, Student Body Committee, Classified Employees Committee, department heads and Managers Committee of the medical center, and Medical School Administrators Group.

Meetings were held with the chancellor/dean, hospital director, academic dean, and provost, all of whom gave the program verbal support. I was encouraged to submit a proposal to administration for funding. The ad hoc Advisory Committee was expanded to include representatives of 25 departments of the medical center, many of whom contributed to the development of the proposal. This participatory planning process gained additional legitimacy for the health promotion concept. The involvement of this number of people was impressive to the administration.

The task of writing the proposal had two phases. The first proposal called for an annual budget of $50,000 to hire both a full-time health educator with expertise in evaluation and a secretarial staff. A two-year program was proposed, which was to include health promotion activities and testing of results, such as changes in attitudes toward work, absenteeism rates, and levels of cardiovascular fitness. It was reasoned that a program of this scope would offer a valuable service to the medical center population and generate evaluation data that would be useful to the administration and to the academic community.

The administration rejected the proposal because of "high" cost, but the Advisory Committee was encouraged to resubmit the plan with a smaller budget. The administration viewed the potential benefits of the program in terms of positive public relations and wanted the maximum amount of activity costing the least number of dollars. The value of the needs assessment efforts of the Advisory Committee was not recognized. Instead, there were clear messages that continued funding for the program would be based on documented high levels of activity. The gang of three and the Advisory Committee recognized that our options were limited. Either we designed a less expensive program or there would be no program. That was the political reality.

Our challenge was what to do with the limited resources we expected to receive in order to salvage any semblance of a disciplined approach to health promotion. We decided to focus during the first year on awareness raising—given adoption-diffusion as our theoretical base. If we succeeded in selling the program to the administration the first year, we could get a data base the second year. Not ideal, but still possible.

Instead of tailoring the program to data-based planning, we placed a premium on generating short-term activities that had high visibility and popularity in the center. The second proposal, developed in cooperation with the Advisory Committee, emphasized a total "service orientation." The cost was $15,000. It was accepted. Half the funding came from the hospital, and half from the school. The administration also agreed to fund the program at this level on an annual basis.

It was soon apparent that additional staff was needed to augment my efforts and those of the Advisory Committee. Agreement was reached that a half-time administrative assistant would be hired. The hiring process was not simple. A temporary freeze on new state positions was in effect. To circumvent this problem, a "temporary employee status" was ascribed to the administrative assistant position. The Personnel Department seemed reluctant to advertise the position outside the medical center, thereby reducing the number of potential candidates who might apply. A conflict resulted over this issue, but confrontation was averted when a woman with many skills in areas related to health promotion expressed interest in transferring from the medical center, where she was a volunteer, to the Health Promotion Program. She was hired for the paid position.

I also executed a number of other administrative tasks to get the program up and running. Cost accounts had to be established to access funds for the purchase of services, materials, and equipment. This involved coordination with the hospital director, academic dean, and Fiscal Affairs Department. The creation of these cost accounts was viewed as a way for the administration to symbolize commitment to the Health Promotion Program. However, more problems developed.

Medical School officials were unable to identify a source of funds that could be committed to the program. Numerous meetings were held with the administrators in the office of the academic dean to address this problem. When these funds were finally made available to the program, I discovered they were restricted for temporary employee salaries or consultant fees. Since the hospital portion of the budget was already being used to pay the administrative assistant, her salary had to be transferred to the medical school. The bureaucratic red tape involved in processing this "personnel action" took nine weeks to unravel and reduced the time I was able to devote to program development.

IMPLEMENTATION STAGE

There were two aspects to the implementation plan: (1) public relations and information dissemination, and (2) activity development. Both aspects addressed the priority objective for the first year—raise awareness and interest in health promotion.

The interests and talents of other members of the Advisory Committee were utilized on task-specific subcommittees. There were four of these: publicity, fitness, nutrition, and education. I consulted with these smaller groups to develop work plans for the first year.

The Publicity Subcommittee wished to give as much visibility as possible to the Health Promotion Program. So a number of strategies were developed. The staff was responsible for a constant stream of announcements in the weekly medical center newsletter, organizing fitness demonstrations in the medical school lobby, inviting the chancellor/dean to award trophies at sporting events and cosponsoring activities with the large sections such as the Personnel, Medicine, and Surgery Departments and the Pain Control Unit. The Publicity Subcommittee was responsible for originating a logo for the program and disseminating posters and pamphlets about ongoing activities. The heart-shaped logo was easily identifiable and appeared on all publicity materials. One of the more successful publicity gimmicks was the awarding of "Health Promotion T-shirts" to participants after they completed an activity. Medical students often wore their shirts to class, and so were walking advertisements for the program. The T-shirts seemed to help build an esprit de corps among particular groups (e.g., bicycle club members). Another effective publicity campaign was the use of posters giving notice of scheduled activities. These posters always showed people having fun and included a simple message such as "Dance for health." They were very striking in comparison to the many other posters around the center that announced scientific seminars, clinical rounds, and so on.

The Fitness Subcommittee responded to needs its members perceived for physical fitness activities among the center's population. Through their efforts and periodic publicity in the center's newsletter, approximately 20 volunteer and paid instructors were recruited so that a number of programs could be offered: exercise to music classes, jogging clinics, weight-lifting classes, walking groups, yoga classes, bicycle maintenance classes and touring club, basketball league, massage classes, aerobic dance classes, and meditation classes.

Work on these activities was divided between

the staff and the subcommittee so that I maintained liaison with the volunteer instructors. The task of scheduling rooms, ordering supplies, coordinating publicity, and documenting attendance was shared with the administrative assistant.

The Education Subcommittee contributed to the awareness-raising objective by sponsoring a "Wellness Jubilee." This was a two-day event that offered demonstrations and exhibits focused on raising awareness about the wellness benefits of physical fitness, nutrition, relaxation, and social support. In keeping with the wellness philosophy, neither disease prevention, screening for disease, nor any other medical care issue was acceptable for presentation. Twenty-five participants, 19 from the medical center and 6 from outside the center took part in the jubilee.

Many persons who had not participated in any other phase of the Health Promotion Program responded to the call for volunteer assistance at the jubilee. For example, the Pediatrics Department had its patients design signs for each exhibit. Exhibitors from the Medical Center were recruited by advertising in the weekly newsletter and in paycheck enclosures. I recruited the "outsiders" (e.g., the Dairy Council and the YMCA). As the organization of the event gained momentum, more and more potential exhibitors came forth with ideas. Together with the Education Subcommittee, I screened all potential entries and provided guidance to the exhibitors in developing their display or demonstration. The exhibitors provided information and demonstrated skills in areas like the following:

"The Foot in Sports"—Podiatry Service

"Healthy Back"—Physical Therapy

"Social Support Systems"—Family and Community Medicine and the Office of Continuing Education

"Yoga and Massage"—Pain Control Unit

"Current Literature on Health Promotion and Wellness"—Library

"Eating More Nutritious Meals"—Food and Nutrition Service

Everyone who came to the jubilee received a button and balloon imprinted with the Health Promotion Program logo. As always, we accentuated the *positive* in our publicity campaigns. These publicity devices contributed to the atmosphere of fun and entertainment.

The jubilee attracted approximately 700 members of the medical center community, which far exceeded the Advisory Committee's expectations. A personal invitation was sent to the chancellor/dean. He came at the height of activity during the first day. A delegation from the Advisory Committee reviewed the attendance figures with him several weeks after the event to reinforce the fact that many people were interested in health promotion activities.

A Nutrition Subcommittee is now organizing a health promotion cookbook. It has begun to solicit contributions of time-honored and healthful recipes from the medical center community. It is anticipated that the book will be sold in the hospital gift shop and that proceeds will help fund the Health Promotion Program.

BARRIERS ENCOUNTERED DURING THE PROGRAM

In all settings, there are constraints to effecting change. Of major importance is the degree of legitimacy the culture attaches to the innovation. A major obstacle in obtaining legitimacy for the Health Promotion Program was the value the medical center placed on cure and treatment of disease rather than on enhancement of well-being. The disease-oriented mind-set pervaded all elements of the center's community, including nonmedical care personnel such as employees in the cafeteria and in environmental building services.

Our gang of three recognized this barrier to the diffusion process. Therefore, at all Advisory Committee and subcommittee meetings, we held the line firmly on wellness—the positive base of the Health Promotion Program. This was not always easy. Many members of the Advisory Committee did not understand why we insisted on the distinction between wellness and disease prevention; and many did not think it was important. The Wellness Jubilee provided a practical application of the difference and helped most members of the Advisory Committee understand the distinction.

Mention has been made of administrative problems in organizing the program. The management of fiscal matters by the administration was a significant barrier to program development. Moreover, during the first year of the program, serious management and labor disputes arose at the medical center. Organized sick-outs and union agitation occurred among several groups of employees. It was difficult to build the Health Promotion Program at a time when low morale and mistrust were so evident in the organization. The challenge to the Advisory Committee and to me was to demonstrate to the employees that the Health Promotion Program was more than an orchestrated publicity stunt to placate them.

The lack of administrative commitment to the program, demonstrated by the limited resources allocated to it, was another barrier. A major problem in obtaining administrative commitment was the frequent turnover of organizational leadership. In the first year of the program, there were changes in the following positions: hospital director, associate hospital director for ambulatory/support services (my supervisor), director of medical records, director of personnel, hospital controller, director of nursing, and group practice administrator. These personnel changes among the executive leadership fostered a climate of organizational instability. I spent an inordinate amount of time developing relationships with new administrative personnel who filled these and other vacated positions.

The administration's inability to locate permanent space for the program hampered our attempts to expand the variety of offerings. The medical center was undergoing rapid growth when the Health Promotion Program was initiated. Indoor space became consumed for offices and new clinical services. As a result, program activities often had to be held in back hallways and employee lounge areas.

Scheduling activities was another difficulty. Many of the employees involved in patient care activities had irregular hours. Some time in the period between 11:00 A.M. and 1:00 P.M. was available to most of the personnel and students. Still, some departments allowed only a half hour for lunch. To respond to the needs of these persons, the program organized offerings after the first shift (3:30 P.M.). This adjustment conveyed the idea that the program was for everyone and not only for those with flexible work/class schedules.

FACTORS FACILITATING PROGRAM DEVELOPMENT

The major factor facilitating the development of the Health Promotion Program was the contribution of the volunteers who assisted staff with many tasks. To a large degree, the program was built on the credibility of the personnel who volunteered their time and expertise. In keeping with diffusion theory, they could be classified as innovators because they adopted certain practices (e.g., aerobic dancing, meditation) long before these were popular with their peers. The program offered them an opportunity to further cultivate and share their skills.

A brief sketch of three of the volunteers illustrates the richness of the resources they brought to the program.

- Mr. A has been a pharmacy clerk in the hospital for seven years. He is an influential member of the small Black population of the medical center and is well liked by classified, as well as professional, employees. A former star basketball player during his high school days, he has been coaching young players from the community for several years. He heard of the Health Promotion Program by word of mouth among his friends and offered his services to staff to organize a summer basketball league. He demonstrated exceptional abilities in working with people. The league became the most popular of the program's events during the summer and expanded greatly during the following season. Mr. A feels coaching offers him an opportunity to be creative and to cope with the stress of his job. His confidence in coaching and managing the basketball league has given him the impetus to pursue a paid coaching career.

- Mr. B is a second-year medical student. Before enrolling in the medical school, he worked in a bicycle repair shop and raced cycles competitively. He is well known and liked by the student body. During the summer, he organized a cycle maintenance class and touring club. He also advocated for the Health Promotion Program within the student population. Mr. B will repeat his popular class and work to expand the medical center's cycle club.

- Ms. C is an administrator in the Department of Medicine. She became acquainted with the program through members of the Advisory Committee and introduced the idea of holding aerobic dance classes at the center. Ms. C used her enthusiasm and administrative clout to bring her idea to fruition. Her department has also cosponsored the aerobic dance class with the Health Promotion Program, adding legitimacy and credibility to the activity.

EXPANDED PROGRAM

Approximately 19 percent of the medical center population participated in the Health Promotion Program during the first year. Fifty percent of all departments were represented, and 35 percent of the first- and second-year students participated in one or more activities. The average number of activities was four and a half per month. There were never less than three activities nor more than seven. Approximately 280 volunteer hours of instruction were provided by employees and students.

Thanks to our successes, we have received a slightly increased budget for a second year of programming. Energies will be directed to a needs assessment and to attracting more "early adopters" into the program. There will be increased activity, with an outreach component identifying and training interested members in the medical center to promote the program in their departments. Specific objectives for a percentage of new participants and retention of first-year participants have been set. An evaluation of one aspect of the program is also planned. Mostly, the organizational climate of the medical center has been showing signs of additional stability and harmony. The administration has held numerous meetings to elicit input from employees on ways to improve working conditions. The turnover rate has also slowed down. Given these changes, it would seem that the Health Promotion Program could find a solid niche within the organization. Progress is already being made to house the program in the financial and administrative arm of the entire medical center rather than in the hospital.

Ultimately, the diffusion of the wellness concept among the students and employees will depend on strong support from the administration as well as from the grass-roots community. It is unclear, at this point, how much support the program will receive from either of these sources.

CONCLUSIONS

The following is a list of subjective conclusions about the planning process of the program during its first year.

1. The diffusion of a health promotion concept in a disease-oriented culture, such as the medical center, is a long-range goal requiring employment of multidimensional educational strategies.
2. The unstable nature of the organization impeded the rate of diffusion of the Health Promotion Program among its population.
3. Awareness- and interest-raising activities were first-stage strategies in diffusing the wellness concept. Selecting and conducting events that had broad-based appeal to the population were crucial in gaining visibility and acceptance within the organization and by the administration.
4. As expected, health promotion activities were most appealing to "innovators" and "early adopters" who already had special interests in fitness, recreation, and health education activities. It was the health educator's role to identify the interest of these people and harness their energy for the Health Promotion Program.
5. Consistent reinforcement, over time, of the basic concept of wellness through activity and publicity was needed to ensure a high level of awareness of the program. The purpose of this consistent reinforcement is to move the client population from the interest stage of adoption to the trial stage.

POSTSCRIPT

At this writing (winter 1983), two powerful clinical departments have offered to collaborate with the staff and Advisory Committee on a project to develop a health and fitness center. A plan was cooperatively written that provides for the following components in the proposed center: (1) rehabilitation for cardiac and orthopedic patients; (2) sports health for athletes; and (3) health promotion activities tailored to the needs of the medical center population, as well as the general community. Space has already been allocated to build the indoor health and fitness center. Approximately half of the space will be devoted to clinical examining rooms and exercise testing functions, while the remaining space will be a multipurpose area that could be used for a variety of activities.

The development of the health and fitness center, as well as an affiliation with the clinical departments, may enable the Health Promotion Program to expand its activities. Opportunities may also exist for more extensive evaluation of the impact of the program on the participants' life-styles. For this effort to be successful, the aggressive organizational work accomplished early on by program staff and volunteers will need to continue. It remains to be seen if the Health Promotion Program can be integrated into the mainstream of activities at the medical center.

REFERENCES

Goodenough, W. H. 1963. *Cooperation and Change.* New York: Russell Sage Foundation.

Green, L.; Kreuter, M.; Deeds, S.; and Partridge, K. 1980. *Health Education Planning: A Diagnostic Approach.* Palo Alto, Calif.: Mayfield.

Rogers, E. M. 1983. *Diffusion of Innovations.* 3d ed. New York: Free Press.

Stewart, G. W. 1975. "The People: Motivation, Education and Action." *Bulletin of the New York Academy of Medicine* 51(1):174–185.

Travis, J. R. 1977. *Wellness Workbook for Health Professionals.* Mill Valley, Calif.: Wellness Resource Center.

Analysis

This case focuses on a health educator as the planner and coordinator of a health promotion program at a university medical center. A major barrier to implementing the program was the fact that medical centers are oriented primarily to treatment of disease. The case offers an example of what can be done despite the barrier of organizational mission and minimal administrative support.

Donnelly mentions that adoption-diffusion theory (Rogers 1983) provided a rationale that allowed the "gang of three" to proceed with the program despite less than adequate support. During the first year a series of activities was offered. The purpose of these activities was to raise the awareness of the medical center community about wellness. By keeping a variety of activities before the community at all times and punctuating these with occasional events such as the Wellness Jubilee, the program staff allowed the diffusion process to work.

However, the philosophical barrier we have referred to cannot be ignored. Despite the best of plans and the most attractive programs, the mind-set of many members of the medical center community was so disease-oriented that the notion of wellness was foreign to them. Festinger's theory of cognitive dissonance applies here (Festinger 1957).

The case offers an example of the use of adoption-diffusion as both a theory and a strategy. The theory explained to the health educators where the population stood in adopting a new behavior and also provided a guide for program planning.

The disease orientation and the underlying apathy of the administration toward the program were formidable barriers to its potential for influencing the health practices of the medical center. It is well accepted that we all need support, particularly moral support, and encouragement in our work situations. We usually look to a supervisor for this, and legitimately so. Donnelly did not get support from those from whom he had a right to expect it, but he did get it from his two colleagues in the gang of three and from the Advisory Committee. Although support should come from those in administrative positions, it often does not. People can and do build their own support systems (Gottlieb 1981; Squyres 1982), as Donnelly has illustrated.

Although the administration did not advocate for the program nor provide adequate financial support, its response to the program was not entirely negative. It did offer a benign tolerance and therefore some support. For example, the dean/chancellor was invited to and did participate in key health promotion events. His presence gave these events a credibility they would not otherwise have had. For instance, at the road race, his presence suggested his approval to the medical students who participated; at the Wellness Jubilee at the height of the activity, it sanctioned this event in the minds of many members of the medical center community.

The maintenance of attendance records at all events provided data on who was attending and the departments they represented. These data indicated the breadth of interest in the program among the medical center community. They were presented to the administration in the budget hearing for the second year of the program and were instrumental in getting a small increase in the budget.

The importance of maintaining records of all health education programs cannot be overemphasized. The time and place, purpose, attendance, and any other pertinent information about an activity should be recorded. Although these types of records may not seem important to health education goals, they are very important in illustrating to others what has been done, that is, the tangible aspects of the health educator's activities. In this instance, they were also useful in identifying where to target programs.

Donnelly refers to two issues, hiring personnel and setting up an account for the Health Promotion Program, that took an inordinate amount of time and caused him considerable frustration. In the best of large organizations, these conditions prevail. In this instance, however, the resistance the health educator confronted was a direct result of the lack of strong administrative support. Had the administration been totally supportive of the health promotion effort, the Accounting and Personnel Departments would have known this and have given a high enough priority to the program's needs so that the time spent and the frustration caused would have been less than it was.

Donnelly points out that the program deliberately emphasized wellness. Disease prevention issues were excluded from the Wellness Jubilee. Many members of the Advisory Committee did not understand the distinction between wellness and disease prevention and thought those who insisted on this were being difficult.

The distinction is, of course, highly important. Wellness is a positive concept; disease prevention is a negative concept. Learning is much more likely to take place in a positive than in a negative atmosphere. The idea of "forcing" the positive concept on the medical center and not allowing disease issues to be discussed was conceptually sound. The purpose was to promote the concept of doing things because you enjoy them, not because you are afraid of getting a disease. The latter concept forces compliance with practices; the former helps people learn that some activities are enjoyable and incidentally may prevent disease.

Will this Health Promotion Program survive in the medical center with only administrative tolerance? If the program can survive in the short run—at least long enough to garner sufficient grass-roots and administrative support—it may well survive in the long run.

References/Select Resources

Festinger, L. A. 1957. *Theory of Cognitive Dissonance.* Stanford: Stanford University Press.

Festinger's famous theory, developed around 30 years ago, has been used to predict and explain the behavior of individuals and groups. The term *dissonance* applies to what happens when a person holds certain beliefs and attitudes and is asked or required to function or behave in a manner contrary to them. According to the theory, the person will act in a way to reduce dissonance between his or her value system and behavior. That is, she or he will respond by, as occurred in the Donnelly case, not carrying out the new behaviors (rejection) or by changing his or her beliefs and attitudes as the new behavior is carried out.

Gottlieb, B. H., ed. 1981. *Social Networks and Social Support.* Beverly Hills: Sage Publications.

This book of readings is directed at mental health workers who are interested in social support issues as they relate to clients. However, a close reading (particularly of part 2, on social network analysis and social support) will provide insight into the health educator's need for and use of his or her own professional support networks. In the final analysis, what we find from these readings is the need for social supports if we are to function effectively as individuals and professionals.

Mink, O. G.; Schultz, M.; and Mink, B. 1979. *Developing and Managing Open Organizations.* Austin, Tex.: Learning Concepts.

This article describes the role of values, power, and influence in the administrative structure of an organization. It provides tools for assessing organizational structures and for examining how these influence the change process. The role of the worksite in shaping individual lives is analyzed historically, and projections are made regarding the future of sociotechnical systems. The authors discuss how models may be useful in coping with internal and external forces of change.

Rogers, E. M. 1983. *Diffusion of Innovations.* 3d ed. New York: Free Press.

For this edition, Rogers reviewed 3,085 studies on diffusion—an indication of the tremendous increase in diffusion research since his first publication in 1962, when he reported on 405 studies. Rogers has extended diffusion theory by including factors that antecede and follow the adoption process, giving rise to the following questions: Where did the diffusion come from? Which comes first, the need or the innovation? What kinds of problems are encountered, and how are they solved as the innovation is implemented?

The fit of diffusion of innovation to the situation the planners encountered in the Donnelly case was fortuitous. Diffusion theory provided a frame of reference for the program. It also gave the planners psychological support. The knowledge that they were implementing the program according to a well-tested theory about the adoption of new practices offset to some degree the frustrations encountered with the program.

Squyres, W. 1982. "The Professional Health Educator in HMOs: Implications for Training and Our Future in Medical Care." *Health Education Quarterly* 9(1):67–80.

The author's frank discussion of the issues of health education practice in HMOs is applicable as well to the practice of health education in all medical care settings. She points out that health educators are poorly prepared to work in these settings because they not only lack knowledge of the system but often lack substantive knowledge about health and disease issues. On the other side of the coin, she says that the medical care environment is difficult for the health educator because it offers a great deal of responsibility but no authority. The Donnelly case offers an excellent example of that difficulty.

Discussion Questions

1. What steps would you take to develop grass-roots support for an employee health promotion program at a medical center?

2. Do you believe that a greater commitment would have been possible from the administration in this case? If so, how do you think it could have been developed? (a) What is the evidence for more administrative support? (b) What is the evidence against more administrative support?

3. Describe an employee program based on the concept of disease prevention and one based on the concept of wellness. Provide a program plan for a specific target population; include theory, methodology, and evaluation procedures.

4. Write an article for the local newspaper describing the difference between a program based on the prevention concept and one based on the wellness concept. How would you use this comparison if you were marketing a program in the employee newsletter?

5. What issues would you raise with the medical center administrator as arguments for support of a health promotion program based on the wellness concept? Defend the validity of your arguments from the perspective of the medical center's philosophy and mission.

Initiating a Health Promotion Program for Public School Personnel

Vilma T. Falck, Ph.D.

Increased demands on public education have produced stressful conditions for school personnel. Stress refers to those pressures and tensions (whether behaviorally, biologically, economically, or environmentally induced) that, unless suitably managed, can lead to psychological or physiological maladaptations (U.S. DHHS 1980). The extent to which stressful conditions represent a hazard for school personnel has not been fully documented, nor has the number within this population who may be particularly vulnerable to this health risk (Brodsky 1977; Hendrickson 1979; Kyriacou and Sutliffe 1978a, 1978b; Needle, Griffin, and Svendsen 1981). However, the American Public Health Association (1980) has specifically addressed the problem of the health of school personnel and has emphasized the importance of promoting health in this workplace.

The promotion of health and the prevention of chronic or disabling disease are part of the "second public health revolution," described and prescribed by the Surgeon General in *Healthy People* (U.S. DHEW 1979). Occupational health has been specifically addressed by the National Education Association, which has expressed concern that adverse and stressful conditions in schools may lead to increased emotional and physical disabilities among teachers and other school personnel. The development of stress management programs that will facilitate the prevention and treatment of stress-related problems has been recommended.

Recently, considerable attention has been given to the occupational role experienced by educators

---

Vilma T. Falck is an Associate Professor at the University of Texas School of Public Health in Houston.

who work with handicapped and health-impaired children (Dixon, Shaw, and Bensley 1980; Shaw et al. 1980; Weiskopf 1980). This group is considered to be especially vulnerable to job-related stress as a result of their responsibilities for children who have extraordinary needs. The experiences of various levels of public school employees have been markedly influenced by Public Law 94–142, the Education for All Handicapped Children Act of 1975. This legislation established the right of handicapped or health-impaired children to have educational opportunities within public schools. Now enrolled in public schools were children who previously would have been left at home or managed in special, more restrictive environments or in hospital-type settings where their health needs, physiological needs, and demands for personalized care would be met by a therapeutically oriented staff. The public schools' admission of such children, who require continuous attention and care as well as education, has resulted in a number of difficulties for the teachers, resource personnel, and administrative staff who serve them.

PHASE 1: PLANNING

In response to the societal trends to promote health in the workplace, a project was planned for a population of educators who were responsible for young handicapped and/or health-impaired children. The project was planned as a result of a Community Forum that was held to define goals and objectives for a collaborative project to meet the health education needs of handicapped children and their parents. However, during the forum, the representatives of local, regional, and state health and education agencies recommended that a program to meet the needs of school personnel who were experiencing burnout also be given high priority. As evidence of burnout, there were reports of requests for transfer, resignations, conflicts with parents, and feelings of alienation and discouragement in the face of increasing workloads.

Following this conference, which had been planned and organized by health education faculty and graduate students at the University of Texas School of Public Health, a decision was made to request funds from the Regional Education Service Center to develop a program that would establish and meet the needs of special-education personnel. The center is a nonprofit educational service delivery system established by the state of Texas to guide, assist, coordinate, and serve schools in a seven-county area.

NEEDS ASSESSMENT

A community involvement process was designed by health educators at the University of Texas School of Public Health to clarify issues and concerns and to ensure cooperation of key individuals before assessing the needs of the population thought to be at high risk for stress-related problems. Included were representatives of local, regional, and state education agencies. Teachers, principals, nurses, and supervising staff were invited to a small conference during which needs for health education in public schools were discussed. This group recommended that educational programs be developed for personnel in addition to those for children. Contacted personally were the superintendent for instruction in the largest school district within the seven-county area, the state director and several other directors of special education, a director for school health services, regional level educational consultants, and the physician who currently served as president of the medical society in the largest county.

The possibility of artificially exacerbating a need by focusing attention on burnout had to be avoided. The burnout phenomenon is currently rife within professional groups and there may be preconceived notions about its existence and inevitability. The project staff did not want to create a situation in which these groups were reinforced and satisfied merely by finding an acceptable label for their condition. The important concept to be developed and sold was prevention. The premise upon which the project was developed was that burnout, even if it exists, is not inevitable. The proposed educational program would be geared to correlate content with an actual needs assessment. The problem was how to verify what real needs, if any, existed within this population relative to the problem of occupational stress for which educational programs might be useful. Verification of needs would help allay fears that resources might be spent on a faddist trend or on a problem that might be more flamboyant than real.

A multilevel verification process was initiated by the project director and her staff (health education faculty and graduate students at the University of Texas School of Public Health) to help assure that decisions for program planning for this population would be based on an accurate information base. The process included five assessment approaches:

1. Document analyses
2. Interagency conference decisions (nominal group process was employed during a conference for representatives of public education and health agencies)
3. Structured interviews with key informants
4. Reports of stressful incidents
5. Self-assessment surveys of a representative sample of the target population

The process was specifically geared for verification of educational needs. It did not attempt to verify the presence or absence of risk factors.

A synthesis of information gained via the multilevel process provided a structure for identifying educational needs in two categories: those needs specific to program content and those to be considered in the provision of educational programs. Noneducational needs were also identified. A needs profile is shown in Table 1 on page 364.

SELECTION OF CONTENT AND PROCESS

Following the needs assessment, an advisory committee, which included representatives of public school administrators, special-education teachers, and public school resource personnel, met with project staff members. They reviewed the results of the needs assessment and determined how lim-

Table 1
Needs Profile

Type of Needs	Data Referent
Educational Needs	
Content	
Increased skills and/or knowledge needed by school personnel	
Classroom management	Document analysis
Coping and stress management	Interagency conference
Interpersonal skills	Structured interviews
Weight control/foods/nutrition	Reports of incidents
Personal fitness	Self-assessment survey
Prevention-oriented behavior	
Delivery System	
Increased opportunity for school personnel to learn preventive skills in school setting	Interagency conference
Improved format and nontraditional approaches to in-service education	Structured interviews
Increased utilization of community resources	Surveys
Noneducational Needs	
Revision of administrative policies and guidelines for program recognition	Document analysis
Revision of organizational structures to facilitate interagency cooperation	Interagency conference
Increased funding for continuing education	Structured interviews
Formation of building-level support teams	Reports of incidents
Increased utilization of technical assistance and community resources	Surveys

ited funding could best be used to address those needs.

The committee decided to develop and implement a prevention-oriented educational program to include five of the six identified content areas:

1. Coping and stress management
2. Interpersonal skills
3. Weight control/food nutrition
4. Personal fitness
5. Prevention-oriented behavior.

Development of four of these would help assure the fifth: prevention-oriented behavior. The sixth identified content area, classroom management, was considered to be unrelated; moreover, addressing this need would require resources in time and funding that would not be available for this project.

The approach to be used to reach the school personnel would be small self-help groups to be established on a building level, led by facilitators who would be trained during a six-day training series. A pilot project was planned to test feasibility; 32 volunteers would receive training that should enable them to conduct programs in each of their schools.

Work began on a training manual to address the identified content areas. Using the manual, each facilitator would train others to further extend the program. The manual was developed by project

Table 2
Prevention-Oriented Educational Program

Interpersonal Skills	Group Process
Self-management	Information sharing
Support system	Problem solving
Goal setting	Decision making

staff at the University of Texas School of Public Health, using recognized authorities as consultants to assure content accuracy in the areas of nutrition, exercise physiology, mental health, and group process. Faculty of the University of Texas, representatives of the Hogg Foundation for Mental Health, and public school leaders served as consultants.

Table 2 presents the educational design that was followed. For instance, an educational program was devised to assist each participant to manage stress and simultaneously develop interpersonal skills that would be enhanced via the small-group process; this approach would serve as a model for replication of the program.

PHASE 2: COORDINATING

During a six-day program, 32 teachers and administrators representing 11 school districts within a seven-county area were trained as facilitators. The intent was to train volunteers who would be highly motivated, choosing to take on what was to be regarded as an extra responsibility with the full consent and endorsement of their school superintendent. A professional-quality brochure was prepared, as requested by the funding agency, to communicate the purpose and scope to potential participants as well as to school administrators.

An interesting outcome of this effort was that the brochure had limited circulation—despite a process of recurrent communication to ensure the content would be acceptable to the funding agency (as well as to the target receivers, including those in the position of approving the project and releasing their representative for the training program). Apparently the brochure was viewed as politically provocative owing to administrative policies in certain areas. Several of the school districts within the region had recently changed policies regarding staff development, in-service time, and designation of those who might attend.

As a result, the 32 anticipated participants were variously recruited. Some were volunteers; others were told to attend. Two-thirds (65 percent) did not know before attending the first training session that they would be asked to replicate the program. In addition, many reported they did not really understand that the program was to help them; they assumed it was a program to help children. This situation created a dilemma when facilitators for the second year of the project were to be selected from the pool of participants.

Fortunately, the high trainer-trainee ratio (3 project staff members to 32 participants) and the intensive workshop training format provided the opportunity to identify those committed persons who met prescribed competencies and who could implement the pilot program in their respective schools. Although all 32 recruited persons received the initial training, only 14 were selected, on the basis of their demonstrated qualifications and their interest in being facilitators for program extension.

PHASE 3: IMPLEMENTING

The 14 facilitators, some functioning as teams, planned and implemented a variety of prescribed activities in their schools. Each was encouraged to use the training materials in ways to meet his/her individualized program. To field-test all training materials, each team was assigned a separate part of the Training Manual to emphasize.

The programs ranged from those offered only to special educators (classroom teachers) to programs that included all levels of educators (school principal, nutritionist, resource person, etc.), for the training materials were proving to be adaptable to all levels and types of school employees. For instance, one facilitator initiated a pilot program for school bus drivers. One selected facilitator, however, withdrew from the project owing to her time constraints, despite active and enthusiastic support of the school administration.

One of the purposes of the project was to implement relatively small self-help groups who would systematically set goals for themselves and develop programs to maintain or improve their health behaviors. However, facilitators were encouraged to develop programs to meet local needs. Only one team thus far has developed a program consisting of a small group of persons who meet regularly together and function as a support group for one another. The others have presented programs to larger groups that are beginning to stimulate organization of small groups who regularly exercise or eat lunch together. It may be that the support group concept will evolve from these initial activities.

PHASE 4: DEVELOPING AN EVALUATION DESIGN

This project is in the second year of a three-year design. The evaluation design for the first year, in addition to the multilevel needs assessment, focused on collecting data that would be useful for assessing the appropriateness of content in the training materials and improving overall educational strategies. Results of multilevel needs assessment defined characteristics of the educational program. But the evaluation design also allows for measuring the following changes resulting from the educational program:

1. *Knowledge change*—the level of knowledge of the participants as they enter and leave the program
2. *Behavioral change*—participants' completion of activities listed in a personal contract
3. *Attitude change*—changes in attitudes and beliefs about preventive behaviors as a result of participation; also attitudinal differences between participants and nonparticipants

KNOWLEDGE CHANGE

A pretest was used to assess the level of knowledge upon entry into the program. This information also served to indicate the appropriateness of program content and to point out needed changes in degree and level of topics that were addressed via modules in the training manual. A posttest was administered during the final training workshop. This information provided objective data that reflected the change in knowledge level resulting from participation in the program; it also indicated which educational units within each module needed revision. Modules addressed the following topics: Taking Charge of Yourself, Coping with Stress, Nutrition and Well-Being, and Energy and Fitness. Separate posttests were prepared for those who would be participants in the extended program, that is, those whom the facilitators would recruit for participation in the individual schools.

BEHAVIORAL CHANGE

As part of the educational program, all participants are asked to complete a Personal Contract for Health. This contract includes two-month and six-month goals and provides behavioral management techniques and management strategies to assist participants in achieving these goals. Of the 32 participants, 12 (38 percent) selected an exercise goal and 14 (44 percent) chose a weight-loss goal, which in most cases included emphasis on nutrition and exercise. Four persons (12 percent) chose goals that were specifically stress-related, and 2 (6 percent) chose only nutritional goals.

In view of the unsatisfactory manner by which the 32 participants had been recruited, the results of the two- and six-month evaluations were not surprising. All participants were sent letters alerting them to the time for review; each letter was followed by a phone call (structured informal survey), which was the strategy used for the review. Twenty-six (81 percent) were reached by phone. Half of the surveyed participants reported that they had achieved their two-month goal; seven had not been successful but were still trying. Three had illnesses or pregnancies that prevented them from keeping to their plan. Three expressed limited or no interest in the program. Nine of the 14 participants who were selected to serve as facilitators during the second year of the project had reached their two-month personal goal. It must be added that this information, obtained from the two-month follow-up, was not a criterion for the facilitator selection process. Selection criteria had been based on expressed interest and concern, administrative support, attendance, scopes on pre- and posttests, and leadership qualities.

ATTITUDE CHANGE

Instruments to assess attitude changes included the Health Locus of Control Scale, the General Well-Being Schedule, the Job Descriptive Index, and other items that addressed occupational stress and were specific to the needs of the project. The evaluation results indicated that changes in attitudes and beliefs occurred. At the end of the six-day training program, participants showed an increase in their belief that the individual has control over his or her own health; an increase in their belief that other people, such as family, friends, co-workers, and health care providers, could affect their health; and a decrease in their belief that chance events were responsible for individual health. On all three measures, participants reported a more positive attitude toward personal control of health than a comparison group of special-education personnel who had been surveyed but were not included in the program.

Surprisingly, in the area of stress, the survey indicated that a relatively low percentage of special-education personnel considered their occupation extremely stressful. This preliminary result is provocative in view of the reason for initiating this project: reported burnout. It should be added that the word *burnout* was avoided throughout the project.

SUMMARY

A prevention-oriented health education program for public school employees has been developed. It is geared to improve adaptive capability; its strategy is to help individuals help themselves and their peers to become more competent in selecting behaviors conducive to good health. This program was designed to meet the expressed needs of a population working in an environment that is considered to be at high risk for stress-related disorders.

This training program promises to be a useful approach to help school employees help themselves to make decisions based on sound information and to set personal goals in the management of perceived stress and in the areas of nutrition and physical fitness. Evaluation is being made of changes that occur in knowledge, attitudes, and specific skills as a result of participation in this type of health education program. Preliminary results are encouraging, but the path is hazardous. Project activities of themselves can contribute to an overload and result in an antithesis of the intent of the program. The participant who dropped out of the program despite administrative encouragement is an example of this phenomenon. Intellectually she knew the prevention-oriented educational program was geared to help her, but she found the best coping mechanism was to eliminate this extra activity.

This case study is a report of an intensive effort with a small group. Issues related to the assessment of changes in knowledge, specific behaviors, and attitudes will continue to be studied, not only for initial participants in the project, but also for those who serve as they extend the prevention-oriented educational program to others during the next two years. Collection of data to examine issues that are reported to be indicative of problems in this population (e.g., requests for transfer, resignations) will be continued. Program evaluation, as is well known, begins at the initiation of a project. What has been described here is a progress report; more careful evaluation and recurrent analyses are necessary and in progress.

REFERENCES

American Public Health Association. School Health Section. 1980. *Health of school personnel.* Washington, D.C.

Brodsky, C. 1977. "Long Term Work Stress in Teachers and Prison Guards." *Journal of Occupational Medicine* 19(2):133–138.

Dixon, B.; Shaw, S.; and Bensky, J. 1980. "Administrators' Role in Fostering the Mental Health of Special Services Personnel." *Exceptional Children* 47(1): 30–36.

Hendrickson, B. 1979. "Teacher Burnout: How to Recognize It; What to Do about It." *Learning* 7(5): 37–39.

Kyriacou, C., and Sutliffe, J. 1978a. "A Model of Teacher Stress." *Educational Studies* 4(1):1–6.

Kyriacou, C., and Sutliffe, J. 1978b. "Teacher Stress: Prevalence, Sources, and Symptoms." *British Journal of Educational Psychology* 48:159–167.

Needle, R. H.; Griffin, T.; and Svendsen, R. 1981. "Occupational Stress: Coping and Health Problems of Teachers." *Journal of School Health* 51(3):175–181.

Shaw, S. F.; Bensky, M.; Dixon, B.; and Bonneau, R. 1980. "Strategies for Dealing with Burnout among Special Educators." *Education Unlimited*, September–October:21–23.

U.S. Department of Health, Education, and Welfare. Public Health Service. Office of the Assistant Secretary for Health and Surgeon General. 1979. *Healthy People: Surgeon General's Report on Health Promotion and Disease Prevention.* DHEW Publication no. (PHS) 79–55071. Washington, D.C.: Government Printing Office.

U.S. Department of Health and Human Services. Public Health Service. 1980. *Promoting Health/Preventing Disease: Objectives for the Nation.* Washington, D.C.: Government Printing Office.

Weiskopf, P. E. 1980. "Burnout among Teachers of Exceptional Children." *Exceptional Children* 47(1): 18–23.

Wertheimer, M. 1972. *Fundamental Issues in Psychology.* New York: Holt, Rinehart & Winston.

Analysis

In this case, the health educator describes the planning, initial implementation, and evaluation of the first year of a three-year project funded to "develop a program that would establish and meet the needs of special-education personnel" in a large metropolitan area.

Several planning models could apply to this case. Falck and her colleagues essentially followed the Mico model, which has horizontal and vertical dimensions (Ross and Mico 1980:213). The horizontal phases are identified by six steps: "(1) initiation of planning activity, (2) needs assessment, (3) goal setting, (4) planning or programming the activity to be carried out, (5) implementing the activity, and (6) evaluating the activity's effectiveness." The three vertical dimensions are content, methodology, and process.

The in-depth needs assessment described in the case should be noted. Five different processes were used to identify needs as perceived by the target population.

The avoidance of the use of the word *burnout* in the needs assessment is an example of not predetermining what the target population sees as a need. The issue of approaching projects with unstated or implicit assumptions and so denying the target population the opportunity to speak for itself is a central issue in the case study by Thomas, Israel, and Steuart (p. 225).

The concept of diffusion of innovation (Rogers 1983) and theories of learning/social change provide a theoretical fit for the educational plan developed for the school personnel. They suggest the strategy of making learning experiences available to the target population and allowing its members to take what they want as they see the need.

This case raises several issues related to the practice of health education: for instance, the need for objectivity by the health educator, the importance of establishing communications among several participating groups, the attempt to meet the different needs of participating organizations, and the predicament of having responsibility but no authority. The last two warrant some discussion.

It is very clear that Falck and her colleagues strove toward excellence in all phases of this case. We've mentioned the needs assessment. The care with which the training manual was developed is a second example. The well-designed educational program and evaluation protocol are other examples. Nonetheless, the project encountered serious barriers in the implementation phase. These had nothing to do with the work of the health educator, but were due to the school system's internal political issues over which the health educator had no control.

Health educators often encounter these kinds of barriers because they cannot always control the behavior of other persons involved in a project. They are therefore often in the position of having a great deal of responsibility but no authority. Squyres (1982) discusses this issue in relation to health educators in HMOs. As can be seen from this case, it is true in other settings as well.

In these situations, health educators must separate the educational component of a project from political, organizational, or other factors that present barriers to goal attainment. An analysis of the situation should be put in writing for administrators and funding agencies. Otherwise, health education may be tagged with program failure when in fact the educational component has been well done, as in this case, and other factors have interfered with successfully implementing the educational program.

The issue of meeting the needs of different participating organizations or systems within organizations is also illustrated by this case. For example, in the needs assessment, the classroom teachers identified classroom management as a problem. Yet Falck states that classroom management "was considered to be unrelated; moreover, addressing this need would require resources in time and funding that would not be available for this project." But with this need being ignored, the question is, Whose needs were being met? The training program treated the problem of personal stress, which may well have been created in part by the classroom management problem. So it would seem that stress could have been alleviated by dealing with the class management problem. Health educators are often caught in this kind of crossfire. In this case, the health educator's options seemed to be limited by the policy "Do what we will accept or do nothing."

This case offers a model of good practice. It illustrates, though, that despite good practice, educational issues are sometimes superseded by organizational and political issues over which the health educator often has no control. Nonetheless, Falck demonstrates that competency and persistence can produce some positive results.

References/Select Resources

Brennan, A. J. 1982. "Health Promotion: What's in It for Business and Industry?" *Health Education Quarterly* 9 (Special suppl.):9–19.

This paper explores the motivations, expected benefits, and rationale for employee health education programs. In describing three programs of large corporations, it points out the special features that have proven viable. The costs and benefits associated with worksite programs are presented. Pitfalls that result from overenthusiasm without realization of economic realities are also described. This paper promises to be a classic resource for practicing health educators.

Huse, E. F. 1980. *Organizational Development and Change.* 2d ed. New York: West.

This well-arranged text explains principles of organizational development to assist organizations to improve productivity and the quality of work life. Using a systems approach, it delineates underlying concepts, principles, and assumptions of organizational development. Especially applicable to the Falck case is chapter 13, which has a section concerning the school system.

Rogers, E. M. 1983. *Diffusion of Innovations.* 3d ed. New York: Free Press.

There has been a tremendous increase in diffusion research since Rogers's first publication in 1962, when he reported on 405 studies on diffusion. For this edition he reviewed 3,085 studies. By now extending diffusion theory to include factors that antecede and follow the adoption process, Rogers poses several questions: Where did the diffusion come from? Which comes first the need or the innovation? What kinds of problems are encountered, and how are they solved as the innovation is implemented?

Rogers identifies factors that influence the diffusion of an innovation at each step in the process. The barriers to the school personnels' participation in the educational programs described in the Falck case offer a good example of Rogers's thesis that the diffusion process does not always move along smoothly.

Ross, H. S., and Mico, P. R. 1980. *Theory and Practice in Health Education.* Palo Alto, Calif.: Mayfield.

This is a useful volume for both the beginner and the seasoned practitioner. It offers a comprehensive listing of theories, models, strategies, and issues for the practicing health educator. The descriptions of each is necessarily brief but most adequate for the novice. The issues are treated from the perspective of the individual, the organization, and the larger society. The book contains a comprehensive section on planning models that is relevant to the planning described in the Falck case.

Squyres, W. 1982. "The Professional Health Educator in HMOs: Implications for Training and Our Future in Medical Care." *Health Education Quarterly* 9(1):67–80.

In this frank discussion of health education practice in HMOs, Squyres says that the medical care environment is difficult for the health educator because it offers a great deal of responsibility but no authority. The Falck case illustrates that this issue is relevant to the practice of health education in other settings as well.

Zaltman, G.; Duncan, R.; and Holbek, J. 1973. *Innovations and Organizations.* New York: Wiley.

This book provides an overview of research on innovations in organizations up to 1973. It examines how innovations are facilitated or inhibited by the characteristics and the environment of organizations. The authors define an innovation "as any idea, practice or material artifact perceived to be new by the relevant unit of adoption." Health educators are regularly faced with influencing the adoption of innovation at the individual level. But it is useful to consider the health educator's role in promoting adoptions within organizations because very often this may be his or her primary role. The organization may be a client such as an industry interested in developing a wellness program. Or the organization may be the health educator's employer, so that the issue of innovation could arise if the health educator's role within the organization is expanded. Understanding the adoption of innovations by organizations can therefore be as important as understanding that adoption by individuals. As the authors point out, although organizations are composed of individuals, their adoption process is quite different.

Discussion Questions

1. What skills are needed by a health educator to coordinate a project, such as this one, sponsored by several agencies.

2. Could there have been any way to avoid the problem of recruiting the first group of trainers from among the classroom teachers?

3. What training methods would you select for training the facilitators?

4. As a health promotion program for wellness in the workplace, how is this case similar to or different from other cases of employee health promotion programs described in Part Four?

5. Prepare a memorandum for your administrator, identifying the health education component of this project and the political issues that impinged on it.

PART FIVE

Professional Development

The preceding cases have given you a panoramic view of the practice of health education. This view may have piqued your interest sufficiently to persuade you to consider health education as a career.

The Green case that follows describes how one health educator set his sights for a career in health education. Green presents many interesting issues and personal anecdotes spanning more than ten years. He chats with the reader about how he developed his career and how *a plan, persistence,* and *belief in himself* enabled him to meet his personal and professional goals. The case also offers a historical view of the development of research and evaluation in health education.

One issue of major importance that Green raises is his perspective on the scope of the health education field. In the sixties, some health educators perceived that the field should be focused on social change. Others, including Green, perceived it as including social change but centering on individual and group change. The latter can lead to social change, but that is not necessarily its purpose.

The case offers gems of insight for the beginner or the seasoned professional. Selecting a career and finding one's niche is not always easy. Green's reflections on his career may enable students to find some direction for theirs.

A Participant-Observer in a Period of Professional Change

Lawrence W. Green, Dr.P.H.

Most of the case studies in this volume are keyed to a community or organizational level of analysis, because those are the levels at which health educators most commonly function and the opportunities for health education are most frequent. Indeed, these levels of health education activity are, in the final analysis, the best hope for the ultimate success of health education. For without community commitment, there can be little continuity of health education programs that are truly responsive to the needs of individuals, families, and locally differentiated groups.

As educators, however, we must be concerned also with the development of people, including ourselves, as individuals and as professionals. I have been asked to write a case study on how health educators get started in a professional track that leads to opportunities to influence policy. I would not presume to assess the careers of others in the context of case studies. The field is too small to disguise an anonymous case. This chapter, therefore will analyze the experience of one person—myself—in relation to the academic, political, scientific, and policy changes occurring during a period in health education. This, then, is a biographical case rather than a program or community case; unlike most case studies, it is more a study of professional socialization and career orientation than a study of a specific problem. It would not qualify as a single case study because the subject is too varied and the period too long, so it is presented as a chronological series of case studies.

My purpose in this analysis is to cast my scattered observations on the careers of many people, including my students, in a single, personalized perspective. I will critically examine my own early efforts as if they were unique, though in reality many of my peers, contemporaries, and students have had similar experiences. The presentation might imply that my efforts had been consciously and systematically planned, but the goals were actually vague in the beginning and the specific activities were often fortuitous. My hope in personalizing this presentation is that I might bring a long and plodding process to life for the young professional embarking on a career with expectations of influencing science or policies in health education.

Lawrence W. Green is Director of the Center for Health Promotion Research and Development at the University of Texas Health Science Center in Houston.

I am indebted to the many professionals and scholars in health education and related fields whose labors and contributions to policy I have tried to reflect in the joys and pains of my own experience. But in doing so, I have regrettably and unavoidably made my experience seem greater than theirs. I am especially grateful for the contributions in general and the specific suggestions on earlier drafts of this paper of Drs. John Allegrante, Sigrid Deeds, Nell Gottlieb, Donald Iverson, Lloyd Kolbe, David Levine, Patricia Mullen, Ian Newman, and Judith Ottoson. They cannot be held accountable for this version, however, as their advice was not unanimous on any single point in previous drafts.

THE STAGE IS SET IN 1970

The 1960s had been a period of great turmoil in the United States and abroad. As students at Berkeley, my classmates and I were properly radicalized and outraged by the conditions in the South that led to the Civil Rights Movement and those in Vietnam and Cambodia that led to the student strikes and destruction of property in protest. I sympathized and even participated, but, after I had had training briefly in local, state, and federal agencies and for two years in Bangladesh, the radical solutions seemed expedient but simplistic. I began to resent the distraction from my studies that I knew I needed to complete in order to make a more thoughtful and basic contribution to the capacity of people and communities to serve their own health needs. Many of my contemporaries joined the Peace Corps; some went to jail in protest or dropped out, disenchanted either with radical causes or with both radical and establishmentarian ways of pursuing them. It was a time, especially in Berkeley, when the traditions of science and professionalism virtually had to go underground in the face of the more-radical-than-thou ethic. Serious research was regarded by many as bourgeois, health education as a sellout.

On the positive side, the elderly were fighting successfully in the early and mid-60s for Social Security reforms that would give them medical benefits. This was also the period of "maximum feasible participation" in health planning and neighborhood health agencies. These two movements were to have a profound impact on the status of health education policy in 1970. They were not so different from the issues today of unemployment, further reforms in Social Security, and the New Federalism.

How does one set priorities at such a time? What social purposes should health education serve, and how can one person make the right choice among the many causes and developmental needs of such a varied field to make the best use of one's training and skills? These are the questions addressed by the first three case studies.

CASE STUDY 1: ASSESSING THE PROBLEMS OF ONE'S TIME

What are the social problems to which health education could be most usefully addressed if one concentrated one's energies on behalf of a particular social cause?

The most significant impact of Medicare and Medicaid, passed in 1966, was the transfer of considerable purchasing power for medical care into the hands of the aged and the poor and medically indigent. This purchasing power, put together with increased federal spending on other New Frontier, Great Society, and War on Poverty initiatives of the Kennedy and Johnson eras, caused the medical care dollar to undergo a more rapid rate of inflation than the rest of the economy. The rapid escalation of medical care costs was regarded by many as the single most urgent problem of the nation with regard to health in 1970, and clearly the issue that new policies in health education were expected to address. It threatened to nullify the advances made in achieving more equitable access to health services.

Other trends were converging in 1970 with more subtle, but nevertheless momentous, force. There was a growing recognition of diminishing returns on morbidity and mortality reductions with the increasing expenditures on medical care and biomedical research. The increased costs of medical care were not yielding commensurate improvements in death and disease rates. There were also broader cultural trends, such as a declining trust in and growing disenchantment with government and professionalism, especially in regard to medical care. There was a growing interest in a return to self-help skills, in community and personal development, in quality of life, and in other aspects of health beyond medical control. The behavioral and social sciences were taking a firm hold in public health, medicine, and education. Nuclear threats seemed beyond the control of self-help, government, medicine, and social services.

There were equally compelling concerns with population control, in which health education was expected to contribute through family planning, population education, and sex education. Some, especially in California, regarded the human potential movement to be even more fundamental as a basis for a new social order: More open and honest communication, more self-realization, more liberated women, assertiveness, parent effectiveness, Black pride, Chicano and Indian nativism, transcendental meditation, all seemed worthy candidates for a new public health in which health education could make a primary and basic difference in the quality of life. Then there was (and still is) world hunger. Some would argue that it is selfish and indulgent for a country, a class of people, or even an individual, to be concerned with quality of life and human potential when others have not even fulfilled a basic human need. And so in 1970, as today, the issues and problems competed for the attention, and appealed to the conscience, of professionals in the human services.

By what standard was a health educator to set priorities? Primacy of causality? One theory held that all other development was retarded by world population growth. Another theory or ideology held that population control could not succeed until more "basic" socioeconomic developments occurred. Yet another set of theories and philosophies held that any socioeconomic development was meaningless without the self-respect, dignity, and cultural pride that could come only with one of the human potential movements, or without the absence of fear that could come only with nuclear arms control and peace.

My own conclusion about "the problem" deserving highest priority was that it could not be defined a priori by professionals or politicians in a pluralistic society. Quality of life is an elusive concept that will vary over time and between cultures, subcultures, families, and individuals. The role of health education is to build the capacity of individuals and communities to assess their own social or quality-of-life concerns, the health needs associated with them, and the actions that they can take individually and collectively to affect those health needs.

CASE STUDY 2: DEFINING THE OPTIONS FOR PERSONAL-PROFESSIONAL ACTION

One could finesse the choices in 1970 between these alternative issues and problems of the time—any one of which would be worthy of a career of professional effort to influence people and policy—by first choosing between institutions and organizations from which to launch a long-term effort and then choosing the strategies one might develop within health education. How does one make such choices? It is hard to say. In retrospect, I believe I chose my strategy first and my place second. By concluding that the social problem should be chosen by the people served, I could devote myself in good conscience to the task of developing the capacity of health education to contribute to a wide range of social problems or quality-of-life concerns. The focus shifted thus from ends to means. My initial decision was not one of selecting the paramount social issue or problem, but rather that of determining how to tackle the generic problem of underdevelopment in health education. It was a matter of first choosing between the types of battle that needed to be fought, including the weapons to be used, and then choosing the battleground best suited for waging the battle. In any era and place, the war will be defined historically and culturally. The battles and the weapons are left for individuals to choose.

The optional battles one could wage for health education included radical politics, professional politics, community development, mainstream consensus politics, and a longer-range strategy of policy development through research to build the evidence and knowledge base required for rational planning in health education. Each of these options was a correct choice for some of my contemporaries. Radical political action was still needed to continue the pressure for redistributing resources to the disadvantaged. Professional political action was needed to upgrade the quality of professional practice on the basis of what was already known. Community development and consensus politics were needed to keep health education in the mainstream of social change.

All of the battles to be fought for health education in the 1970s, it appeared to me, would have to be waged with more scientific weapons than had been used in the past. The 1960s and earlier decades had already seen a period of rapid social change and vast development and redistribution of health resources in the United States. Health education had made its way on the strength of obvious and self-evident truth and logic about the necessary relationship between education and the ability of people to take full advantage of the health resources they were being offered. New vaccines, new screening tests, and other medical procedures were being offered, but the message was that they could be used most effectively if people consulted regularly with medical practitioners. The objective of most programs calling for health education was to increase the availability and utilization of services. The successful increase in health screening, immunization, prenatal care, family planning, maternal and child care, neighborhood health centers, Pap smears, and other services for early detection and treatment of suspicious symptoms was a mixed blessing. It reduced the gap in access to medical care between the affluent and the poor, but it also inflated the cost of all health care services. It also might have given people a false sense of security that their health needs were met so long as their medical needs were met.

The issue of the '70s, it appeared, would be defined more by the increasing scarcity of resources, the need to control costs, the need to limit utilization of services, and the need to be sure that those services used were the most cost-effective and beneficial from a larger social and economic perspective than the narrow and provincial medical objectives of the past. These were not entirely new issues in 1970, but it was apparent that they would be moved higher on the agenda of important issues, and that health education would have to compete for resources on the strength of its scientific credibility and its effectiveness in communicating its cost-containing capacity as well as its social benefits.

When examined from this perspective, Johns Hopkins University appeared to be a strong scientific fortress in which I could hope to develop policy-relevant health education research and evaluation. Its proximity to Washington made it an attractive staging ground for the political use of data as a weapon to further policy. Johns Hopkins had notable strengths in health economics, health services research, health policy, and health administration, all of which would be useful allies in the battle of the '70s, as I had defined it.

CASE STUDY 3: DEVELOPING A PLAN

The stage was set by 1970, both for global changes and for the elements of a personal plan for the 1970s that was only a vague intellectual notion at the time, although it began to take more concrete form within my first few years at Johns Hopkins. This plan sustained my professional and scientific efforts in a cohesive and cumulative way through the decade.

The plan consisted essentially of a series of priorities or steps for health education research and development if the field was to compete effectively for resources in times of increasing scarcity. The steps or priorities were as follows:

1. Address the social, economic, and quality-of-life concerns of the time and of specific populations or communities.
2. Identify the health problems imposing the greatest burden on the social and economic concerns of the time.
3. Identify the health-related behaviors most important and most amenable to change through health education.
4. Design and then carry out rigorous, credible evaluations of health education strategies targeted on the factors influencing the priority behaviors and their associated health problems.
5. Disseminate the findings of research and evaluation through professional training, continuing education, publication, consultation, speaking, correspondence, and testimony to governmental agencies, legislative groups, foundations, and professional associations.

Such priorities imply a sequence of action, although the sequence may be repeated with each successive redefinition of social problems or concerns. As Sir Godfrey Vickers once observed, "The history of public health is a history of successive redefining of the unacceptable."

These priorities became the objectives of the Division of Health Education at Johns Hopkins and were elaborated in their first published form in the article "Toward Cost-Benefit Evaluations of Health Education: Some Concepts, Methods and Examples," which appeared in a 1974 supplement of *Health Education Monographs*. These concepts eventually became the organizing framework for the curriculum of the division, for the annual continuing education workshop on "Educational Diagnosis and Evaluation in Public Health and Medical Care," for a health education information retrieval system, and for much of my own research and writing. Developing a long-range plan for a cohesive program of any kind requires such organizing concepts.

CASE STUDY 4: DEFYING PROFESSIONAL NORMS

The research and curriculum we developed at Johns Hopkins were by no means revolutionary, but they departed in their emphasis from some professional norms of the time. It was not the first time professional ranks had been broken by a health educator, nor the first time anyone felt the sting of professional criticism for embarking on a program that ran counter to professional norms. Innovation is unavoidably counternormative.

Professional norms are not to be disregarded or discounted simply in the name of innovation and change without considering the function they serve in assuring the public of the self-regulation, peer review, and quality control that distinguish the professions from governmentally regulated trades and commercial services. What are the conditions and consequences of professional deviance and sanction?

One condition for deviance is to find another organization in which such "deviance" is sanctioned. Johns Hopkins had been a bastion of scientific respectability and, in that sense, a haven for an academic refugee from Berkeley. I realize in retrospect, however, that this feeling was attributable no more to the difference between Berkeley and Johns Hopkins than to the problem of any young graduate who drifts from the dominant paradigms of the place where he or she trained. In any case, the consequence for me was some degree of guilt feeling and some perceived, if not actual, criticism from the profession for "abandoning" or "betraying" elements of the ideology of health education. I feared I had abandoned the Nyswander philosophy ingrained in Berkeley students, as expressed in the emphasis on group dynamics and Lewinian psychology. By laying the emphasis on scientific rather than group dynamics methodology and criteria for decision making, and by emphasizing economic, medical, and behavioral rather than more strictly perceptual or consumer satisfaction criteria of success, I flirted with the possibility that I was forsaking the Nyswander ideology, or at least the latter-day Berkeley representation of it. Others of my contemporaries also have expressed difficulty in living up to the ideals of Dorothy Nyswander, or of Lucy Morgan if they graduated from the University of North Carolina, or of Mabel Rugen if from the University of Michigan.

I would suggest to any student, as you depart from the fold of your professional training, that you will experience some sense of infidelity to your teachers and peers as you take on new challenges in new places. If you do not feel this, it may be a sign that you are not addressing the problems of your time, your new community or organization, and your new role, but rather importing ritual and doctrine from your previous professional home. In retrospect, I see that my peers and I have all carried the Nyswander, Morgan, and Rugen concepts forward in different ways.

If I have presented the experience of running against the grain of some professional norms in mostly negative personal terms, the obvious truth is that I avoided far more unnecessary conflicts than I engaged in and that there were more rewards and satisfactions than sticks and stones. There was, for example, the inherent reward of being able to offer policy-relevant data that others could use. It is always intrinsically satisfying to see someone else apply one's own ideas, data, or methods. That is an inherent reward of teaching, but it is multiplied many times when the users are numerous practitioners and government and other officials, and many more times when the users are legislators and policymakers. One also observes the multiplier effect when one is training doctoral students and postdoctoral fellows who go on to train yet larger numbers of students than one could ever hope to admit to a single graduate program. The expectation that they would elaborate and apply the concepts they learned from me was very satisfying. But it was an expectation that I had to suppress for fear that I would set up unreasonable pressures for them to export "the Hopkins model" and feel guilty when they found it unusable or inappropriate in their new situations, as I found the Berkeley model to be when I arrived at Johns Hopkins.

In the final analysis, the innovator must make room for others to challenge the professional norms that build up around the models or methods he/she has offered. We strived to create this climate of innovation and challenge at Hopkins by building an interdisciplinary faculty and accepting postdoctoral fellows who would bring contradictory points of view, and by pushing our own graduates out to plow new fields. But ultimately I knew it was I who had to go away to make room for both Johns Hopkins and myself to grow in health education.

POSSIBLE LESSONS FOR THE YOUNG PROFESSIONAL WHO HOPES TO INFLUENCE POLICY

I conclude this series of case studies with a few suggestions drawn from my experience. I would presume to offer these as guides to the young professional embarking on a career in health education in which he or she hopes to make a difference in policy. I believe these suggestions should apply as much to influencing local policy as to state, federal, or international policy.

First, I would suggest three paths to policy influence. These are not mutually exclusive, although the aggressive pursuit of one may tend to preclude or dampen success in another. The first is the expertise, research, and credentials route. This path depends on academic and professional training or learning by some other mechanism, plus intensive investigation, communication of what one has learned, and the gradual development of ability, insight, and a reputation for integrity, knowledge, objectivity, and dependability. Credentials, in the form of degrees and positions, can substitute for some of this background and can facilitate obtaining some of it, but steadfast patience and consistent pursuit of a narrow range of objectives is the key ingredient for successful pursuit of this path to policy influence.

The second path is political representation. On this route, one begins by representing the interest of a few people in a negotiation or other action on their behalf. Successful representation in any community leads to a larger number of people, often friends of the first party, who are willing to have you represent them similarly. Running for office in professional associations is a way to start. The political representative can extend the number and type of people he or she is representing and/or broaden issues on which he or she offers representation. As the numbers increase and the issues broaden, the representative often steps upward in the levels of decision making at which representation is offered. The source of power for the political representative is not necessarily expertise, although it may include that. It is rather the number of constituents whose votes or purchasing power he or she can bring to bear on the sway of decisions.

The third route to policy influence is one that I have come to appreciate as much as the first two as a result of my federal experience. This is the route of the diligent and faithful civil servant. Many of the people in Washington who helped or blocked me most effectively were neither politicians nor experts, but rather people whose power had been accumulated gradually or abruptly as a reward for their faithful service to an individual, a community, or a cause. In some rare instances these faithful civil servants had served a series of directors with widely divergent political views, but had survived because of their ability to see beyond the short-range political expediency.

My first suggestion, then, is to pick a route, a path to follow, for your first ten years of professional life and to pursue it diligently, resisting the temptation in the early stages of your career to try pursuing more than one path simultaneously.

My second suggestion is take a long-range view. Resist the temptation to back down from your long-range objective when criticism begins to mount and doubt begins to creep in. Your first impulse and the vision that grew out of it were probably correct and valid, but problems, barriers, and criticisms can undermine your self-confidence and deflect you from the path you chose. People who accomplish less than they expected of themselves often seem to have been detracted and deflected, pursuing too many paths at once, diffusing their energy, and undermining the concentration of efforts required to achieve anything more than a series of flashes in the pan. I am not referring to the choice between career and family or between work and the nurturance of friends. These need not be competitive and indeed should be complementary and mutually supportive sides of an integrated life. Moreover, it is not so much the singularity of the career goal that is important. Indeed, many goals may be achieved on the same path. It is rather the cumulative building of one development upon another so that each succession is stronger and more significant than the preceding one, building on the strength of the foundation upon which it rests. This is what granting agencies call the "track record" of the applicant.

The third suggestion I have for young professionals who hope to influence policy is to develop an acute sensitivity to what people need to know to further the cause. What do your colleagues and staff need to know, what do your constituents need to know, what do policymakers above you need to know in order to support your efforts, to understand your purpose, to accept your methods, and to believe in your cause?

The fourth suggestion I have drawn from this postmortem on my experience of the past decade is that you have fidelity to an irreducible set of principles that give meaning and integrity to your cause. I hesitate to state what these principles are for me personally because they might be too helpful, in the sense of offering a cookbook approach to what must be a deeper, personal, existential commitment. I will give only one example to illustrate the kind of principle I have in mind, but even this example is not intended to represent truth for everyone. The principle that has guided most of my decisions when in doubt has been *experiment*. The experimental method has been an ideal for ascertaining truth that I have emulated in my work, not only in research but in administrative and teaching practices as well. I carried this so far as to establish, as a motto of our master's training program at Johns Hopkins, that we were training an "experimenting practitioner." A small number of other principles guided my actions and continued to direct my planning for the future. These are somewhat less methodological and more ideological and therefore less universally applicable.

Finally, I suggest to the young professional who hopes to influence policy that he or she maintain flexibility on virtually everything else. It is enough that I have suggested selecting a single path among three, setting a limited number of long-range goals and maintaining fidelity to a finite set of principles. I do not intend to advocate a style of rigidity beyond that. Indeed, in everyday interactions and movement, flexibility and going with the flow are necessary, not only to maintain your own mental health but also to continue growing and learning from others and from new experiences that may not have been built into your long-range plans.

Analysis

The cases in this book offer a sense of what health educators do, the settings in which they work, and the issues that affect their daily activities. The student may ask: Where do I want to make my contribution to health education? What aspect of this field do I wish to work in and why? Green's case offers guidelines students can use in answering these questions.

Green describes the process by which he decided what he wanted to do and the contribution he wanted to make to health education. He traces the course of his decision for ten years, indicating that his plan began with vague outlines but took shape over time. It is significant for the beginner to note how the plan developed and to recognize the role of fortuitous events in its development. Without a plan Green could not have taken advantage of these events.

Green indicates that his "advice" is for those interested in influencing health education policy but points out that policy is developed by organizations and by local and state governments as well as the federal government. For example, many departments within large organizations develop policy on given issues. Therefore all health educators need to be concerned about policy because organizational policy affects what a health educator can do in that organization. Further, as Steckler and Dawson (1982) note, policy development will have much to do with determining the viability of health education as a profession.

Green advises the young professional to focus on a single path "for the first ten years of professional life and to pursue it diligently," while "setting a limited number of long-range goals and maintaining fidelity to a finite set of principles." His own career attests to the efficacy of his advice. Green has contributed more to the research and evaluation literature in health education than any other individual. His career thus serves as an excellent example to new professionals.

References/Select Resources

"Health Education Policy Issues." 1978. *Health Education Monographs* 6 (Suppl. 1).

This issue of the monographs presents a collection of policy papers that have stimulated much discussion and activity in regard to policy formation. Paul Mico presents the introduction to policy formation. Scott K. Simonds looks at ethical issues as they relate to policy. Lawrence W. Green reviews recent research in health education and shows how it should influence federal policy. H. Ogden describes policy development at the federal level up to 1978. Maurice Reizen and colleagues explore policy development at the state level. Finally, Jeanette Simmons, in her commentary on the preceding papers, stresses the importance of the consumer's role in policy formation.

Kahn, A. J. 1969. *Theory and Practice of Social Planning*. New York: Russell Sage Foundation.

This classic text in social planning provides an excellent introduction to policy issues, particularly in chapters 5 and 6. Although the policy issues are explored within the context of social welfare, health educators will find the mechanics of policy formulation to be useful in considering how best they may influence policy decisions.

Steckler, A., and Dawson, L. 1982. "The Role of Health Education in Public Policy Development." *Health Education Quarterly* 9(4):275–292.

As the authors note, health educators must become involved in policy formation if the profession is to remain viable. With this premise in mind, the authors present a lucid discussion of how health educators can become involved at the various levels of government and in nongovernmental organizations. Included here are basic definitions that are of particular use to those who are unfamiliar with the process of policy formation.

Discussion Questions

1. Outline a path you would like to follow during your professional career for the next ten years. What are some of the barriers and problems you might encounter along the way?

2. Identify some of the professional norms that appear to operate in health education today.

3. Provide some examples of how policy at the state and federal level may influence personal health behavior.

4. What are some ways you could influence policy at the local level to help achieve health education goals?

5. Provide some examples of how you could implement Green's concept of the "experimenting practitioner" (p. 380).

Glossary

Accountability
Accepting responsibility for one's actions to another.

Administrative Style
Personal attributes that individuals apply to the management of personnel and programs.

Adoption
The decision to make full use of a new idea as the best course of available action.

Change Agent
An individual, organization, or group that assists a client or client system to identify issues of concern and the means of dealing with these concerns. Involvement can be intensive or minimal. The change agent's role can include functions such as diagnosis, planning, facilitating, and evaluating.

Communication
The process by which messages are transferred through a channel to a receiver.

Community Development
Approaches and techniques that rely upon local communities as units of action; attempt to combine outside assistance with organized, local self-determination efforts; and correspondingly seek to stimulate local initiative and leadership as the primary instrument of change.

Community Organization
By this process, a community identifies its needs, develops the abilities and finds the resources to meet these needs, and develops cooperative and collaborative attitudes and practices in the community.

Conflict Resolution
This is a process used to resolve differences. All parties accept the agreed-upon decision and work together toward a solution.

Consultation
By this process, a third party assists a person, group, or organization to use internal and external resources to make decisions and effect change.

Counseling
The process by which a counselor assists an individual or group to identify and deal with situations or information related to interactions with others and enables the individual(s) to make effective decisions.

Culture
The ideas, customs, values, and practices that influence the behavior of a group, organization or society during a given period.

Decision Making
The process by which an individual, organization, community, or society agrees upon a course of action or a solution to an issue.

Diffusion
Innovations spread to members of a social system by the process of diffusion.

Evaluation
A systematic approach used to determine the extent to which target goals have been achieved and whether program inputs are causally related to outputs. This evaluation can also involve an examination to determine how activities are carried out to achieve the goals.

Health Belief Model
As originally developed, a composite of theories that predicts or explains a given individual's willingness to accept a procedure used to detect or prevent disease.

Health Education
The process by which individuals, organizations, communities, and societies learn to make informed decisions about issues related to health and disease. The process can be either planned or unplanned. The planned process includes a variety of scheduled activities to assist target populations in making decisions.

Health Promotion
Any combination of health education and related organizational, political, and economic interventions designed to facilitate behavioral and environmental adap-

tations to improve or protect health (from L. W. Green, 1979, "National Policy in the Promotion of Health," in the *International Journal of Health Education* 12(3), 161–168.)

Learning
A process concerned with the acquisition of knowledge, attitudes, skills, and experience, resulting in behavioral change and enabling individuals to function within a social context.

Management
The art and science of directing, coordinating, and controlling resources—human and material—focused on an objective within a group, organization, community, or society.

Methods
In health education, this term refers to discrete communication techniques, such as printed and electronic media, group discussion, counseling, gaming, group instruction, role playing, and story telling. These methods are used as tools to assist in the learning/social change process.

Model
A composite of theories that delineates and organizes relevant facts and determines the sequence of activities.

Needs Assessment
The process by which both perceived and unperceived deficiencies of individuals, groups, communities, and societies are identified.

Organizational Development
A process of change in an organization's culture through the application of behavioral science knowledge, most often based on a systems perspective.

PRECEDE
A seven-phase, diagnostic health education planning model to organize relevant facts and determine a sequence of activities to facilitate program planning. The PRECEDE model can be used in any setting for any type of program.

Prevention of Disease
Primary Prevention: Protection against disease.
Secondary Prevention: Early detection and prompt treatment of disease.
Tertiary Prevention: Minimizing and controlling the effects of disease.
These three levels of disease prevention are effected through various interventions, including economic, social, medical, behavioral, and environmental prevention methods.

Self Care
By this process, consumers assume responsibility for making decisions affecting their health. These decisions can be related to self-limiting or life-threatening ill-

nesses and can include diagnosis, determination of the severity of symptoms, and selection of treatment.

Self-Help Group

Usually refers to individuals with a common problem who come together to assist one another in dealing with that problem.

Social Change

The process by which the structure and function of a social system is transformed as a result of individual and/or group learning.

Social Support

Personal relationships that can be depended upon to provide emotional or material aid in times of need.

Strategies

A combination of methods planned to complement, supplement, and reinforce each other, to assist in the learning/social change process.

Theory

A systematic formulation of principles and concepts used to predict and explain behavior.

Wellness

A positive attitude demonstrated by behavior that focuses on maintaining health through exercise, nutrition, meditation, laughter, stress control, and similar modalities.

Author Index

Acheson, E. D., 319
Aguilera, D. C., 30
Aiken, L. 145
Ajzen, I., 209
Alderman, M. H., 103
Allison, G. T., 307
Anderson, T., 274
Annel, M., 202
Argyle, M ., 325
Argyris, C., 50, 51–52, 152, 153, 222, 223, 247, 248
Arnold, M., 312
Arole, M., 203
Arole, R., 203
Athos, A. G., 175, 176
Averill, B. W., 120
Avery, C. H., 123

Bailey, J., 21
Baker, S., 279
Baldridge, J. V., 307
Bandura, A., 7, 86, 91, 205–206
Baranowski, T., 132, 287
Barry, M. C., 74, 76, 296, 297, 298–299
Bates, I., 125
Bateson, G., 209
Baumgartel, H., 297, 299
Bean, C. A., 299
Becker, M., 276, 277, 325
Belle, S., 319

Benne, K. D., 109, 271
Benne, R., 299
Bennis, W. G., 271
Bensley, M., 362
Berkman, L. F., 210
Berman, H. J., 159
Bernheimer, R. E., 103, 110
Berson, A., 260
Bigge, M. L., 9
Bivins, E. C., 178, 237
Blalock, H. M., 224
Bloom, B., 226
Boissioneau, R., 248
Bonaguro, J., 325
Bower, B., 201
Boyce, J., 274
Brammer, L. M., 28–29, 30, 39, 40
Brennan, A. J., 369
Brewster, B. S., 201
Brewster, T., 201
Brodsky, C., 362
Broskowski, 159
Brown, E. R., 197–198
Bruner, J. S., 7, 8, 9, 100, 101, 108, 110, 151, 154, 236, 237, 339
Burke, A., 23

Campbell, D. T., 278, 279
Carey, R. G., 166
Carlaw, R. W., 1
Cassel, J., 210

Cathcart, R. S., 110
Chadwick, J. H., 314
Chin, R., 271
Clark, N., 132, 287
Clarke, E., 274
Clever, L. H., 103, 109–110
Cohen, E., 21
Cohen, J. D., 309
Coombs, J. A., 316
Comstock, L., 121
Cook, T. D., 278, 279, 286
Cordello, D., 314
Corey, K. E., 271
Cornacchia, H. H., 23
Cosper, B., 101
Cottle, W. C., 31
Cottrell, L., 226
Cox, T., 209
Crapo, L., 210
Crawford, R., 197–198
Cullen, J., 276
Cutler, G. R., 132, 279, 280, 281, 287

Dalis, G. T., 19
Darkenwald, G. G., 7
Davis, P., 166
Dawson, L., 380, 381
Deeds, S. G., 115, 157, 172, 224, 287
DeJoseph, J. G., 166
Dewey, J., 23, 197

Dixon, B., 362
Donnelley, J., 157
D'Onofrio, C., 158, 175, 176
Dosch, P., 80, 83
Downie, N. M., 31
Drolet, J., 80, 83
Drucker, P. F., 175, 176
Duncan, R., 7, 8, 9, 64, 67, 139, 141, 142, 236, 238, 247, 249, 297, 300, 370
Durham, M. L., 141

England, A. L., 103
Ensor, P., 23
Estabrook, B., 120, 124
Estler, S. E., 307

Festinger, L. A., 6, 358, 360
Finnegan, M., 172
Fishbein, M., 209, 322
Fodor, J. T., 19
Foltz, A., 274
Fox, B., 276
Freire, P., 191, 196–197, 198
French, J. R. P., 138
Fries, J. F., 210
Fruchter, R., 274
Fry, R. F., 110

Gaby, D. M., 214, 215
Gaby, P. V., 214, 215
Gapinski, P. A., 39, 40
Gibson, J., 157
Gilmore, G. D., 188, 189
Giloth, B., 132
Glogow, E., 158, 175, 176
Goldfarb, D. L., 137
Goldsmith, S., 156, 157
Gottlieb, B. H., 65, 66, 359, 360
Grabbe, P., 84, 86, 296, 299
Green, L. W., 1, 2, 75, 76, 114, 120, 122, 123, 160, 180, 222, 224, 274, 276, 285, 286–287, 315, 321, 325, 338, 339–340
Greenberg, J. S., 21, 23
Griffin, T., 362
Griffiths, W., 217
Guzick, D., 274

Hall, E. T., 91
Hall, J. H., 134
Hamburg, M., 1
Hamburg, M. W., 1
Handelman, I., 159, 172
Haynes, R. B., 9, 93

Hebert, B. J., 157
Hecht, A. B., 321
Henderson, A., 125
Hendrickson, B., 362
Herbert, B. J., 157
Hillman, S., 101–102
Hilton, D., 202
Hochbaum, G. M., 217
Holbek, J., 139, 370
Holst, E., 123, 215
Horne, P. J., 7, 10, 236, 238, 258
Howard, B., 42
Howard, G. S., 83, 86
Hoyman, H. S., 49
Hunt, M., 274
Huse, E. F., 50, 52, 369

Iscoe, I., 226
Isom, R., 276
Ivancevich, J., 157
Iverson, D. C., 76

James, W., 276
Jenkins, D. H., 107, 110
Jones, S., 322

Kahn, A. J., 381
Kahn, R. L., 66, 141
Kalmer, H., 89, 277
Kaplan, B. H., 210
Kassim, K., 325
Katz, A. H., 123, 215
Katz, D., 66, 141
Katz, E., 6
Katz, H. J., 316
Kelly, G., 213
Kelman, H. C., 9
Kelsey, J., 274
Kenegan, A., 314
Kidd, J. R., 7, 189
Kime, R. E., 17, 50, 52
Klein, D., 226
Klein, N., 52
Kleinman, J., 274
Klotz, A., 118
Knowles, M., 7, 39, 40, 210, 260
Knowles, W. C., 42
Knutson, A. L., 217
Koontz, H., 156
Kopstein, A., 274
Kouzes, M., 90, 151, 154
Kreider, S., 123
Kreuter, M. W., 224, 287
Kronenfeld, J., 275, 276, 280
Kyriacou, C., 362

Lazarsfeld, P. F., 6, 270, 271
Leaville, L. W., 209
Lebo, J., 310
Lenrow, P., 232
Leventhal, H., 322
Levin, H. M., 166
Levin, L. S., 123, 215
Lewin, K., 5, 7, 9, 74, 76, 86, 107, 110, 296, 299
Lewis, C. E., 211
Lieberman, S., 276
Likert, R., 175, 176
Linn, L. S., 211
Lippitt, G., 152, 153, 154
Lippitt, R., 50, 52, 152, 153, 154, 315
Lorig, K., 209, 210
Lynton, R. P., 85, 86, 189, 247, 248

Mager, R., 102
March, J. G., 307, 309
Margo, G. E., 197–198
Marshall, C., 276
Martindale, D., 7
Maslow, A. H., 6
Mathews, B. P., 65, 66, 102, 115, 172, 339, 340
May, J. T., 141
McCammon, C., 319
McGuire, W. J., 276, 322
McKay, S. R., 294
McLuhan, M., 85
Means, R. K., 10, 11, 23
Merriam, S. B., 7
Merton, R. K., 91, 270, 271
Messick, J. M., 30
Metsch, J. M., 260
Miaoulis, G., 325
Mico, P. R., 1, 2, 6, 64, 66, 90, 121, 122, 123–124, 151, 154, 179, 237, 348, 350, 368, 370
Miles, R., 120
Milham, S., 319
Milio, N., 215
Miller, G., 209
Mink, B., 360
Mink, O. G., 360
Mullane, M., 125
Mullen, P. D., 6, 114, 115, 116, 120, 158, 166, 172
Murphy, J., 172

Needle, R. H., 362
New, P. K., 141
Nuckolls, K. B., 210

Numbers, R. L., 209
Nyswander, D. V., 178, 259, 260

O'Donnell, C., 156
Olsen, J. P., 307
Olsen, L. K., 23

Pareek, U., 85, 86, 189, 247, 248
Parkinson, R., 315, 326
Parlette, N., 158, 175, 176
Partridge, K. B., 224, 287
Pascale, R. T., 175, 176
Patton, M. Q., 84, 87, 131, 132, 214, 215
Payton, C., 80, 83
Peters, T. J., 331
Pigg, R. M., 18, 23–24
Pine, G. J., 7, 8, 236, 238, 258, 260
Plovnick, M. S., 110
Posavac, E. J., 166
Powell, H. B., 103

Rakich, J. S., 157
Rash, J. K., 18, 24
Ratcliffe, J., 208
Raven, B., 138
Redican, K. J., 23
Redman, B. K., 92
Reynolds, R., 205, 206
Richards, R. F., 89
Richardson, W. C., 166
Risse, R., 209
Robbins, L. C., 142
Robinson, C., 319
Robinson, V. M., 85, 87
Roemer, M. I., 125
Rogers, C., 85
Rogers, E. M., 6, 7, 74, 76–77, 114, 116, 138, 151, 154, 205, 206, 222, 224, 235, 238, 269, 270, 271, 276, 296, 299–300, 348, 350, 358, 360, 368, 370

Rosen, G., 177, 178
Rosenstock, I. M., 217, 285, 287, 322
Ross, H. S., 1, 2, 6, 24, 64, 66, 121, 122, 123, 179, 237, 348, 350, 368, 370
Ross, M. G., 77, 179
Rossi, P. H., 138
Rubin, I. M., 110
Rutstein, D. D., 274

Sackett, D. L., 93
Schaller, W. E., 22, 24
Schauffler, H. H., 120
Schlaadt, R. G., 17, 50, 52
Schon, D. A., 248
Schultz, M., 360
Schwartz, R., 132
Shaw, S. F., 362
Sheats, P., 109
Shepard, D. S., 166
Shoemaker, F. F., 276
Shortell, S. M., 166, 314
Sieten, A. M., 124
Silverberg, E., 274
Silversin, J. B., 316
Simmons, J., 1
Singer, R., 322
Skiff, A., 120
Sliepcevich, E., 125
Spector, R., 52
Spencer, M. E., 11
Squyres, W., 152, 154, 316, 360, 369, 370
Srinivasan, L., 198, 206
Stanley, J., 278, 279
Staton, W. M., 23
Steadham, S. V., 188, 189
Steckler, A., 380, 381
Stephens, G. G., 134
Sutliffe, J., 362
Svendsen, R., 362

Swanson, G. M., 319
Syme, S. L., 210

Taba, H., 7, 8, 9, 87
Taylor, D. W., 93
Taylor, J. B., 172
Thomas, R., 225
Thompson, G. E., 159, 172
Thompson, M. S., 166
Tritsch, L. E., 17, 50, 52
Turner, C. E., 11

Ulich, R., 5

Velder, M., 21
Vosen, B., 166

Wakefield, J., 276
Waterman, R. H., 331
Watson, J., 50, 52, 315
Waxweiler, R. J., 319
Weber, M., 7
Weeks, H. A., 218
Weeks, L. E., 159
Weiskopf, P. E., 362
Weitzner, M., 260
Werlin, S. H., 120
Werner, D., 201
Westley, B., 50, 52, 315
Whorf, B. L., 210
Williams, L. S., 313, 314
Windsor, R. A., 132, 275, 278, 279, 280, 281, 287
Wolfe, D., 160
Wolle, J. M., 110, 157

Zaltman, G., 7, 8, 9, 64, 66, 67, 139, 141, 142, 236, 238, 247, 249, 297, 300, 370
Zander, A., 238
Zapka, J. G., 116, 121, 124, 132, 158, 166, 172
Zweiner, J. D., 134

Subject Index

Accountability, 246
Accreditation Council for Psychiatric Facilities, 95
Administrative structure, 144, 152
Administrative style, 63–64
Administrative support, 65, 108, 109, 144, 338
 Environmental, 337, 339
 Financial, 334, 339
 Lack of, 57 ff, 135–137, 244, 248, 353, 355, 356
Administrators', perception of health education, 92
Advisory committees, 56, 68 ff, 301, 302, 341–342, 348–349, 353–355, 357, 359
American Cancer Society, 278, 333
American Diabetes Association, 44
American Heart Association, 44, 333
American Hospital Association, 266
American Lung Association, 21, 89, 262, 288, 333 (National Association for the Study and Prevention of Tuberculosis, 178)
American Medical Association, 15
American Public Health Association, 362
American Red Cross, 289
American School Health Association, 15, 18

Arizona State University, 42
Arthritis Foundation, 212
AT & T communication, 314, 327

Bangor-Brewer Tuberculosis and Health Association, 288

Cardiopulmonary resuscitation (CPR) training, 69
Change agent, 79
Child Health Organization, 177
Columbia University, 11
 School of Public Health, 250
Communicating with patients
 Definition of, 151
Communication
 Channels, 277
 Facilitation of, 193, 194
 Multiple methods, 118, 285
 Theory, 6, 210
Community development, 226
 Neighborhood, definition of, 227
Community health education, 177 ff
Community organization, 2, 68 ff, 74–75, 259, 285, 288 ff, 297, 301 ff
Competition among agencies, 181
Comprehensive health planning, 250 ff
Conflict resolution, 63–64, 292, 293, 295

Consumer education, 191 ff, 199 ff, 208 ff, 225 ff, 250 ff, 288 ff
Continuing education, 250 ff
Continuity of staff, 75, 298
Cornell University Medical School, 263
Cost analysis, 120, 166
 Cost benefit analysis, 122
 and health education, 122
Counseling definitions, 29, 30
Credibility of health educators, 3, 4, 138, 145, 183, 185, 222, 322, 323
Culture
 Corporate, 315, 323, 324, 327, 330
 Definition, 327
 Ethnic, 191 ff
 Influence on decision making, 46, 48
 of medicine, 93–94, 149, 355
Curriculum development process, 18, 20 ff, 32 ff, 35–36, 42 ff, 54–56, 253
 Hoyman spiral approach, 44
 Traditional approach, 44

Data
 Access to, 57, 329, 330
 Automation, 172
 Decisions on what to collect, 159
 Definition of, 159
 Problems with analysis, 57

Decision making, 306, 342
  Analysis of process, 316–317
  Children, 21, 22
  Corporate, 334
  Cultural and organizational influences, 46, 48
  Garbage can theory, 307–309, 311
  Organized anarchy theory, 307–309
  Task force or council, 288 ff, 304 ff
Disease detection Pap smear, 216 ff, 274
Disease prevention (See *Prevention*.)
Diseases
  Arthritis, 208
  Bladder cancer, 319
  Breast cancer, 328
  Cervical cancer, 216, 273 ff
  Chronic obstructive pulmonary disease (COPD), 126
  Colon cancer, 319, 328
  Diabetes, 42 ff
  Diarrheal dehydration, 199
  Hematopoietic cancer, 319
  Hypertension, 103 ff, 126, 181
  Lead poisoning, 250
  Leukemia, 319
  Nasopharyngeal cancer, 319
  Rectal cancer, 328
  Stomach cancer, 319
  Tuberculosis, 250, 262 ff
Drug education, elementary school, 20 ff

Education
  for economically deprived, 191
  Non-formal, 206
Education Commission of the States, 16, 19
Evaluation design and techniques
  Cost analysis, 120
  Data collection, 126
  Data triangulation, 84
  Design, 366
  Document review, 131
  External, 255, 260
  Interim, 333, 337
  Internal validity, 278–283
  Interviewing, 81
  Planning/evaluation, 126, 184, 232, 237, 278–279
  Process, 290, 345–347

  Qualitative, 131
  Questionnaires, 81
  Response shift bias, 84
  Structured interviews, 127
  Then/post design, 83
Evaluation of programs
  Community health education, 180
  Consumer education, 255–256
  Problems, 60–62
  Training, 80–83
  Undergraduate course, 37–38

Family practice, 134
Federal Risk Reduction Grant, 48, 341
Ford Motor Company, 319 ff

Group dynamics, 324 (See also *Group Process*.)
Group process, 84, 104–107, 201
Groups, 179
  Cohesiveness, 186, 194
  Informal structure, 194

Harlem Health Alliance, 252 ff
Harvard-MIT School of Public Health, 11
Health belief model, 277, 285, 324
Health care costs
  Control of, 315
  to employees, 314, 327
  and health promotion, 314
  Potential savings (table), 328
  Reimbursement, 314
Health/disease concept, 3
Health education
  Courses of instruction, 10–11
  Discipline of, 10
  Historical summary, 10–11, 177–178
  Research, 79 ff, 119, 135, 208 ff, 273 ff, 374 ff
  Value of, 123
Health Education (HE) framework, 2–4, 285
Health education methods (See *Methods*.)
Health educator
  Certification, 18, 65
  Integrated skills, 39–40
  Need for objectivity, 106–107, 368
  Process vs. task, 179

  Professional development, 374 ff
  Professional norms, 377–378
  Professional preparation, 18, 70, 72
  Survival, 325
Health educator's functions, 178
  Change agent, 232, 237
  Community organization, 84
  Consulting, 42 ff, 50, 64, 68–69, 288, 316, 333
  Coordinating, 22, 71–73, 95, 121, 216, 221, 348, 364
  Counseling, 16, 25 ff, 39
  Curriculum development, 16, 17, 294
  Direct service, 316, 348
  Evaluating, 83, 99, 120, 132, 221, 241, 348
  Facilitating, 106, 193, 225, 256, 258, 266–267, 294, 316, 348, 362
  Liaison role, 112–114, 121
  Planning, 121, 213, 221, 241, 332, 362
  Program design, 322
  Program manger, 338
  Project director, 348
  Research, 213
  Staffing, 100, 122, 250, 263
  Staffing support, 305, 310, 316
  Training, 45–46, 56, 64, 79 ff, 98, 294, 341, 365
Health educator's, role in
  Community, 178–180
  Medical care, 90–91
  School, 16–17
  Worksite, 316
Health hazard appraisal, 134, 328, 330
Health insurance
  WELLCHEC plan, 82
Health Insurance Institute of America, 313
Health maintenance organizations, 369 (See also *Medical care settings*.)
Health programs
  Cardiac care, 126
  Childbirth classes, 126
  Fitness, 333
  Healthy back, 333
  Maternal and child health, 288 ff
  Nutrition awareness, 333
  Parenting course, 289

Prenatal care, 126
Smoking cessation, 126, 333
Stress management, 333, 362
Weight control, 126, 333
Health promotion, 314–316, 329, 332, 341 ff, 352, 363 ff
  Environmental support, 337
  Record system, 336
  Surgeon General's report, 18
Health worker (paraprofessional), 199, 203
Home health agencies, 182

Implementation
  Logistics, 184, 185, 211
Infant and maternal mortality rates (table) 251, (table) 291
Institute of Cultural Action, 191
International Childbirth Education Association, 290
Interpersonal relations
  Among staff members, 183, 188
  with target group, 229, 324
  Trust, 257

The Johns Hopkins University, 241
Joint Commission on Accreditation of Hospitals, 146

La Leche League, 290
Lamaze training, 289, 291
Learning vs. compliance, 8
Learning/social change
  Applied principles, 140, 151, 187, 191, 236, 238, 244, 296, 311, 339, 348
  Comparison and application, 8–9
  Definitions, 6–8
  Imposed learning, 9, 74, 297, 311, 359
  Informal learning, 84, 151, 220
  Learned learning, 9, 74, 359
  Planned change, 50
  Readiness to learn, 151, 236–237
  Reinforcement, 184, 201, 222
Legislation, 68 ff, 73
Lobbying
  Informal, 73, 306

Management
  and health education, 156 ff
  Resource allocation, 112
  Role in health promotion, 315

Management information systems
  Components of, 159
  Departmental master calendar, 166
  Relation to management functions, 172
  Reporting forms, for specific activities, 169
  Staff activity log, 161
  Staff needs, 172
  Theory, 6
Maternal and child health, 178, 192, 289–290
Medical care provider
  Educational component of role, 91–92, 130
  vs. role of health educator, 92
Medical care settings
  Acute care hospitals, 89, 143 ff
  Ambulatory care centers, 125 ff, 134 ff
  Chronic care hospitals, 89, 143 ff
  Health centers, 125 ff
  Health maintenance organizations (HMOs), 89, 103 ff, 112 ff, 117 ff
  Psychiatric hospitals, 95 ff
Medical datamation, 134
Medically indigent patients, 216
  Medicaid, 126
  Referral methods, 218
Medical records
  Audit or review, 149
  Health education program notes, 170
Mental health, 225 ff
Methods of health education (See also *Strategies*.)
  Closed circuit TV, 242
  Contract, 113, 115
  Drama, 192, 201
  Film discussion, 219
  Group orientation, 335
  Group sessions, 98–99, 147–148, 184–186, 192–194, 220, 289–290, 333–337
  Jokes and proverbs, 193
  Media, 211, 335
  Medical record insert or audit, 149, 170, 219
  Multiple, 75, 98, 199, 210
  Pamphlets and films, 146
  Screening, 219

Short stories, 193
Statements, documents, and guidelines, 264, 265, 267
Success stories, 193
Survey, 341, 342
Training manual, 364–365
Models
  Health belief model, 277, 285, 324
  Model for change, 238
  PRECEDE (Health Education Planning Model), 274, 285, 315
Motivating participation
  Group belongingness, 84
  Marketing, 335
  Personalizing, 335
  Social events, 223
  Use of fun, 85

National Cancer Institute, 273
National Commission on Excellence in Education, 18, 19
National Education Association, 15
National Foundation/March of Dimes, 289
National Health Planning and Resources Development Act, 125
National Institute of Arthritis, Metabolism and Digestive Diseases, 42
National Institute of Occupational Safety and Health (NIOSH), 319–320
Needs assessment, 22, 57, 128, 129, 184, 188, 193, 348
  Informal procedures, 352
  Medical record audit, 149
  Multi-level, 208, 363

Occupational health nurses, 321, 335, 344
Occupational Safety and Health Administration (OSHA), 320
Organizations
  Dissonance of, 54 ff
  Stability of, 298
Organizational change
  Political model for, 307–309 (See also *Domain Theory*, 90, 151.)
Organizational development, 50, 237

Patient education, 95 ff

Subject Index   393

Patient education (*continued*)
  Ambulatory care, 125
  Acute care hospitals, 143, 146
  Community based, 208
  Counseling, 127, 147, 150
  Directed to specific problems, 220
  Group sessions, 98–99, 147–148
  Health centers, 125
  Planned, 127
  Program effectiveness, 128
  Program efficiency, 128
  Providers, 127
  Reimbursement, 131
Pattern Maker's League (AFL-CIO), 319
Peer education, 184, 186, 203
Perception
  Change of, 209
  Patient vs. physician, 209
  Role of language in, 210
Physicians
  Consultation with, 212
  as gatekeepers, 214, 218
  as opinion leaders, 222
Pilot programs, 328, 333, 365
Planning, 193, 226 *ff*, 242 *ff*, 263 *ff*, 274 *ff*, 334, 353, 362
  Objectives, 97, 106, 149, 226
  Problems with, 129
  Program, 149
  Selection of content and process, 363
  Workshops, 184
Planning committees, 97, 100
Policy development, 378–380
Policy statements, 271, 286
Political issues
  Within a community, 305–307
  Within an organization, 129–130
Practice management techniques, 4
Prevention of Disease, 134 *ff*, 199 *ff*, 202, 216 *ff*, 273 *ff*, 288 *ff*
  Physician attitudes, 218
Primary care, 134
Professional operating procedures, 3
Professional Standards Review Organization, 146
Public health education (See *Community health education*).
Public Health Service, 89

Research, 79 *ff*, 117 *ff*, 135, 208 *ff*, 273 *ff*

Responsibility for health status, 120, 196
Risk Reduction Grant, 48, 341
Role delineation project, 2, 248, 348
  Role refinement and verification, 249
Rural Health Initiative Act, 125

Safety program, 332, 336
School health curriculum project, 43–44, 45, 51
School health education, 15–19, 178
  How health should be taught, 17
  Role of school health educator, 16–17
  State of the art, 15
  What should be taught, 18
  Who should teach health, 17–18
  Why teach health in schools, 18–19
Seaside Health Education Conference, 79
Self-care, 117 *ff*, 122, 208
  Cold self-care, 118 *ff*
Self-help, 229
  Courses, 329
Social support, 65, 192, 200, 316
  Networking, 194, 210
  in training, 85
Society of Public Health Educators, 178
South Carolina Department of Health and Environmental Control, 240
Southern New England Telephone (SNET), 332 *ff*
Strategies for health education (See also *Methods*.)
  Consultation, 152
  Consultation teams, 343
  Direct staff assistance, 343
  Discharge planning, 146–147
  Group process, 259, 365
  Indirect assistance, 343
  Information, 320–322
  Modeling, 85, 231
  Nominal group process, 147
  Political, 307
  Reinforcement of, 104, 184
  Role modeling (social learning), 17
  Role playing, 21
  Selection of, 180

Team building, 104
  Workshops, 344
Surgeon General's Report, on Health Promotion and Disease Prevention, 18

Teaching tools (see *Methods*).
Theories
  Adoption/diffusion, 6, 74, 114, 138, 139, 151, 205, 235, 238, 269, 278, 290, 296, 297, 348, 353, 357, 358, 368
  Adult learning theory, 39, 258
  Andragogy, 260
    vs. pedagogy, 39
  Barriers to diffusion, 355
  Cognitive dissonance, 6
  Domain theory, 90, 151
  Field theory, 7
  Force field analysis, 107, 108, 270
  Hierarchy of needs, 6
  Homophily, 270
  Intervention theory and methods, 50
  Related to change, 104, 106, 108, 114, 188, 269
  Role theory, 91, 92, 297
  Social learning theory, 7, 85, 91, 258
    Modeling, 202, 205
  Theory of instruction, 7, 100, 339
  in use, 247
Title I-A, Higher Education Act of 1965, 225
Training, 179, 183, 240 *ff*
  Allied health personnel, 148
  Consumer advisory groups, 260
  of nurses, 148
  Phases of, 247
  of physicians, 148
Tuberculosis Control Division (U.S. Public Health Service's Center for Disease Control), 262

University of Alabama at Birmingham, 273
University of Maine, School of Nursing, 289
University of Massachusetts Health Services at Amherst, 117
University of Massachusetts Medical Center, 352

University of North Carolina,
    School of Public Health, 1, 225
University of Texas, School of
    Public Health, 365

Veterans administration, 89
Volunteers, 73, 210, 214, 256, 291,
    341 *ff*, 356, 357, 365

Organization of, 293
Recruitment of, 210

Wellness, 79–81, 327, 352
    Involvement of school district,
        82–83
    Philosophy of, 85–86
    Reinforcement of, 357

Wellness vs. disease prevention,
    355, 359
Women, 191
    Health conference, 192–196
    Health course, 32 *ff*
    Self-empowerment, 191